Essentials of Implant Dentistry

Essentials of Implant Dentistry

Edited by Preston Bailey

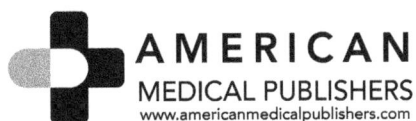

AMERICAN
MEDICAL PUBLISHERS
www.americanmedicalpublishers.com

American Medical Publishers,
41 Flatbush Avenue,
1st Floor, New York,
NY 11217, USA

Visit us on the World Wide Web at:
www.americanmedicalpublishers.com

ISBN: 978-1-63927-053-8

Cataloging-in-Publication Data

Essentials of implant dentistry / edited by Preston Bailey.
 p. cm.
Includes bibliographical references and index.
ISBN 978-1-63927-053-8
1. Dental implants. 2. Dentistry. 3. Dental therapeutics. I. Bailey, Preston.
RK667.I45 I46 2022

617.693--dc23

Table of Contents

Preface

Dentistry is a branch of medicine that deals with the study, prevention, diagnosis and treatment of diseases and disorders of the oral cavity. The surgical component which interfaces with the bone of the jaw or skull in order to support a dental prosthesis is known as dental implant. Modern dental implants are based on a biological process named as osseointegration. It is used to tightly fuse the bone to the surface of certain materials such as titanium and ceramics. The success of the dental implant depends on the health of the person who is receiving the treatment and the health of the tissues in the mouth. This book contains some path-breaking studies in the field of clinical dentistry. The topics included herien on implants are of utmost significance and bound to provide incredible insights to readers. The extensive content of this book provides the readers with a thorough understanding of the subject.

Various studies have approached the subject by analyzing it with a single perspective, but the present book provides diverse methodologies and techniques to address this field. This book contains theories and applications needed for understanding the subject from different perspectives. The aim is to keep the readers informed about the progresses in the field; therefore, the contributions were carefully examined to compile novel researches by specialists from across the globe.

Indeed, the job of the editor is the most crucial and challenging in compiling all chapters into a single book. In the end, I would extend my sincere thanks to the chapter authors for their profound work. I am also thankful for the support provided by my family and colleagues during the compilation of this book.

Editor

Thickness of the Schneiderian membrane and its correlation with anatomical structures and demographic parameters using CBCT tomography

Demos Kalyvas[1*], Andreas Kapsalas[1], Sofia Paikou[1] and Konstantinos Tsiklakis[2]

Abstract

Background: The aims of the present study were to determine the thickness of the Schneiderian membrane and identify the width of the maxillary sinus, which is indicated by the buccal and lingual walls of the sinus angle between. Furthermore, to investigate the possibility of a correlation between the aforementioned structures and also other anatomical and demographic parameters using CBCTs for dental implant surgical planning.

Methods: The study included CBCT images of 76 consecutive patients with field-of-view 15×12 or 12×8cm. Reformatted cross-sectional CBCT slices were analyzed with regard to the thickness of the Schneiderian membrane designated by the medial and the lateral walls of the sinus, in three different standardized points of reference. Age, gender, and position of the measurement were evaluated as factors that could influence the dimensions of the anatomical structures, using univariate and multivariate random effects regression model.

Results: The mean thickness of the Schneiderian membrane was 1.60 ± 1.20 mm. The average thickness revealed now differentiation by age ($p = 0.878$), whereas gender seemed to influence the mean thickness ($p = 0.010$). Also, the thickness of the Schneiderian membrane increased from medial to distal ($p = 0.060$). The mean value of the angle designated by buccal and lingual walls of the sinus was $73.41 \pm 6.89°$. The angle measurements revealed no correlation with age, but a tendency towards lower mean angles in females ($2.5°$ on average, $p = 0.097$). According to the anatomical position of the measurement, a differentiation was also detected. No correlation between thickness of the Schneiderian membrane and the angle of the walls of the sinus was concluded ($p = 0.662$).

Conclusions: This study demonstrated that the thickness of the Schneiderian membrane and the width of the maxillary sinus can only be affected by gender and anatomical position, but not by the age of the patient.

Keywords: Schneiderian membrane, Sinus, Thickness, Width, CBCT

* Correspondence: demkal@dent.uoa.gr
[1]Department of Oral and Maxillofacial Surgery, School of Dentistry, National and Kapodistrian University of Athens, Greece, Thivon 2 str, 11527 Athens, Greece
Full list of author information is available at the end of the article

Background

The maxillary sinus is the largest of the paranasal air-filled spaces, and it develops firstly in utero [1, 2]. Anatomically, the maxillary sinus is a pyramid-shaped cavity located in the facial skull with a mean volume of 12.5 mL (min 5 mL and max 22 mL) [2–6]. The size, the shape, and the wall thickness of every maxillary sinus not only vary among the population, but also between the two sides of an individual skull [6].

The Schneiderian membrane is the mucous membrane that covers the inner part of the maxillary sinus cavity [7]. Histologically, it consists of an overlaid periosteum with a thin layer of a pseudo-stratified ciliated epithelium and highly vascularized connective tissue [1, 7]. According to Kim et al. 2009, it has been proved that mesenchymal stem cells from the sinus membrane have an ability of bone formation, which plays a vital role in sinus floor elevation procedures [8]. Many studies have measured the thickness of the Schneiderian membrane using different methods such as cadaver examinations, CTs, and CBCTs. Normally, the thickness of the Schneiderian membrane is approximately 1 mm [6, 9]. However, in everyday clinical practice, mucosal thickening of the maxillary sinus is a common radiographic finding in asymptomatic patients; therefore, mucosal lining of more than 4 mm is considered to be pathological [6, 9].

When planning any surgical treatment for the maxilla that includes the posterior region, not only the dimensions and abilities of the Schneiderian membrane, but also the anatomical variations of the maxillary sinus are very significant for every clinician. Cone-beam computed tomography provides essential three-dimensional information regarding the inner part of the maxillary sinus in order to increase the success rate of every surgical procedure and, simultaneously, in order to limit the intra- and post-operative complications.

In the international literature, there is a limited number of studies that quantify the dimensions of the Schneiderian membrane using CBCTs. Therefore, the aim of the present retrospective study is to measure the thickness of the Schneiderian membrane and to identify the width of the maxillary sinus, which is indicated by the angle between the buccal and lingual walls of the sinus in a given height, using CBCT imaging. Furthermore, the present study detects possible

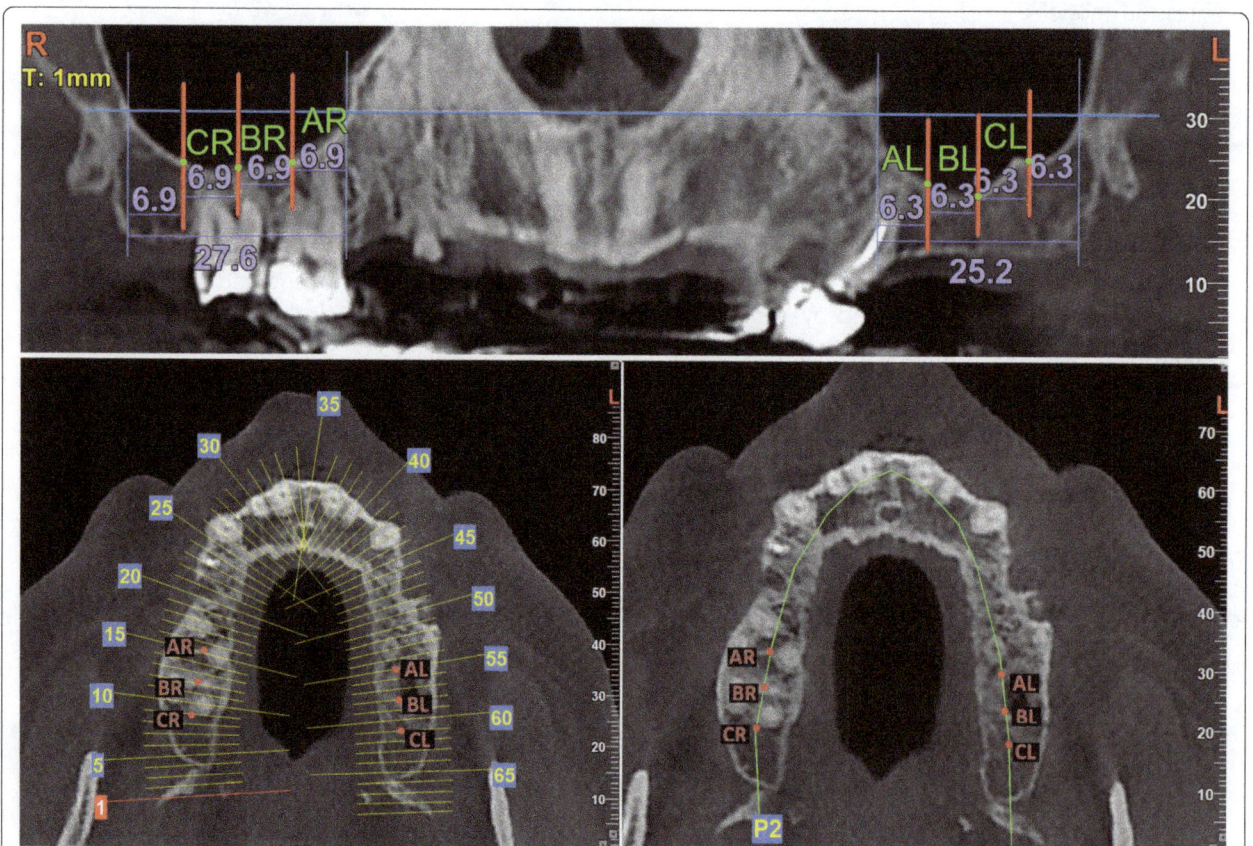

Fig. 1 Demonstration of the method used in the panoramic image to divide the sinus in four equal parts and find three fixed points for the measurements. Also, these fixed points in the horizontal plane with and without sections

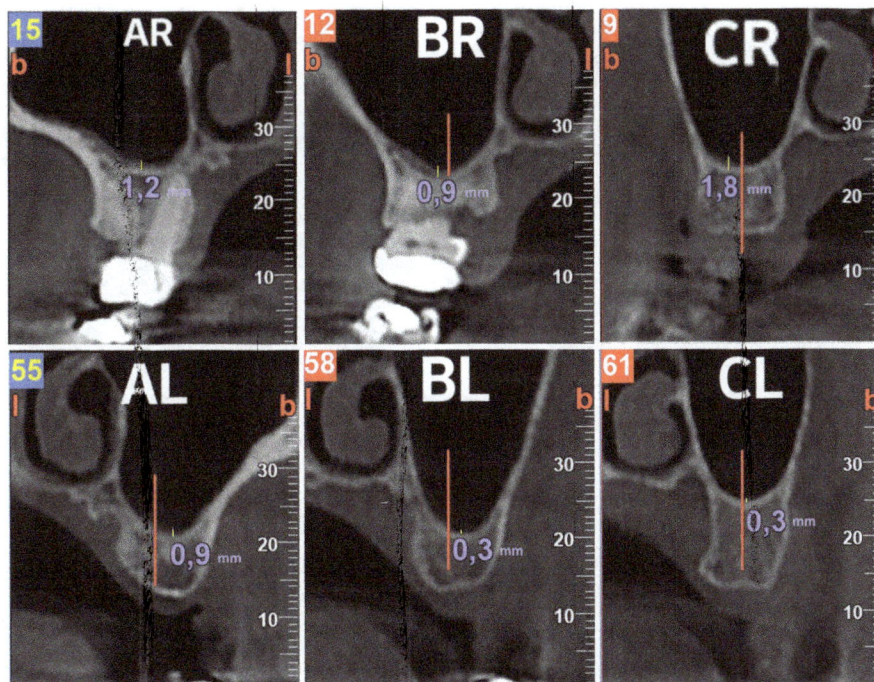

Fig. 2 Demonstration of the method used to measure the thickness of the Schneiderian membrane in the cross-sectional images for each of the three fixed points

correlations between the aforementioned factors and also between each of these factors with anatomical locations and demographic parameters.

Methods
Patient selection
The study sample included 76 patients, of which 39 were females and 37 were males. In total, 120 sinuses (44 both left- and right-sided, 21 right-sided, and 11 left-sided) were evaluated as suitable for the present study and were measured. The total sample was classified in four age groups (below 45 years, 45–54 years, 54–64 years, and over 65 years of age). The mean age value of the sample is 58 years (ranging from 19 to 65 years of age).

All patients were Greek adults, and all CBCT examinations were performed to evaluate the posterior maxilla for future implant surgery. All patients were either patients of our clinic or had been referred to our clinic by their private dentist for implant or other pre-implant surgery. The minimum acceptable alveolar process was 5 mm. Patients with previous implant therapy or/and maxillary sinus augmentation in their history as well as patients with active periodontal disease, cysts, polyps, sinusitis, allergic rhinitis, or other pathological entities in their maxillary sinuses were excluded from our study. Other exclusion

criteria were the presence of systematic diseases impacting the metabolism and quality of the bones in patients' history, such as thyroid disease, hyperparathyroidism, diabetes, chronic renal disease, osteoporosis, and no development or acquired craniofacial or neuromuscular deformities. None of the patients previously or currently received medication including vitamin D, human growing hormone (HGH), or bisphosphonates. All the collected data were anonymous.

Imaging procedure
The CBCT images were obtained with NewTom VGI Tomograph (NewTom, Verona, Italy) with a voxel size of 0.3 mm. Operating parameters were set at 5.28 mA, 110 kV, exposure time 3.60 s, and field of view (FOV) of 15×12 or 12×8 cm. Panoramic reformatted images with thickness of 1 mm were chosen for the present study.

All measurements were performed in millimeters using the ruler contained in the NNT Viewer®.

The distance between the medial and the lateral walls of the maxillary sinus in the panoramic reformatted images was divided in four equal segments. Thus, three points were created; AR, BR, and CR for the right sinus and AL, BL, and CL for the left sinus (Fig. 1). For each of the aforementioned points, a cross section of 1 mm thickness was performed in

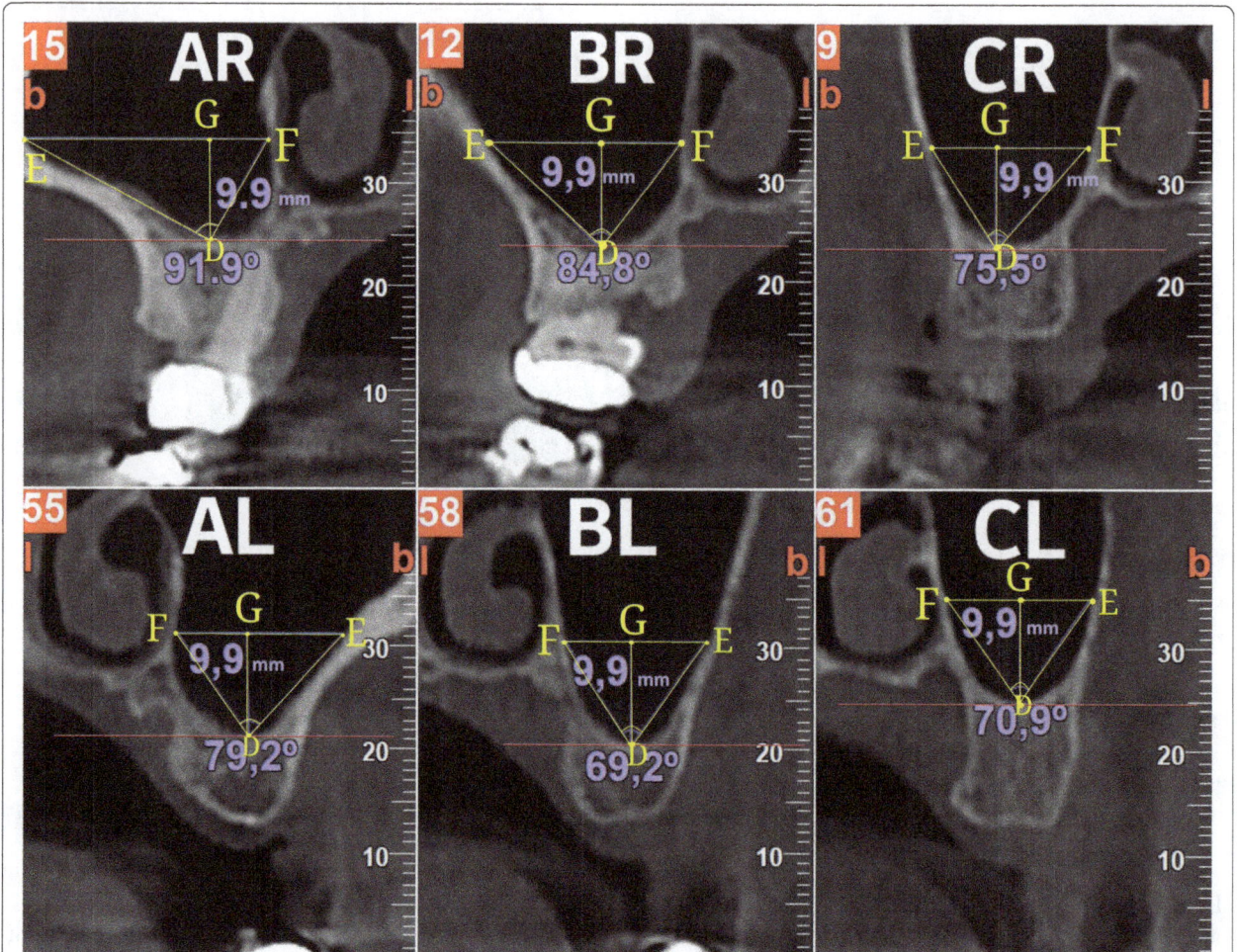

Fig. 3 Demonstration of the method used to measure the angle designated by the buccal and lingual walls of the sinus angle for each of the three fixed points in a given height

the middle of the alveolar bone. In the cross-sectional images, the thickness of the Schneiderian membrane was measured in the deepest point of the sinus floor (point D). Thus, three different measurements were performed for each sinus (Fig. 2).

These three cross-sectional images, in which the thickness of the Schneiderian membrane was previously measured, were also used for the measurement of the angle of the maxillary sinus. A segment DG (point D is the deepest point of the floor of the

Table 1 Sinuses' thickness by gender and overall

| | Sex | | | |
| | Male | Female | Overall | |
	Mean (SD)	Mean (SD)	Mean (SD)	p value
Thickness (mm)-AR	2.06 (1.54)	1.36 (2.09)	1.73 (1.84)	0.131
Thickness (mm)-BR	1.77 (1.43)	1.00 (0.82)	1.40 (1.23)	0.010
Thickness (mm)-CR	1.54 (1.06)	0.77 (0.61)	1.17 (0.95)	0.001
Thickness (mm)-AL	2.13 (1.96)	1.64 (2.54)	1.88 (2.28)	0.431
Thickness (mm)-BL	2.02 (2.09)	1.46 (1.08)	1.72 (1.64)	0.210
Thickness (mm)-CL	1.72 (1.58)	1.26 (1.18)	1.48 (1.39)	0.226
Average thickness (mm)—all points	1.95 (1.28)	1.24 (1.02)	*1.60 (1.20)*	*0.010*

Significant entries are in italic

Table 2 Average thickness by age group

	Age (years)					
	< 45	45–54	55–64	65+	Overall	
	N (%)	N (%)	N (%)	N (%)	N (%)	p value
Total	14 (100.0)	14 (100.0)	28 (100.0)	20 (100.0)	76 (100.0)	
	Mean (SD)	Mean (SD)	Mean (SD)	Mean (SD)	Mean (SD)	p value
Average thickness (mm)—overall	1.55 (1.21)	1.86 (1.57)	1.61 (1.25)	1.45 (0.86)	1.60 (1.20)	0.878

maxillary sinus) is created, vertical to the horizontal plane with stable length equal to 9.9 mm. The mean of 9.9 mm was chosen, because of a limitation of the NNT® software's limitation. A linear segment EGF (point E is the point where the segment EGF intersects with the buccal wall of the maxillary sinus, and point F is the point where the segment EGF intersects with the lingual wall of the maxillary sinus) is created which vertical to segment DG and parallel to the horizontal plane. The points D, E, and F designate a triangle named DEF. The angle which is measured is EDF (Fig. 3).

Using the built-in ruler of the NNT Viewer®, we measured the angle EDF for each cross-sectional image created by the aforementioned method. This angle indicates the width of the maxillary sinus in each location. As this angle increases, so does the width of the maxillary sinus.

According to the value of this angle, the sinus width was classified in one of the three following groups (small-, moderate-, and large-sized sinus):

- Angle ≤ 65°: small
- 65° < angle < 80°: moderate
- Angle ≥ 80°: large

Evaluation of the images
The CBCT images were initially evaluated by an oral surgeon and then they were re-evaluated and measured by two experienced dentists who were involved in the patients' treatment and follow-up. In case of any disagreement, both parties re-evaluated and remeasured the related CBCT imaging.

Statistical analysis
All analyses were performed using Stata version 13.1 (Stata Corp., TX, USA).

Results
The mean value of the overall average thickness is 1.60 ± 1.20 mm (males 1.95 ± 1.28 mm and females 1.24 ± 1.02 mm) (Table 1).

The average thickness of the membrane also showed no tendency for differentiation by age group ($p = 0.878$) (Table 2).

The statistical analysis also shows a clear tendency towards lower values when checking from point AR to point CR and from point AL to point CL, which means that the average thickness of the membrane increases from medial to distal. ($p = 0.060$) (Table 3).

The average mean value of the angle of the maxillary sinus in cross sections was $73.41 \pm 6.89°$, revealing high prevalence of moderate-shaped sinuses (average mean angle value 74.65 ± 8.08 for the male group and 72.11 ± 5.17 for the female group) (Table 4).

The angle of the sinus also shows no association with age (Table 5).

On the contrary, it was proven that there is a tendency towards lower angle values in the female group ($2.5°$ on average, $p = 0.097$). It was also shown that at the points BR and BL, the angles were statistically significantly higher than those at the points AR and AL, of the order of $10°$ ($p < 0.001$), but at the points CR and CL the difference is of $2.2°$ ($p = 0.051$). No association between thickness of the membrane and the angle (width) of the current position in the sinus was detected ($p = 0.662$) (Table 6).

Table 3 Thickness by point of measurement (all measurements)

	Position				
	1 (AR/AL)	2 (BR/BL)	3 (CR/CL)	Overall	
	N (%)	N (%)	N (%)	N (%)	p value
Total	120 (100.0)	120 (100.0)	120 (100.0)	360 (100.0)	
	Mean (SD)	Mean (SD)	Mean (SD)	Mean (SD)	p value
Thickness (mm)	1.8 (2.0)	1.6 (1.4)	1.3 (1.2)	1.6 (1.6)	0.060

Table 4 Sinuses' angles by gender and overall

	Gender			
	Male	Female	Overall	
	N (%)	N (%)	N (%)	p value
Sinuses measured	21 (53.8)	23 (62.2)	44 (57.9)	
	Mean (SD)	Mean (SD)	Mean (SD)	p value
Angle (°)-AR	71.79 (16.56)	64.13 (12.09)	68.14 (14.99)	0.039
Angle (°)-BR	80.34 (9.56)	78.60 (5.63)	79.51 (7.92)	0.380
Angle (°)-CR	71.06 (6.82)	71.64 (6.02)	71.34 (6.41)	0.719
Angle (°)-AL	73.87 (14.70)	69.08 (12.43)	71.34 (13.64)	0.197
Angle (°)-BL	80.34 (8.21)	79.25 (7.83)	79.77 (7.96)	0.616
Angle (°)-CL	72.33 (8.15)	72.59 (6.04)	72.47 (7.05)	0.890
Average angle (°)—all points	74.65 (8.08)	72.11 (5.17)	73.41 (6.89)	0.109

Discussion

It is very important to pre-operatively evaluate the thickness of the Schneiderian membrane to plan the surgical procedure in the region that involves the membrane, such as a sinus lift augmentation, which increases the possibility of membrane perforation or other complications.

The present study assumed that the average thickness of the Schneiderian membrane is 1.60 ± 1.20 mm.

There are many studies which estimate the average thickness of the mucosa of the maxillary sinus, some of which have used CBCTs while others have not. These studies are presented in Table 7. These values are not completely different to the results of the present study. From these studies, we can conclude that, clearly, there is variability regarding the thickness of the Schneiderian membrane. This means that a clinician cannot collect information about the thickness of a sinus membrane by patient sex, side, or age.

In this study, it was detected that 27.5% of the measurements made (99 out of 360) were more than 2 mm. However, all X-ray examinations that showed a visually detectable pathology were excluded from our study. For this reason, our study cannot conclude

that the limit of 2 mm is an accurate limit to evaluate a sinus membrane as healthy or pathological. The limit of 2 mm as a criterion is used by Shanbhag et al. 2014, Ji-Young Yoo et al. 2011, Janner et al. 2011, and Cagici et al. 2008 [10–13]. On the contrary, Eggesbo et al. 2006 and Cakur et al. 2011 set the limit of 4 mm as a safe threshold to evaluate a sinus membrane as pathological [9, 14]. Furthermore, Lozano-Carrascal et al. 2017 accept a threshold of 3 mm of membrane thickness for pathology existence [15]. In our study, the membrane thickness of 6.94% of our sample was over 4 mm. For this reason, we can accept a thickness over 4 mm as a safer limit to evaluate if there is a pathology in the sinus or not.

Comparing the thickness of the membrane between the two genders, males seem to have thicker membranes than females. Vallo et al. 2010, Janner et al. 2011, Ji-Young Yoo et al. 2011, Cakur et al. 2013, and Jildirim et al. 2017 [9, 11, 12, 16, 17] also come to this conclusion. Our study assumed that this difference is of the order of 40%. On the contrary, Pazera et al. 2010 concluded that there is no significant difference between thickness of the mucosa and gender ($p = 0.294$) [18].

Table 5 Angle of the walls of the sinus by age groups

	Age (years)					
	< 45	45–54	55–64	65+	Overall	
	Mean (SD)	Mean (SD)	Mean (SD)	Mean (SD)	Mean (SD)	p value
Angle (°)-AR	70.05 (17.57)	68.92 (15.67)	67.43 (12.05)	67.29 (17.30)	68.14 (14.99)	0.958
Angle (°)-BR	80.63 (8.11)	78.50 (10.66)	78.58 (5.70)	80.74 (8.43)	79.51 (7.92)	0.766
Angle (°)-CR	70.80 (7.38)	71.31 (7.73)	69.57 (5.31)	73.93 (5.69)	71.34 (6.41)	0.190
Angle (°)-AL	76.95 (9.55)	67.30 (12.39)	73.75 (14.11)	66.01 (14.75)	71.34 (13.64)	0.136
Angle (°)-BL	79.35 (6.37)	82.81 (10.87)	79.61 (7.65)	78.67 (8.11)	79.77 (7.96)	0.694
Angle (°)-CL	73.71 (8.66)	74.44 (4.38)	71.27 (7.52)	72.19 (6.50)	72.47 (7.05)	0.671

Table 6 Results from a multivariable random effects regression model of all angles on age (in groups) gender and point of measurement

Factor	Difference	95% CI	p value
Age (years)			
< 45[a]	0		
45–54	− 0.9	(− 5.7, 3.9)	0.724
55–64	− 1.4	(− 5.5, 2.8)	0.520
65+	− 0.6	(− 5.0, 3.9)	0.806
Gender			
Male[a]	0		
Female	− 2.5	(− 5.4, 0.5)	0.097
Position			
1 (AR/AL)[a]	0		
2(BR/BL)	10.0	(7.8, 12.3)	< 0.001
3 (CR/CL)	2.2	(−0.0, 4.5)	0.051

[a]Reference category

The aforementioned differences can be attributed to the fact that every study has evaluated different populations and has also set different criteria in the selection of their sample.

In our study, there is no statistically significant influence when comparing the thickness of the mucosa and age ($p = 0.878$). Janner et al. 2010, Vallo et al. 2010, and Jildirim et al. 2017 also come in accordance with our results [12, 16, 17]. The age factor does not seem to affect the anatomical characteristics of the sinus. Unlike a state of inflammation, allergy, smoking of the patient does not affect the sinus thickness or wideness [6].

As regards the width of the maxillary sinus, the mean angle value was found to be 73.4 ± 6.9 °. It seems that there is a tendency towards greater angle values in the male group, but the difference is not statistically significant in order to conclude that wider angles and widths exist in male patients. The aforementioned results can be also associated with the results of the study of Gosau et al. 2009, which showed that female sinuses tend to have lower average volume values than male sinuses [4]. The study of Lozano-Carrascal et al. 2017 also measured the same angle but only in the region of the upper first molar and found a mean value of 73.39 ± 15.23 ° [15]. The present study is more accurate because the mean angle results from three different measurements taken from three different points of the maxillary sinus.

In the present study, it was also concluded that the width of the sinus increases from mesial to distal. Male sinuses had higher prevalence of high angle values compared to female sinuses, but the majority of angle values and widths was characterized as moderate.

In an attempt to correlate the membrane biotype regarding thickness with the sinus width, it was proven that there is no correlation between the thickness and width of the sinus ($p = 0.695$).

Conclusions

In conclusion, the present study demonstrated that male patients tend to have a thicker membrane than female patients. The angles of the sinus seemed to increase in

Table 7 All studies measuring the thickness of the Schneiderian membrane [5, 7, 9, 12, 15, 17–25]

Authors	Year of study	Method of study	Results
Tos and Mogesen et al.	1979	Cadavers	0.3–0.8 mm
Aimetti et al.	2008	Endoscopically	0.97 ± 0.36 mm
Pommer et al.	2009	Cadavers	0.09 ± 0.045 mm
Janner et al.	2010	CBCTs	2.16–3.11 mm (mid-sagittal regions) and 0.9–1.84 mm (lateral-median regions)
Pazera et al.	2010	CBCTs	1.58 mm (95% CI 1.17–1.98)
Cakur et al.	2011	CBCTs	0.5 ± 0.49 mm
Pommer et al.	2012	CTs	0.8–1.99 mm
Anduze-Acher et al	2012	CTs	1.99 ± 2.10 mm
Zheng-Ze Guo et al.	2015	CBCTs	1.93 ± 2.00 mm
Shih-Cheng Wen et al.	2015	CBCTs	1.78 ± 1.99 mm
Yen-Hua Lin et al.	2015	CBCTs	1.32 ± 0.87 mm
Insua et al.	2017	Cadavers	1.36 ± 0.42 mm
Lozano-Carrascal et al.	2017	CBCTs	1.82 ± 1.59 mm
Talo Jildirim et al.	2017	CBCTs	4.19 ± 5.84 mm
Present study	2017	CBCTs	1.60 ± 1.20 mm

width from mesial to distal, and they have no significant correlation with any of our parameters. Thickness of the mucosa and width of the maxillary sinus did not seem to correlate. Future studies including larger groups of participants should be necessarily conducted in order to establish additional possible correlations between the anatomical structures of the maxillary sinus and their variations.

Authors' contributions
DK evaluated and selected the CBCT images for the present study. AK and SP conducted all the required measurements. All four authors interpreted and analyzed the data collected. KT critically revised and approved the article. All authors read and approved the final manuscript.

Competing interests
Authors Demos Kalyvas, Andreas Kapsalas, Sofia Paikou, and Konstantinos Tsiklakis declare that they have no competing interests.

Author details
[1]Department of Oral and Maxillofacial Surgery, School of Dentistry, National and Kapodistrian University of Athens, Greece, Thivon 2 str, 11527 Athens, Greece. [2]Oral Diagnosis & Radiology Clinic, School of Dentistry, National and Kapodistrian University of Athens, Greece, Thivon 2 str, 11527 Athens, Greece.

References
1. Testori T. Maxillary sinus surgery: Anatomy and advanced diagnostic imaging. J Implant and Reconstructive Dent. 2011;2:6-14.
2. Sargi ZB, Casiano RR. Surgical anatomy of the paranasal sinuses. In: Kountakis SE, Onerci TM, editors. Rhinologic and sleep apnea surgical techniques. New York: Springer; 2007. p. 17–26.
3. Bergh van den JPA, Bruggenkate ten CM, Disch FJM, Tuinzing DB. Anatomical aspects of sinus floor elevations. Clin Oral Impl Res. 2000;11: 256–65.
4. Gosau M, Rink D, Driemel O, Draenert FG. Maxillary sinus anatomy: a cadaveric study with clinical implications. Anat Rec (Hoboken). 2009; 292(3):352–4.
5. Guo Z-Z, Liu Y, Qin L, Song Y-L, Xie C, Li D-H. Longitudinal response of membrane thickness and ostium patency following sinus floor elevation: a prospective cohort study. Clin. Oral Impl. Res. 2015;00:1–6.
6. D R, Borgonovo AE, Cicciù M, Re D, Rizza F, Frigo AC, Maiorana C. Maxillary sinus septa and anatomic correlation with the Schneiderian membrane. J Craniofac Surg. 2015;26(4):1394–8.
7. Lin Y-H, Yang Y-C, Wen S-C, Wang H-L. The influence of sinus membrane thickness upon membrane perforation during lateral window sinus augmentation. Clin. Oral Impl. Res. 2015;00:1–6.
8. Kim SH, Kim KH, Seo BM, et al. Alveolar bone regeneration by transplantation of periodontal ligament stem cells and bone marrow stem cells in a canine peri-implant defect model: a pilot study. J Periodontol. 2009;80(11):1815–23.
9. Cakur B, Sümbüllü MA, Durna D. Relationship among Schneiderian membrane, Underwood's septa, and the maxillary sinus inferior border. Clin Implant Dent Relat Res. 2013;15(1):83–7.
10. Shanbhag S, Karnik P, Shirke P, Shanbhag V. Cone-beam computed tomographic analysis of sinus membrane thickness, ostium patency, and residual ridge heights in the posterior maxilla: implications for sinus floor elevation. Clin Oral Impl Res. 2014;25:755–60.
11. Yoo JY, Pi SH, Kim YS, Jeong SN, You HK. Healing pattern of the mucous membrane after tooth extraction in the maxillary sinus. J Periodontal Implant Sci. 2011;41(1):23–9.
12. Janner SFM, Caversaccio MD, Dubach P, Sendi P, Buser D, Bornstein MM. Characteristics and dimensions of the Schneiderian membrane: a radiographic analysis using cone beam computed tomography in patients referred for dental implant surgery in the posterior maxilla. Clin. Oral Impl. Res. 2011;22:1446–53.
13. Cagici CA, Yilmazer C, Hurcan C, Ozer C, Ozer F. Appropriate interslice gap for screening coronal paranasal sinus tomography for mucosal thickening. Eur Arch Otorhinolaryngol. 2009;266(4):519–25.
14. Eggesbø HB. Radiological imaging of inflammatory lesions in the nasal cavity and paranasal sinuses. Eur Radiol. 2006;16:872–88.
15. Lozano-Carrascal N, Salomó-Coll O, Gehrke SA, Calvo-Guirado JL, Hernández-Alfaro F, Gargallo-Albiol J. Radiological evaluation of maxillary sinus anatomy: a cross-sectional study of 300 patients. Ann Anat. 2017;214:1–8. https://doi.org/10.1016/j.aanat.2017.06.002. Epub 2017 Jul 29
16. Vallo J, Suominen-Taipale L, Huumonen S, Soikkonen K, Norblad A. Prevalence of mucosal abnormalities of the maxillary sinus and their relationship to dental disease in panoramic radiography: results from the health 2000 Health Examination Survey. Oral Surg Oral Med Oral Pathol Oral Radiol Endod. 2010;109(3):e80–7.
17. Yildirim TT, Güncü GN, Göksülük D, Tözüm MD, Colak M, Tözüm TF. The effect of demographic and disease variables on Schneiderian membrane thickness and appearance. Oral Surg Oral Med Oral Pathol Oral Radiol. 2017; 124:568–76.
18. Pazera P, Bornstein MM, Pazera A, Sendi P, Katsaros C. Incidental maxillary sinus findings in orthodontic patients: a radiographic analysis using cone-beam computed tomography (CBCT). Orthod Craniofac Res. 2011;14:17–24.
19. Tos M, Mogensen C. Mucus production in the nasal sinuses. Acta Otolaryngol Suppl. 1979;360:131–4.
20. M A, Massei G, Morra M, Cardesi E, Romano F. Correlation between gingival phenotype and Schneiderian membrane thickness. Int J Oral Maxillofac Implants. 2008;23(6):1128–32.
21. Pommer B, Unger E, Suto D, Hack N, Watzek G. Mechanical properties of the schneiderian membrane in vitro. Clin Oral Implants Res. 2009;20:633–7.
22. Pommer B, Dvorak G, Jesch P, Palmer RM, Watzek G, Gahleitner A. Effect of maxillary sinus floor augmentation on sinus membrane thickness in computed tomography. J Periodontol. 2012;83:551–6.
23. Anduze-Acher G, Brochery B, Felizardo R, Valentini P, Katsahian S, Bouchard P. Change in sinus membrane dimension following sinus floor elevation: a retrospective cohort study. Clin. Oral Impl. Res. 2013;24:1123–9.
24. Wen S-C, Lin Y-H, Yang Y-C, Wang H-L. The influence of sinus membrane thickness upon membrane perforation during transcrestal sinus lift procedure. Clin. Oral Impl. Res. 2015;26:1158–64.
25. Insua A, Monje-Gil F, García-Caballero L, Caballé-Serrano J, Wang HL, Monje A. Mechanical characteristics of the maxillary sinus Schneiderian membrane ex vivo. Clin Oral Investig. 2017; https://doi.org/10.1007/s00784-017-2201-4.

Short-term follow-up of masticatory adaptation after rehabilitation with an immediately loaded implant-supported prosthesis

Mihoko Tanaka[1,2*], Collaert Bruno[2], Reinhilde Jacobs[3,4], Tetsurou Torisu[1] and Hiroshi Murata[1]

Abstract

Background: When teeth are extracted, sensory function is decreased by a loss of periodontal ligament receptions. When replacing teeth by oral implants, one hopes to restore the sensory feedback pathway as such to allow for physiological implant integration and optimized oral function with implant-supported prostheses. What remains to be investigated is how to adapt to different oral rehabilitations.

The purpose of this pilot study was to assess four aspects of masticatory adaptation after rehabilitation with an immediately loaded implant-supported prosthesis and to observe how each aspect will recover respectively.

Methods: Eight participants with complete dentures were enrolled. They received an implant-supported acrylic resin provisional bridge, 1 day after implant surgery. Masticatory adaptation was examined by assessing occlusal contact, approximate maximum bite force, masticatory efficiency of gum-like specimens, and food hardness perception.

Results: Occlusal contact and approximate maximum bite force were significantly increased 3 months after implant rehabilitation, with the bite force gradually building up to a 72% increase compared to baseline. Masticatory efficiency increased by 46% immediately after surgery, stabilizing at around 40% 3 months after implant rehabilitation. Hardness perception also improved, with a reduction of the error rate by 16% over time.

Conclusions: This assessment demonstrated masticatory adaptation immediately after implant rehabilitation with improvements noted up to 3 months after surgery and rehabilitation. It was also observed that, despite gradually improved bite force in all patients, masticatory efficiency and food hardness perception did not necessarily follow this tendency. The findings in this pilot may also be used to assess adaptation of oral function after implant rehabilitation by studying the combined outcome of four tests (occlusal contact, maximum bite force, masticatory efficiency, and food hardness perception).

Keywords: Physiologic adaptation, Masticatory function, Immediate loading, Dental implants

Background

Tooth loss represents a major oral disability comparable to an amputation, with severe impairment of oral functions [1]. While denture wearers can rely on mucosal sensors, anchoring prosthetic teeth to the bone via osseointegrated implants has been assumed to create a (partial) sensory substitution for missing periodontal ligament receptors from stimuli transmitted via the bone [2]. The restoration of the sensory feedback pathway is necessary for the physiological integration of implant-supported prostheses in the human body. It helps to optimize essential oral functions, such as chewing and biting. Studies on such functions usually report an improvement of oral functions with implant-supported prostheses as opposed to conventional dentures [3–9]. Improved oral function also impacts on quality of life [10], often scored with ratings for function, pain,

* Correspondence: mihobonn@nagasaki-u.ac.jp
[1]Department of Prosthetic Dentistry, Graduate School of Biomedical Science, Nagasaki University, 1-7-1 Sakamoto, Nagasaki 852-8588, Japan
[2]Centre for Periodontology and Implantology Leuven, IJzerenmolenstraat 110, B-3001 Heverlee, Belgium

discomfort, and psychosocial factors using the GOHAI system [11]. However, one should realize that such rehabilitation may also create some patient-related masticatory and other problems or complications [12]. Such complaints could be related to uncomfortable occlusion, accidental biting of the cheek or tongue, or problems during speech. Other complications might include fractures of prosthetic or implant components. For adequate mastication, the ability to adapt to food of various levels of hardness and various volumes is important. In individuals with natural dentition, such information is processed by the periodontal ligament receptors [13–15]. Since patients with implant-supported prostheses lose the periodontal ligament and its elaborate associated peripheral feedback mechanism, it is possible that they are not able to differentiate food hardness and texture. In this context, it is important to mention that some studies reported no significant improvement of masticatory function after implant treatment [3, 16, 17]. Jacobs et al. [3] indeed noticed that some of these patients might realize that the peripheral feedback mechanism is no longer assisting them, rendering some of them afraid of biting too hard. [3] Instead, these anxious patients are found to bite submaximally with implant-supported prostheses [3].

In addition, it also remains to be demonstrated how a potential compensatory mechanism might work, with one of the options being osseoperception [2, 18–23]. In this context, it is also important to consider the adaptation time needed after oral rehabilitation. Some studies have performed longitudinal evaluations of masticatory function for more than 3 years [24, 25]. However, there are limited data available on short-term adaptation to mastication, especially in the first months after being fitted with a prosthetic appliance. Although approximately 2 months are generally required for adaptation to a new removable denture, the time needed to adapt to a new implant-supported prosthesis has not been established [26]. Furthermore, adaptation is likely to be more difficult with full fixed implant prostheses [27].

In a functional magnetic resolution imaging (fMRI) study of patients with implants, it was demonstrated that punctate mechanical stimulation of oral implants activates both primary and secondary cortical somatosensory areas and was suggested that brain plasticity occurs when extracted teeth are replaced by endosseous implants [28]. In another fMRI study, it was suggested that the time after tooth extraction may affect neural plasticity, which in turn can influence osseoperception, with the amount of time possibly being an indicator for prosthetic treatment planning [23]. The lack of peripheral feedback mechanisms in patients with implant-supported full fixed prostheses may lead to a lack of control over the biting force [3, 29]. Such control is needed for refinement and control of the biting force for various types of food [7, 30–32]. While patients with implant-supported bridges are able to bite food with varying levels of hardness, it could be questioned whether they are able to differentiate between the hardness variations and thus apply an adapted chewing pattern [33]. Although some studies have demonstrated the tactile function of patients with oral implants [18, 19], the perception of food hardness is yet another sensory function that should be evaluated in order to obtain more information on modulation and masticatory adaptation. However, there have been few studies on this issue. Although adaptation to food texture during mastication by dentate subjects has been tested [34], it has not yet been followed up in patients receiving implant placement. In a recent cross-sectional study, mastication adaptability in patients with implant-supported bridges was assessed with soft and hard food models using an electromyogram (EMG) [7]. Patients with implants showed a significantly weaker increase in EMG activity with increased food hardness. In addition, muscular work performance (bite-force ratio and muscle activity) was found to be lower in patients with implants [35]. Furthermore, less coordinated masticatory muscle activity was found in patients with implant-supported prostheses [36].

The purpose of this pilot investigation was to use testing methodologies involving four aspects of masticatory adaptation after rehabilitation with an immediately loaded implant-supported prosthesis and to observe the recovery of each aspect respectively. Our hypothesis is that bite force may recover quickly, but other aspects will require monitoring and recording in order to form an overall judgment on the oral adaption to implant rehabilitation.

Methods

Six females and 2 males (average age 66.4 years, range 52–85 years) with upper ($n = 7$) or lower ($n = 1$) complete dentures participated in this study. Inclusion criteria were (1) an opposite jaw that included natural dentition at least to the second premolar on both sides, (2) a need for fixed rehabilitation, (3) no medical contraindication to the placement of implants, (4) no need for augmentation procedures, and (5) willingness to participate in this study. The only exclusion criterion was temporo-mandibular dysfunction, since it may interfere with chewing and biting patterns and abilities. In the mandible 5 and in the maxilla, 6 OsseoSpeed implants and Uni Abutments 20° (Astra Tech, Mölndal, Sweden) were used to provide support for fixed rehabilitation. All participants were treated at the Center for Periodontology and Implantology, Leuven, Belgium, by the same surgeon (BC). Informed written consent with regard to treatment and masticatory function and follow-up procedures was provided to each participant. The study was approved by the ethics committee of the Catholic University of Leuven (B322201319432).

The day after implant surgery, implants were loaded with screw-retained implant-supported acrylic resin provisional restoration (immediate loading) as previously described [37, 38]. All provisional bridges extended to the second premolar or first molar region.

Occlusal contact area and approximate maximum bite force measurements

Patient's head was positioned with the Frankfort plane parallel to the floor. After opening the mouth, a pressure-sensitive sheet (Dental Prescale, 50H, type R, 97 µm thick, GC, Tokyo, Japan) was inserted on the occlusal plane. Patients were instructed to bite onto the test sheet as hard as possible for 3 s in the intercuspal position. This was repeated three times in each patient. The sheets were analyzed using special analytical equipment (Occluzer FPD-707, GC, Tokyo, Japan), namely, an analyzing device that could calculate bite force (N) and occlusal contact area (mm^2) from the degree of discoloration of the pressure-sensitive sheets. Values from three sheets were averaged for each measurement, as described in a previous study [39]. In a pilot study, dentate patients ($n = 14$, mean age 58.4 ± 12.6 years) showed an occlusal contact area of 20.79 ± 8.10 mm^2 and a maximal bite force of 696.8 ± 237.5 N.

Measurement of masticatory efficiency

To assess the masticatory efficiency, we used glucose extraction in the filtrate obtained after chewing the specimen. After rinsing the mouth with tap water, a gum-like specimen mixed with 5% glucose with a height of 10 mm (Glucosensor Gummy, GC, Tokyo, Japan) was placed on patient's tongue with chopsticks. Patients were requested to chew on the cube for 20 s, after which, they expectorated all the chunks of the cube into a cup equipped with a mesh filter to hold the debris. Thereafter, they rinsed their mouth again with 10 ml of water and expectorated into the same cup. The amount of glucose extraction in the filtrate obtained after chewing the specimen was used as a measure of masticatory efficiency. Glucose concentration in the filtrate (mg/dl) was measured using a calibrated Glucose Sensor Set (Glucosensor GS-1, GC, Tokyo, Japan), which utilizes a glucose sensor for diabetics (Accu-check Comfort, Roche Diagnostic, Basel, Switzerland) to measure masticatory efficiency according to a previous study, which reported its reliability for the evaluation of masticatory function [40]. For reproducibility, we tested the glucose concentration of control glucose solutions (500, 250, 125, 100, and 50 mg/dl) with the glucose sensor. The linear

relationship that was observed between the glucose density of the solution (x) and the masticatory efficiency (the value of the glucose sensor) (y) is displayed in a scatter diagram (Fig. 1). The linear regression equation and Pearson's correlation coefficient were as follows: $y = 0.599 + 1.066x$, $r = 0.99$ ($n = 50$, $p < 0.0001$). The intra-class correlation coefficient (ICC) is a prominent statistic to measure the test-retest reliability of data. The ICC (1, 3) of the data by Glucosensor was $p = 1.000$ ($n = 5$).

Food hardness assessment

Three types of chewing specimen with different levels of hardness (hard, medium, and soft), with the same size and taste, were produced from sucrose (800 g), glucose (870 g), sorbitol (1000 g), gelatin (hard, 390 g; medium, 240 g; and soft, 150 g), Arabia gum (hard, 36 g), citric acid (42 g), lemon juice (15 g), and water and were 15 × 15 ×10 mm in size. The hardness of each type was determined under maximal stress during compression of 9 mm with a crosshead speed of 100 mm/min with a tooth-shaped jig using a texture analyzer (EZ test, Shimadzu Co., Kyoto, Japan). The hardness results were 73 ± 1.5 N for the soft, 88 ± 1.5 N for the medium, and 171 ± 1.9 N for the hard specimens.

To assess the hardness differences, the examiner placed each test specimen on the tongue with chopsticks, and then the participants chewed on all sides and swallowed. They were asked to remember the hardness of the first specimen, which always had medium hardness and served as a control, and then to determine the level of hardness (hard, medium, or soft) of four consecutive and randomly administered specimens by comparing them with the first one. This test was conducted in a double-blind manner to eliminate examiner bias.

The number of correct answers of hardness was used as a measure of hardness recognition. The subjects were allowed to expectorate any specimen that could not be

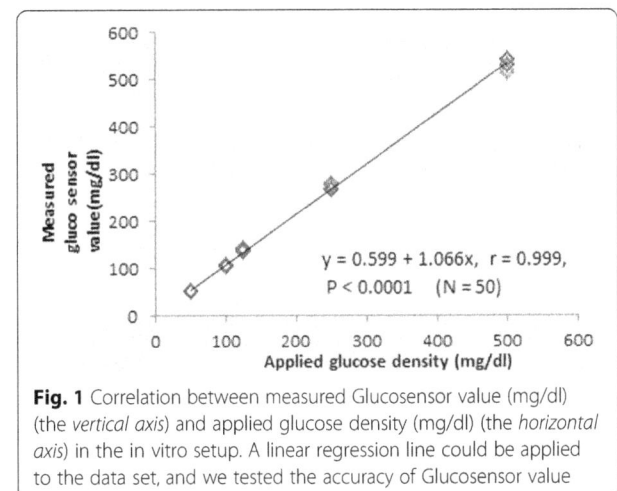

Fig. 1 Correlation between measured Glucosensor value (mg/dl) (the *vertical axis*) and applied glucose density (mg/dl) (the *horizontal axis*) in the in vitro setup. A linear regression line could be applied to the data set, and we tested the accuracy of Glucosensor value

chewed well enough to be swallowed and could change their answers until the last specimen was chewed.

Data collection
Occlusal contact area, maximum bite force measurements, masticatory efficiency, and discriminating hardness assessments were performed on four occasions: (1) before implant surgery with the complete denture in situ, (2) 3 h after surgery, (3) 1–2 weeks, and (4) 3 months after insertion of the provisional screw-retained restoration.

Statistical analysis
Considering the small sample size in the present psychophysical experiments, the option was taken to report mainly the descriptive statistics, in terms of average (SD, range) values for bite force, occlusal contact area, glucose concentration, and number of correct answers regarding hardness. Some nonparametric analyses were added in the difference between baseline prior to surgery and the follow-up data (Wilcoxon test, SPSS for Macintosh ver.21, SPSS, Chicago, USA). A p value <0.05 was considered to be statistically significant.

Results
Two participants were unavailable to attend the testing at 1–2 weeks after the provisional restoration had been inserted, which resulted in missing data.

Overall descriptive analyses yielded the following observations for the four tests.

Occlusal contact area and maximum bite force
Occlusal contact and approximate maximum bite force were significantly increased 3 months after implant rehabilitation because of the adjustment of provisional occlusion, with the bite force gradually building up by 72% compared with that at stage one (prior to implant rehabilitation). Prior to implant surgery, when participants were wearing complete dentures for the lower or upper jaw, none expressed satisfaction with their dentures when we asked about them. However, occlusal contact and approximate maximum bite force varied widely among subjects but steadily increased in the individual participants (bite force, range 16.4–339.80 N, SD = 103.89; occlusal contact area, 0.4–9.63 mm^2, SD = 3.31). The occlusal contact area was increased right after implant surgery ($p < 0.005$) and 3 months after wearing implants ($p < 0.005$). At the same time, maximum bite force also increased on these occasions ($p < 0.001$ and $p < 0.005$) (Fig. 2a, b). There was a positive and significant correlation between occlusal contact area and approximate maximum bite force ($r = 0.91$, $p < 0.001$). Our findings on occlusal contact and bite force were

7.96 ± 3.55 mm^2 and 254.3 ± 76.4 N, respectively, after 3 months of wearing implant-support prostheses.

Measurement of efficiency of specimen mastication
The obtained glucose data varied considerably between before and immediately after implant surgery (before, 0–180.7 mg/dl, SD = 62.9 mg/dl; day 0, 23.0–258 mg/dl, SD = 73.92 mg/dl). In contrast, masticatory efficiency was not significantly different among the four periods (Wilcoxon test) (Fig. 2c). Overall, the masticatory efficiency increased by 46% immediately after surgery, stabilizing at around 40% 3 months after implant rehabilitation. This parameter was decreased in two participants at 3 months after wearing implants, one of whom also showed decreases in both occlusal contact and bite force.

We also obtained data on the healthy control group ($n = 11$), with an age similar to that of the experimental participants (age average ± SD, 65 ± 9; glucose data average ± SD, 25.5 ± 77.6). The findings for our experimental participants under all conditions were lower than those for the control group (Fig. 2c).

Hardness assessment
Hardness perception became better after implant rehabilitation, with a reduction of the error rate by 16% (Fig. 3). While five out of eight participants performed better in this test after rehabilitation, the results in the others were less clear. More detailed analysis showed that, despite wearing dentures, four participants were 100% successful in recognition of hardness before implant surgery, while four others had a 50% success rate, implying a response by chance. Noteworthy, three patients were able to chew and swallow a hard specimen immediately after implant rehabilitation.

Discussion
Occlusal contact was significantly increased 3 months after implant rehabilitation when compared to stage one (prior to implant rehabilitation). We assumed the reason was that some participant's occlusion was worn down because the material of provisional restoration was resin. To observe the adaptation of masticatory function after rehabilitation with an immediately loaded implant-supported prosthesis, we compared the data of four stages (before and after implant surgery) using four tests (occlusal contact, approximate maximum bite force, masticatory efficiency, and recognition of hardness threshold). The present method was simple and acceptable for use in a clinical patient setting, as the specimens had characteristics similar to typical sweets that contain glucose. In a previous study, the present method for masticatory efficiency was validated and found to be comparable to a sieve method [40].

Short-term follow-up of masticatory adaptation after rehabilitation with an immediately loaded... 13

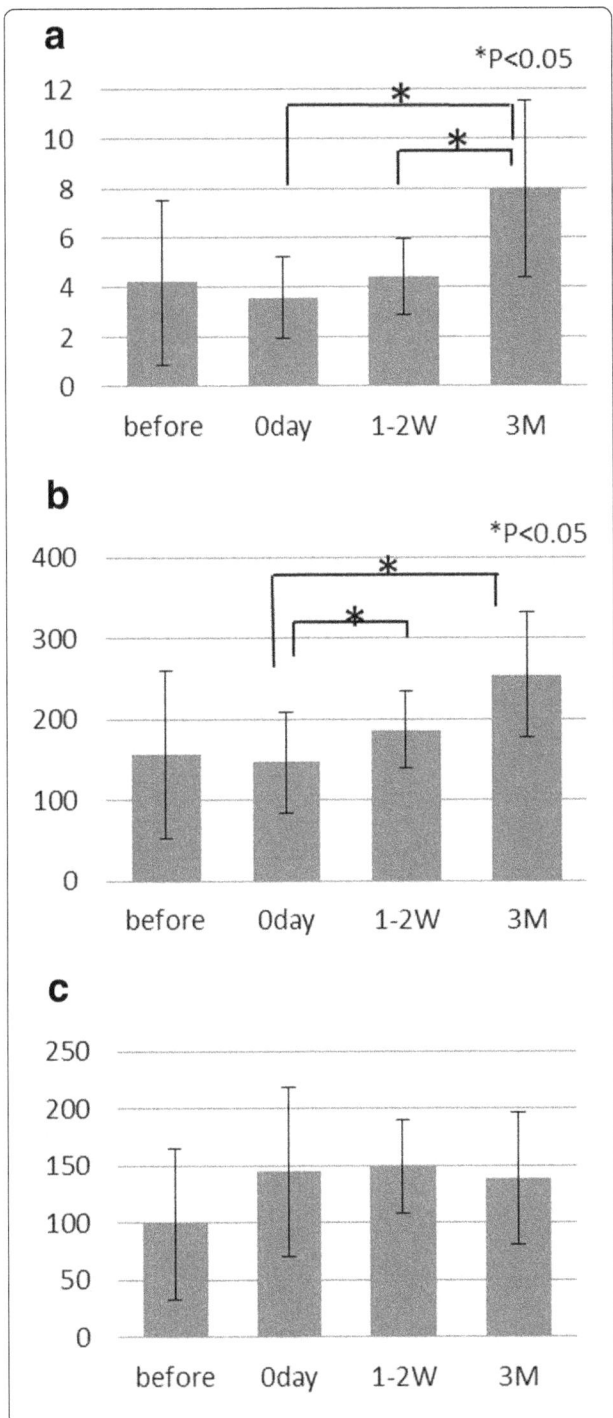

Fig. 2 a Mean and standard deviation (SD) of occlusal contact area at each of the four times. The *horizontal label axis* was the time stage (1) before implant surgery with the complete denture in situ and (2) right after with provisional implant, (3) 1–2 weeks and (4) 3 months after insertion of the provisional screw-retained restoration, and the label to the *vertical axis* was contact area (mm²). The occlusal contact area was increased at 3 months after wearing implants (paired *t* test, *p* < 0.005). *p < 0.005, significant difference between conditions. **b** Mean and standard deviation (SD) of bite force at each of the four times. The *horizontal label axis* was the time stage, and the label to the *vertical axis* was bite force (N). The approximate maximum bite force was increased at 3 months after wearing implants (paired *t* test, *p* < 0.005). *p < 0.005, significant difference between conditions. **c** Mean and standard deviation (SD) of glucose data at each of the four times. The *horizontal label axis* was the time stage, and the label to the vertical axis was glucose data of Glucosensor value (mg/dl)

In this study, we measured occlusal contact and maximum bite during a 3-month follow-up period in patients with implant-supported prostheses. Generally, maximum bite force was increased after 3 months, with a positive correlation to occlusal contact, in accordance with the literature [41].

We found no differences regarding the masticatory efficiency of the specimen among the different time periods, even when bite force and occlusal contact area were significantly increased. Although the present sample is small, masticatory performance seemed to be influenced by the motivation of the participants, with more improvement immediately after implant treatment. However, that is mere surmise.

Recognition of hardness threshold

In the present study, there were no differences regarding the recognition of hardness threshold among the hardness levels at each stage. Edentulous patients with implant-supported dentures showed improved tactile discrimination ability and motor function in contrast to patients with complete dentures [42, 43] However, it is important to

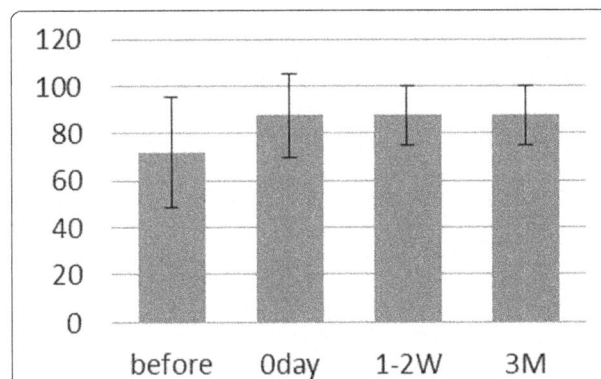

Fig. 3 Mean and standard deviation (SD) of percentage of correct answers regarding hardness at each of the four times. The *horizontal label axis* was the time stage, and the label to the *vertical axis* was percentage of correct answers regarding hardness (%)

compare these results with those from patients with implant-supported prostheses in both jaws, lacking any kind of periodontal feedback. Trulsson [13] reported that the periodontal ligament had the highest sensitivity to changes in tooth load at low forces (below 1 N for anterior teeth and 4 N for posterior teeth). In dentate people, this may help in modulating the jaw muscles, especially when dealing with a rapid force build up, in relation to hard food.

Conclusions

The present pilot study could not confirm an immediate rise in bite force after implant rehabilitation. Instead, improvements were mainly noted up to 3 months after surgery and rehabilitation. Furthermore, it became evident that despite gradually improved bite force in all patients, masticatory efficiency and food hardness perception did not necessarily follow the same trend. The present findings may be used to adapt oral function after implant rehabilitation by studying the combined outcome of four tests (occlusal contact, maximum bite force, masticatory efficiency, and food hardness perception). Studies with a longer follow-up time and larger sample sizes are needed to verify the present results.

Acknowledgements

The authors are grateful to the volunteers who participated in this study. This work was supported by JSPS Grant-in-Aid for Scientific Research (C), grant number 23592860.

Authors' contributions

MT, CB, and RJ conceived and designed the experiment. MT and CB performed the experiments and analyzed the data with R J. TT and HM helped to draft the manuscript. All authors read and approved the final manuscript.

Competing interests

Mihoko Tanaka, Collaert Bruno, Reinhilde Jacobs, Tetsurou Torisu, and Hiroshi Murata states that there are no competing interest.

Author details

[1]Department of Prosthetic Dentistry, Graduate School of Biomedical Science, Nagasaki University, 1-7-1 Sakamoto, Nagasaki 852-8588, Japan. [2]Centre for Periodontology and Implantology Leuven, IJzerenmolenstraat 110, B-3001 Heverlee, Belgium. [3]OMFS IMPATH, Department of Imaging & Pathology, University of Leuven, Kapucijnenvoer 33, BE-3000 Leuven, Belgium. [4]Oral and Maxillofacial Surgery, University Hospitals Leuven, Kapucijnenvoer 33, BE-3000 Leuven, Belgium.

References

1.   Klineberg IJ, Trulsson M, Murray GM. Occlusion on implants—is there a problem? J Oral Rehabil. 2012;39:522–37.
2.   Feine J, Jacobs R, Lobbezoo F, Sessle BJ, Van Steenberghe D, Trulsson M, Fejerskov O, Svensson P. A functional perspective on oral implants—state-of-the-science and future recommendations. J Oral Rehabil. 2006;33:309–12.
3.   Jacobs R, van Steenberghe D, Naert I. Masseter muscle fatigue before and after rehabilitation with implant-supported prostheses. J Prosthet Dent. 1995;73:284–9.
4.   Fontijn-Tekamp FA, Slagter AP, Van Der Bilt A, Van 'T Hof MA, Witter DJ, Kalk W, et al. Biting and chewing in overdentures, full dentures, and natural dentitions. J Dent Res. 2000;79:1519–24.
5.   Stellingsma K, Slagter AP, Stegenga B, Raghoebar GM, Meijer HJ. Masticatory function in patients with an extremely resorbed mandible restored with mandibular implant-retained overdentures: comparison of three types of treatment protocols. J Oral Rehabil. 2005;32:403–10.
6.   Dierens M, Collaert B, Deschepper E, Browaeys H, Klinge B, De Bruyn H. Patient-centered outcome of immediately loaded implants in the rehabilitation of fully edentulous jaws. Clin Oral Implants Res. 2009;20:1070–7.
7.   Grigoriadis A, Johansson RS, Trulsson M. Adaptability of mastication in people with implant-supported bridges. J Clin Periodontol. 2011;38:395–404.
8.   Okoński P, Mierzwińska-Nastalska E, Janicka-Kostrzewa J. Implant supported dentures: an estimation of chewing efficiency. Gerodontology. 2011;28:58–61.
9.   Müller F, Hernandez M, Grütter L, Aracil-Kessler L, Weingart D, Schimmel M. Masseter muscle thickness, chewing efficiency and bite force in edentulous patients with fixed and removable implant-supported prostheses: a cross-sectional multicenter study. Clin Oral Implants Res. 2012;23:144–50.
10. Awad MA, Lund JP, Dufresne E, Feine JS. Comparing the efficacy of mandibular implant-retained overdentures and conventional dentures among middle-aged edentulous patients: satisfaction and functional assessment. Int J Prosthodont. 2003;16:117–22.
11. Hägglin C, Berggren U, Hakeberg M, Edvardsson A, Eriksson M. Evaluation of a Swedish version of the OHIP-14 among patients in general and specialist dental care. Swed Dent J. 2007;31:91–101.
12. Goodacre CJ, Bernal G, Rungcharassaeng K, Kan JY. Clinical complications with implants and implant prostheses. J Prosthet Dent. 2003;90:121–32.
13. Trulsson M, Johansson RS. Encoding of amplitude and rate of forces applied to the teeth by human periodontal mechanoreceptive afferents. J Neurophysiol. 1994;72:1734–44.
14. Hidaka O, Morimoto T, Masuda Y, Kato T, Matsuo R, Inoue T, et al. Regulation of masticatory force during cortically induced rhythmic jaw movements in the anesthetized rabbit. J Neurophysiol. 1997;77:3168–79.
15. Hidaka O, Morimoto T, Kato T, Masuda Y, Inoue T, Takada K. Behavior of jaw muscle spindle afferents during cortically induced rhythmic jaw movements in the anesthetized rabbit. J Neurophysiol. 1999;82:2633–40.
16. Garrett NR, Kapur KK, Hamada MO, Roumanas ED, Freymiller E, Han T, et al. A randomized clinical trial comparing the efficacy of mandibular implant-supported overdentures and conventional dentures in diabetic patients. Part II. Comparisons of masticatory performance. J Prosthet Dent. 1998;79:632–40.
17. Haraldson T, Jemt T, Stålblad PA, Lekholm U. Oral function in subjects with overdentures supported by osseointegrated implants. Scand J Dent Res. 1988;96:235–42.
18. Enkling N, Heussner S, Nicolay C, Bayer S, Mericske-Stern R, Utz KH. Tactile sensibility of single-tooth implants and natural teeth under local anesthesia of the natural antagonistic teeth. Clin Implant Dent Relat Res. 2012;14:273–80.
19. Jacobs R, Van Steenberghe D. From osseoperception to implant-mediated sensory-motor interactions and related clinical implications. J Oral Rehabil. 2006;33:282–92.
20. Abarca M, Van Steenberghe D, Malevez C, Jacobs R. The neurophysiology of osseointegrated oral implants. A clinically underestimated aspect. J Oral Rehabil. 2006;33:161–9.
21. Klineberg I, Calford MB, Dreher B, Henry P, Macefield V, Miles T, et al. A consensus statement on osseoperception. Clin Exp Pharmacol Physiol. 2005;32:145–6.
22. Trulsson M. Sensory and motor function of teeth and dental implants: a basis for osseoperception. Clin Exp Pharmacol Physiol. 2005;32:119–22.
23. Yan C, Ye L, Zhen J, Ke L, Gang L. Neuroplasticity of edentulous patients with implant-supported full dentures. Eur J Oral Sci. 2008;116:387–93.
24. Naert I, Alsaadi G, Quirynen M. Prosthetic aspects and patient satisfaction with two-implant-retained mandibular overdentures: a 10-year randomized clinical study. Int J Prosthodont. 2004;17:401–10.
25. Bakke M, Holm B, Gotfredsen K. Masticatory function and patient satisfaction with implant-supported mandibular overdentures: a prospective 5-year study. Int J Prosthodont. 2002;15:575–81.
26. Miyaura K, Morita M, Matsuka Y, Yamashita A, Watanabe T. Rehabilitation of biting abilities in patients with different types of dental prostheses. J Oral Rehabil. 2000;27:1073–6.
27. Peyron MA, Blanc O, Lund JP, Woda A. Influence of age on adaptability of human mastication. J Neurophysiol. 2004;92:773–9.
28. Habre-Hallage P, Dricot L, Jacobs R, van Steenberghe D, Reychler H, Grandin CB. Brain plasticity and cortical correlates of osseoperception revealed by punctate mechanical stimulation of osseointegrated oral implants during fMRI. Eur J Oral Implantol. 2012;5:175–90.
29. Jacobs R, van Steenberghe D. Qualitative evaluation of the masseteric poststimulus EMG complex following mechanical or acoustic stimulation of osseointegrated oral implants. Int J Oral Maxillofac Implants. 1995;10:175–82.

30. Svensson KG, Trulsson M. Impaired force control during food holding and biting in subjects with tooth- or implant-supported fixed prostheses. J Clin Periodontol. 2011;38:1137–46.

31. Svensson KG, Grigoriadis J, Trulsson M. Alterations in intraoral manipulation and splitting of food by subjects with tooth- or implant-supported fixed prostheses. Clin Oral Implants Res. 2013;24:549–55.

32. Trulsson M, van der Bilt A, Carlsson GE, Gotfredsen K, Larsson P, Müller F, et al. From brain to bridge: masticatory function and dental implants. J Oral Rehabil. 2012;39:858–77.

33. Luraschi J, Schimmel M, Bernard JP, Gallucci GO, Belser U, Müller F. Mechanosensation and maximum bite force in edentulous patients rehabilitated with bimaxillary implant-supported fixed dental prostheses. Clin Oral Implants Res. 2012;23:577–83.

34. Woda A, Foster K, Mishellany A, Peyron MA. Adaptation of healthy mastication to factors pertaining to the individual or to the food. Physiol Behav. 2006;89:28–35.

35. Heckmann SM, Heussinger S, Linke JJ, Graef F, Pröschel P. Improvement and long-term stability of neuromuscular adaptation in implant-supported overdentures. Clin Oral Implants Res. 2009;20:1200–5.

36. Gartner JL, Mushimoto K, Weber HP, Nishimura I. Effect of osseointegrated implants on the coordination of masticatory muscles: a pilot study. J Prosthet Dent. 2000;84:185–93.

37. Collaert B, Wijnen L, De Bruyn H. A 2-year prospective study on immediate loading with fluoride-modified implants in the edentulous mandible. Clin Oral Implants Res. 2011;22:1111–6.

38. Collaert B, De Bruyn H. Immediate functional loading of TiOblast dental implants in full-arch edentulous maxillae: a 3-year prospective study. Clin Oral Implants Res. 2008;19:1254–60.

39. Matsui Y, Ohno K, Michi K, Suzuki Y, Yamagata K. A computerized method for evaluating balance of occlusal load. J Oral Rehabil. 1996;23:530–5.

40. Kobayashi Y, Shiga H, Yokoyama M, Arakawa I, Nakajima K. Differences in masticatory function of subjects with different closing path. J Prosthodont Res. 2009;53:142–5.

41. Hatch JP, Shinkai RS, Sakai S, Rugh JD, Paunovich ED. Determinants of masticatory performance in dentate adults. Arch Oral Biol. 2001;46:641–8.

42. van der Bilt A, van Kampen FM, Cune MS. Masticatory function with mandibular implant-supported overdentures fitted with different attachment types. Eur J Oral Sci. 2006;114:191–6.

43. Mioche L, Peyron MA. Bite force displayed during assessment of hardness in various texture contexts. Arch Oral Biol. 1995;40:415–23.

3

Clinical outcomes following surgical treatment of peri-implantitis at grafted and non-grafted implant sites

Ausra Ramanauskaite[1,2*], Kathrin Becker[3], Gintaras Juodzbalys[4] and Frank Schwarz[5]

Abstract

Background: This retrospective analysis aimed at comparing the clinical outcomes following combined surgical therapy of peri-implantitis at initially grafted and non-grafted (i.e., pristine) implant sites.

Methods: A total of 39 patients exhibiting 57 implants diagnosed with peri-implantitis (i.e., 16 implants at grafted and 41 implants at non-grafted sites) were included. Each subject had received a combined (i.e., implantoplasty and augmentative therapy) surgical treatment procedures at respective implants (grafted sites: 10 patients, 16 implants, non-grafted sites: 29 patients, 41 implants). A chi-squared test (χ^2) was used to assess whether the initial grafting procedure did affect the treatment outcomes (i.e., disease resolution, bleeding on probing (BOP), probing pocket depths (PD)). The mean follow-up period was 41.9 ± 34.75 months.

Results: At the patient level, disease resolution (i.e., absence of BOP and PD $\geq$ 6 mm) was obtained in 4/10 (40%) at grafted and in 7/27 (24.1%) at non-grafted implant sites ($p = 0.579$). BOP reductions was found to be $60.64 \pm 40.81\%$ at non-grafted and $77.45 \pm 30.92\%$ at grafted sites ($p = 0.778$). PD reductions amounted to 2.20 ± 2.22 mm at non-grafted and 1.57 ± 1.54 mm at grafted sites ($p = 0.969$).

Conclusions: The initial bone-grafting procedures at the implant sites did not influence the effectiveness of combined surgical therapy of peri-implantitis.

Keywords: Peri-implantitis, Diagnosis, Treatment

Background

Peri-implantitis is caused by a bacterial challenge and characterized by inflammation in the peri-implant soft tissues and a progressive loss of supporting bone [1, 2]. Consequently, its treatment is cause-related and primarily aimed at arresting disease progression [3].

Based on the currently available evidence, non-surgical mechanical debridement alone seems to have a limited efficacy for the management of peri-implantitis [4, 5]. While adjunctive (i.e., local antibiotics, antimicrobial photodynamic therapy) or alternative measures (e.g. air

abrasive devices, Er:YAG laser monotherapy) may improve the efficacy of non-surgical therapy, the obtained clinical outcomes appeared to be limited to a period of 6 to 12 months and were particularly compromised at advanced defect sites [4, 5]. In contrast, the efficacy of treatment was commonly improved subsequent to a surgical intervention combining open flap debridement either with adjunctive resective (e.g., apical flap, osteoplasty, implantoplasty (IP)), augmentative (e.g., bone fillers/autografts, guided bone regeneration), or a combination of resective (i.e., IP) and augmentative (refers to as combined therapy) measures [6]. Nevertheless, the reported outcomes following surgical therapy of peri-implantitis varied considerably and appeared to be influenced by a variety of different prognostic factors, such as the configuration of the bony defect [7], the physicochemical properties of the

* Correspondence: ausra.ramanauskaite@med.uni-duesseldorf.de
[1]Department of Oral Surgery, Westdeutsche Kieferklinik, Universitätsklinikum Düsseldorf, D-40225 Düsseldorf, Germany
[2]Clinic of Dental and Oral Pathology, Lithuanian University of Health Sciences, Kaunas, Lithuania

bone filler [8, 9], or the surface characteristics of the affected implants [10, 11].

Previous clinical data provide some evidence that ridge augmentation using either autogenous bone or different bone filler materials may constitute a potential risk indicator for the onset of peri-implant diseases [12, 13]. Consequently, it might be hypothesized that initial bone-grafting procedures at implant site may also influence the effectiveness of peri-implantitis treatment. Therefore, this retrospective analysis aimed at comparing the clinical outcomes following combined surgical treatment of peri-implantitis at initially grafted and non-grafted (i.e., pristine) implant sites.

Methods
Study design and participants
For this retrospective analysis, standardized clinical record forms of a total of 39 partially/fully edentulous patients (25 female and 12 male) exhibiting 57 implants were screened. All patients had attended the Department of Oral Surgery, Heinrich Heine University, Düsseldorf, Germany for the treatment of peri-implantitis between 2007 and 2010, and were under regular implant maintenance care. The mean follow-up time was 41.9 ± 34.75 months (range 6 to 126 months). Some patients were also participating in a randomized prospective clinical study, which aimed at investigating the effects of two surface decontamination methods on the clinical outcomes following combined therapy [14].

A data extraction template was generated and used for the anonymous acquisition of demographic study variables/implant site characteristics and baseline as well as follow-up clinical measurements after surgical therapy. The study was in accordance with the Helsinki Declaration, as revised in 2013 and approved by the local ethics committee.

Patient selection
For patient selection, the following inclusion criteria were defined:

(1) Partially or fully edentulous patients rehabilitated with fixed or removable implant-supported prostheses;
(2) Presence of at least one screw-type (one or two part) titanium implant diagnosed with peri-implantitis;
(3) Respective implants had received a combined surgical peri-implantitis treatment;
(4) No implant mobility;
(5) Presence of at least 2 mm of keratinized mucosa;
(6) Treated chronic periodontitis and proper periodontal maintenance care;
(7) A good level of oral hygiene as evidenced by a plaque index (PI) at the implant level < 1;
(8) No systemic diseases which could influence the outcome of the therapy (i.e., diabetes (HbA1c < 7), osteoporosis, antiresorptive therapy);
(9) No history of malignancy, radiotherapy, chemotherapy, or immunodeficiency within the last 4 years and;
(10) Non-smoker or light smoking habits (< 10 cigarettes per day);
(11) Complied with at least 6 months of follow-up;
(12) Information on the initial bone grafting procedure and protocol at the respective implant site was available.

Patients whose data files lacked information on the bone grafting procedures at the implant site or lacked information on augmentation protocols (i.e., lateral ridge augmentation or sinus floor elevation; one- or two-stage approach), and patients who did not comply with at least 6 months of follow-up were not included in the analysis.

Case definition
Peri-implantitis was defined as bleeding on probing (BOP) with or without suppuration (Supp) in addition to changes in the radiographic bone level. Interproximal bone level changes were estimated on intraoral radiographs. In the absence of available baseline radiographs taken at prosthesis installation, "a threshold vertical distance of 2 mm from the expected marginal bone level" was used to assess bone loss [3].

Initial grafting procedures
The identified patients with a history of grafting had received the following treatment protocols:

Lateral ridge augmentation

- Simultaneous grafting (one stage) of dehiscence-type defects, employing a particulated bone substitute, and collagen membrane (2 patients; 3 implants)
- Grafting and staged implant placement at 6 months (two stage) employing a particulated bone substitute and collagen membrane (3 patients; 3 implants)

Sinus floor elevation

- External grafting (lateral window) employing a particulated bone substitute and collagen membrane and implant placement (2 patients; 3 implants)
- External grafting (lateral window) employing a particulated bone substitute and collagen membrane and staged implant placement at 6 months (4 patients; 7 implants)

To be included, the radiographic bone loss at baseline (i.e., prior to treatment) in respective patients had to extend to the formerly grafted area.

Treatment procedures

After an initial course of non-surgical therapy, each subject had received a combined (i.e., implantoplasty + augmentative therapy) surgical treatment procedure [14] at respective implant sites (Fig. 1). This procedure included open flap debridement and a meticulous granulation tissue removal using conventional plastic curets (Straumann Dental Implant System; Institut Straumann AG, Basel, Switzerland) and an implantoplasty at both buccally (i.e., Classes Ib and Ic) and supracrestally (i.e., class II) (Fig. 1) exposed implant surfaces. This was accomplished using diamond burs (ZR Diamonds; Gebr. Brasseler GmbH & Co. KG, Lemgo, Germany) and Arkansas stones under copious irrigation with sterile saline. The remaining unmodified implant surfaces at the respective intrabony defect areas (i.e., classes Ib, Ic, and Ie) were decontaminated using either an Er:YAG laser device (energy density of 11.4 J/cm2, 10 Hz) (elexxion delos; elexxion AG, Radolfzell, Germany) or debrided using plastic curetes and cotton pellets soaked in sterile saline (Straumann Dental Implant System). Respective intrabony defect compartments were homogeneously filled using NBM (BioOss spongiosa granules, particle size 0.25–1 mm; Geistlich, Wolhusen, Switzerland) and were covered with CM (Bio-Gide; Geistlich). Transmucosal healing was supported by a peri- and postoperative antibiotic medication for 5 days.

Clinical examination

For all patients, the following clinical parameters were available: BOP (as measured within 60 s after probing) and PD (as measured in millimeters from the mucosal margin to the bottom of the probeable pocket). BOP and PD were assessed at six aspects around the implant: mesio-buccal, mid-buccal, disto-buccal, mesio-oral, mid-oral, and disto-oral. Maximum PD values (max PD) and mean BOP scores were evaluated before the surgical intervention and at the final follow-up.

The primary outcome variable was disease resolution (i.e., the composite outcome of the absence of BOP and probing pocket depths (PD $\geq$ 6 mm). Reduction of mean BOP and maximum PD values were defined as secondary outcome variables.

Data analysis

Commercially available and open source software programs (SPSS Statistics 23.0: IBM Corp., Ehningen, Germany and R Development Core Team) were used. Mean values, standard deviations (SD), medians, minimums, and maximums were calculated for mean BOP and maximum PD scores.

The analyses were performed at both patient and implant levels. Prior to this analysis, clinical parameters were pooled according to the grafting procedure (grafted or non-grafted), considering the patient as statistical unit. The differences in the baseline maximum PD values between the grafted and non-grafted implant sites were assessed using Wilcoxon rank-sum test. To evaluate disease resolution, changes in mean BOP and maximum PD between the groups (i.e., non-grafted vs. grafted) chi-square test (χ^2) were applied. For the evaluation of disease resolution, if patients exhibited multiple implants with different treatment outcomes, they were assigned to a group according to the worst one. Based on the sample size calculation, for a large effect size ($w = 0.5$, df $= 1$, alpha $= 0.05$, power $= 0.8$), a minimum of 32 patients were needed [15].

The results were considered statistically significant at $p < 0.05$.

Results

The present analysis was based on 39 patients diagnosed with peri-implantitis in 57 implants. The patients were

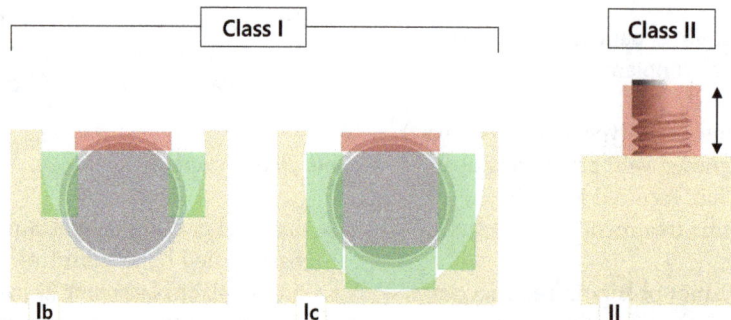

Fig. 1 Combined surgical therapy of peri-implantitis at respective defect sites: class I: intrabony component showing either a buccal dehiscency with a semicircular component (Ib) or a buccal dehiscency with a cicumferential component (Ic). Class II: supracrestal component. The red rectangles indicate the surface areas undergoing an implantoplasty, while the green areas indicate the defect areas undergoing augmentative therapy

divided into 2 groups according to the grafting of the site: non-grafted implant sites (29 patients/41 implants) and grafted implant sites (10 patients/16 implants).

The characteristics of the implant sites are presented in Table 1. In total, 26 implants (45.6%) were located in the maxilla and the remaining 31 (54.4%) were located in the mandible. Out of these implants, 15 (26%) were located in the anterior (incisor and canine area) and 42 (74%) were located in the posterior regions (premolars and molars). All the studied implants (100%) presented with BOP, and only 1 implant had BOP in fewer than 6 sites.

At the baseline, the maximum PD values at the grafted and non-grafted sites 6.25 $\pm$ 0.45 mm and 6.77 $\pm$ 1.61 mm, respectively (Table 1, Fig. 2). The Wilcoxon rank-sum test did not show a significant difference in the baseline maximum PD values between the groups ($p = 0.353$) (Table 1).

Disease resolution

In general, disease resolution (i.e., the absence of BOP and PD $\geq$ 6 mm) was achieved in 19 out of 57 (33%) implants and in 11 out of 39 (28%) patients. At the patient level, disease resolution was obtained in 4 out of 10 patients (40%) at grafted sites and in 7 out of 29 patients (24.1%) at non-grafted sites. The chi-square test ($\chi2$) demonstrated no significant difference between the two patient groups ($p = 0.579$, df = 1, $\chi2 = 0.307$) (Table 2, Fig. 3a). However, the results of the implant-level analysis revealed a significant difference between the two groups, indicating a higher disease resolution at grafted implant sites (9/16 (56%) compared to non-grafted sites (10/41 (25%)) ($p = 0.048$, df = 1, $\chi2 = 3.921$) (Fig. 3b).

BOP reduction

Mean and median BOP reduction values (%) for the 2 groups are presented in Table 3. At the patient level, mean BOP reduction amounted to 77.45% (minimum 0%;

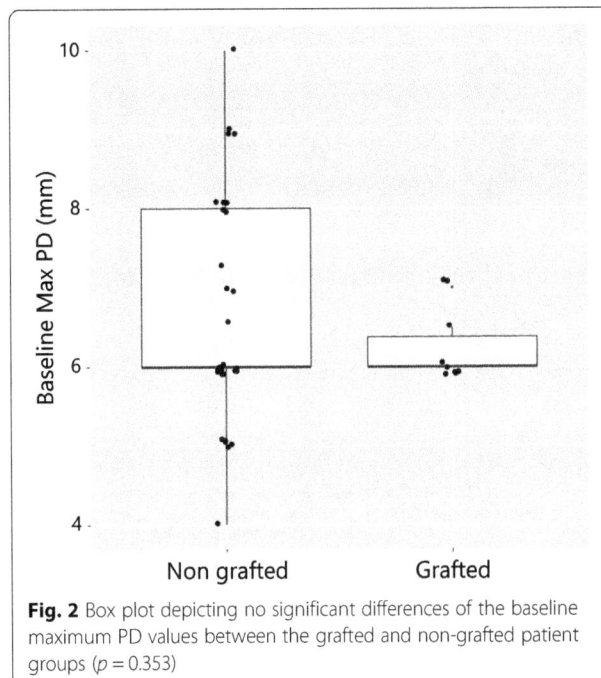

Fig. 2 Box plot depicting no significant differences of the baseline maximum PD values between the grafted and non-grafted patient groups ($p = 0.353$)

maximum 100%) and 60.64% (minimum 0%; maximum 100%) at grafted and non-grafted sites, respectively.

At the implant level, BOP reduction was noted to be 74.96% (minimum 0%; maximum 100%) at grafted implant sites and 54.88% (minimum 0%; maximum 100%) at non-grafted implant sites. According to the results of the chi-square test, the mean BOP reduction did not differ significantly between the groups at either the patient ($p = 0.778$, df = 1, $\chi2 = 0.079$) or the implant ($p = 0.515$, df = 1, $\chi2 = 0.422$) level (Fig. 4).

PD changes

The reduction in the maximum PD (mm) values between the 2 groups is presented in Table 4. At the patient level, reduction in the maximum PD values amounted to 1.57 mm (minimum – 1.0 mm; maximum 4 mm) and 2.20 mm (minimum: – 4.0 mm; maximum 6.0 mm) at grafted and non-grafted sites, respectively. At the implant level, the corresponding reduction in the maximum PD values were calculated to be 1.31 mm (minimum

Table 1 Implant site characteristics

	Non-grafted sites	Grafted sites
Implant number	41	16
Maxilla/mandible	19/22	7/9
Anterior/posterior	10/31	5/11
Baseline max PD* values (mm)		
Mean	6.77	6.25
SD	1.61	0.45
Median	6.0	6.0
Minimum	3.0	6.0
Maximum	10.0	7.0

*No significant difference in baseline maximum PD values between the groups was found (Wilcoxon $p = 0.353$)

Table 2 Disease resolution between the non-grafted and grafted implant sites

	Non-grafted sites	Grafted sites	Total
Patient level	7/29 (24.1%)	4/10 (40%)	11/39 (28%)
Implant level	10/41 (25%)	9/16 (56.3%)	19/57 (33%)

No significant difference between the groups was found at the patient level ($p = 0.579$, chi-square test). Significantly higher disese resolution was achieved in grafted implant sites at the implant level ($p = 0.048$, chi-square test)

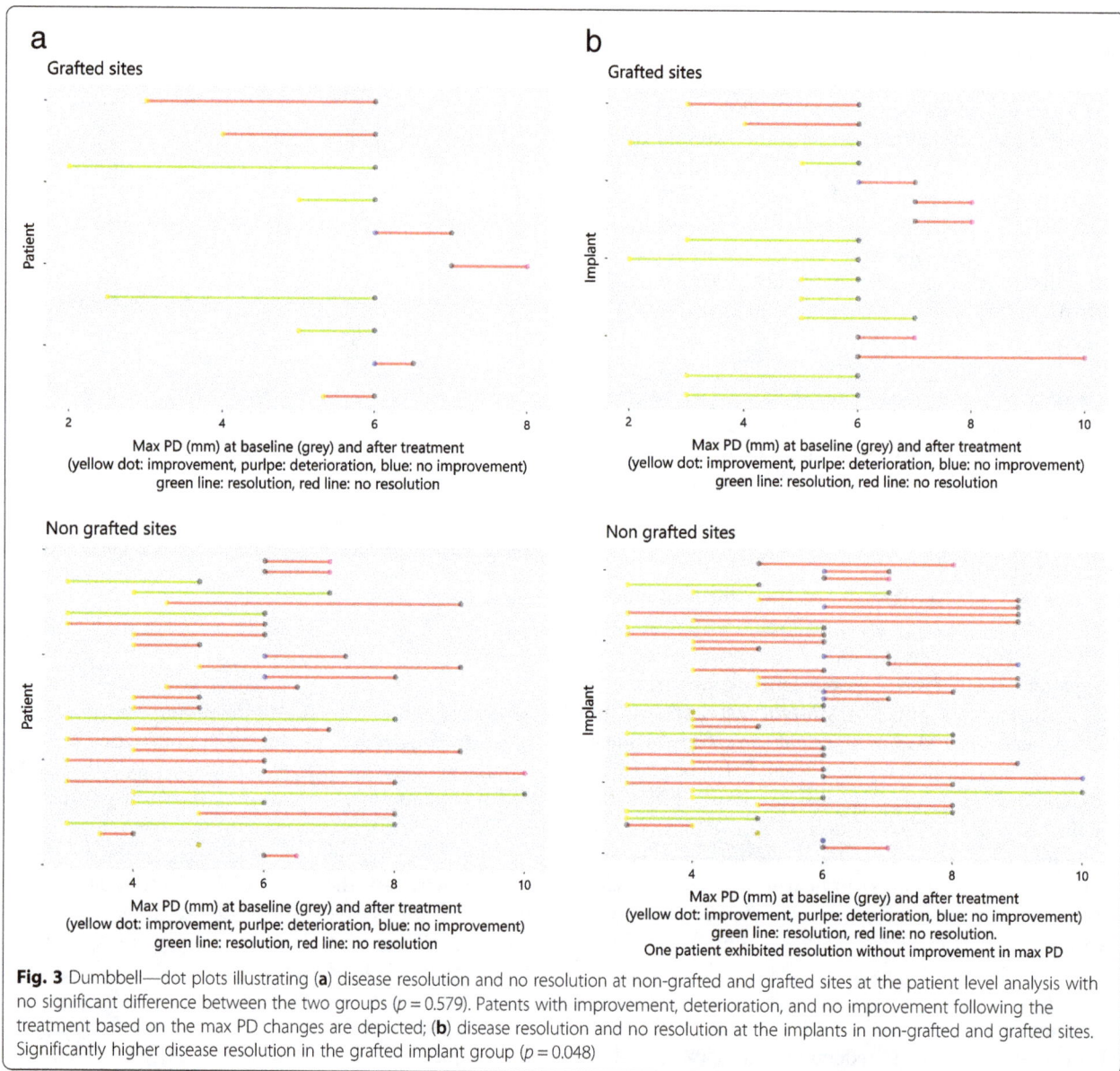

Fig. 3 Dumbbell—dot plots illustrating (**a**) disease resolution and no resolution at non-grafted and grafted sites at the patient level analysis with no significant difference between the two groups ($p = 0.579$). Patents with improvement, deterioration, and no improvement following the treatment based on the max PD changes are depicted; (**b**) disease resolution and no resolution at the implants in non-grafted and grafted sites. Significantly higher disease resolution in the grafted implant group ($p = 0.048$)

– 4.0 mm; maximum 4.0 mm) at grafted implant sites and 2.10 mm (minimum – 4.0 mm; maximum 6.0 mm) at non-grafted implant sites. For the between-group comparison, no significant difference could be detected between the groups at both the patient ($p = 0.968$, df = 1, $\chi2 = 0.002$, chi-square test) and implant ($p = 1$, df = 1, $\chi2 = 0.00026$, chi-square test) level (Fig. 5).

Discussion

According to the eighth European Workshop of Periodontology (EFP), evaluation of the effectiveness of different peri-implantitis therapies should be based on a composite outcome of disease resolution, including resolutions of mucosal inflammation, reductions in probing pocket depths, and no further bone loss [3].

Table 3 Reduction of mean BOP (%)

Group	Patient level					Implant level				
	mean	SD	median	min.	max.	mean	SD	median	min.	max.
Non-grafted sites	60.64	40.81	67.0	0	100	54.88	43.65	67.0	0	100
Grafted sites	77.45	30.92	87.25	0	100	74.96	38.95	100	0	100

The differences between the groups did not yield a significant difference (patient level $p = 0.778$, implant level $p = 0.515$, chi-square test)

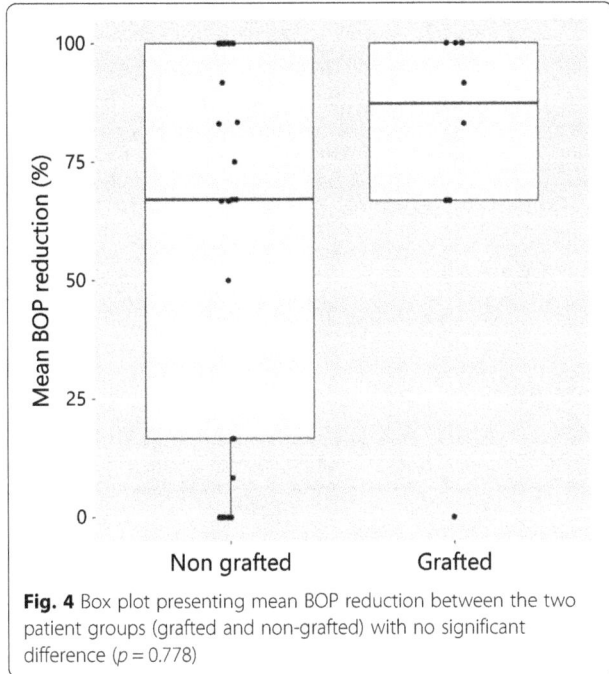

Fig. 4 Box plot presenting mean BOP reduction between the two patient groups (grafted and non-grafted) with no significant difference (p = 0.778)

The current retrospective clinical investigation evaluated treatment outcomes following combined surgical therapy for peri-implantitis at formerly grafted and non-grafted implant sites. A composite outcome of disease resolution as the absence of BOP and PD ≥ 6 mm was considered. Accordingly, peri-implantitis resolution was achieved in 33% of the treated implants, corresponding to 28% of the patients. Although no significant difference regarding grafting of the implant site was detected at the patient level (grafted sites 4/10 (40%), non-grafted sites 7/29 (24.1%), p = 0.579), implant-level analysis pointed to a higher disease resolution at the grafted implant sites (9/16 (56%) at grafted sites, 10/41 (25%) at non-grafted sites, p = 0.048).

The disease resolution noted in the present analysis is in line with the data reported in previous clinical studies. In particular, the treatment success (defined as absence of BOP) following combined surgical therapy was obtained in 60% (9/15) of the patients in the 7 years of clinical investigation [16]. Additionally, according to the results of the studies reporting on the composite treatment outcomes following surgical regenerative peri-implantitis therapy, treatment success was achieved in 35% (9/26) (treatment success defined as PD < 5 mm, absence of BOP/suppuration, no further bone loss) [17] to 51.1% (23/45) of the implants (treatment success defined as evidence of ≥ 25% bone fill, PD < 5 mm, BOP score ≤ 1) at 5 and 7 years of follow-up, respectively [18]. However, in this context, it should be realized that these studies used different criteria to define treatment success; hence, clinical outcomes cannot be compared directly.

In the present study, mean BOP reduction ranged from 60.64 to 77.45% at the patient level and from 54.88 to 74.96% at the implant level, with no significant difference between the grafted and non-grafted implants sites. Slightly higher mean BOP reduction values, ranging from 75.5 to 90%, were indicated in the long-term (7 years) clinical investigations following regenerative surgical therapy of peri-implantitis [16, 17]. It is interesting to note that BOP reduction was found to be significantly influenced by the implant-surface characteristics [17]. This observation is in agreement with the data presented in a 3-year randomized controlled clinical trial, where superior treatment outcomes were noted for implants with non-modified surface implants compared to modified surfaces [11].

The further evaluation of maximum PD reduction did not indicate a significant difference between the two groups (i.e., grafted vs. non-grafted), with the range of 1.57 to 2.20 mm at the patient level analysis and 1.31 to 2.10 mm at the implant level. These results are in concurrence with data from the previous studies, where mean PD reduction amounted from 0.74 to 2.55 mm [16], up to 3 [18], and > 4 mm [17] following surgical regenerative peri-implantitis therapy. To the authors' best knowledge, this is the first clinical study to evaluate peri-implantitis treatment outcomes at formerly grafted and non-grafted implant sites. Therefore, the results (e.g., disease resolution, changes in mean BOP, and maximum PD) cannot be compared to those from previous studies.

A recent systematic review and meta-analysis indicated lateral bone grafting procedures (both simultaneous with implant placement and staged) to be associated with peri-implant tissue stability [19]. Particularly, the results, which were based on eight clinical investigations, addressed that different surgical interventions (i.e., GBR and autogenous, allogeneic, or xenogeneic bone blocks) resulted in low and similar BOP values, along with

Table 4 Reduction of maximum PD (mm)

Group	Patient level					Implant level				
	Mean	SD	Median	Min.	Max.	Mean	SD	Median	Min.	Max.
Non-grafted sites	2.20	2.22	2.0	−4.0	6.0	2.10	2.35	2.0	−4.0	6.0
Grafted sites	1.57	1.54	1.0	−1.0	4	1.31	2.18	1.5	−4.0	4.0

No significant difference between the groups was observed (patient level p = 0.968, implant level p = 1, chi-square test)

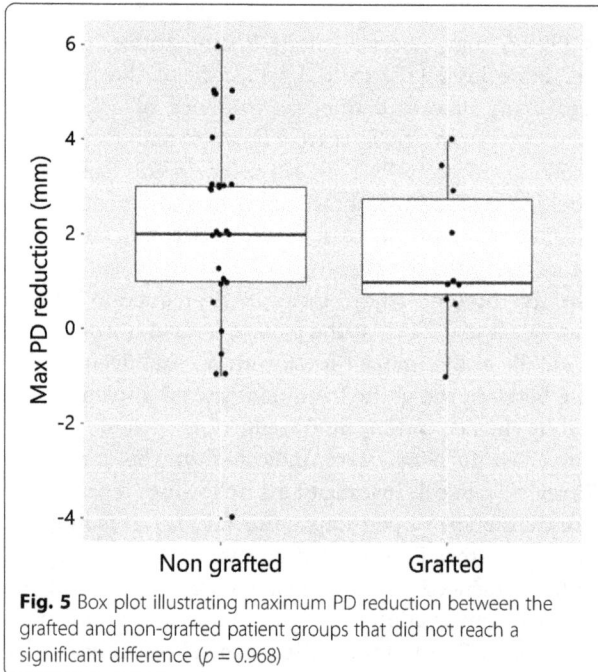

Fig. 5 Box plot illustrating maximum PD reduction between the grafted and non-grafted patient groups that did not reach a significant difference ($p = 0.968$)

Funding
The study was self-funded by the authors' own departments.

Authors' contributions
AR and FS have made substantial contributions to study conception and interpretation of data as well as manuscript drafting. KB was involved in the data management as well as the statistical analysis. GJ contributed to the data interpretation. All authors read and approved the final manuscript.

Competing interests
Ausra Ramanauskaite, Kathrin Becker, Gintaras Juodzbalys, and Frank Schwarz declare that they have no competing interests.

Author details
[1]Department of Oral Surgery, Westdeutsche Kieferklinik, Universitätsklinikum Düsseldorf, D-40225 Düsseldorf, Germany. [2]Clinic of Dental and Oral Pathology, Lithuanian University of Health Sciences, Kaunas, Lithuania. [3]Department of Orthodontics, Westdeutsche Kieferklinik, Universitätsklinikum Düsseldorf, D-40225 Düsseldorf, Germany. [4]Department of Oral and Maxillofacial Surgery, Lithuanian University of Health Sciences, LT-46383 Kaunas, Lithuania. [5]Department of Oral Surgery and Implantology, Carolinum, Johann Wolfgang Goethe-University Frankfurt, D-60596 Frankfurt am Main, Germany.

References
1. Lindhe J, Meyle J, Working Group D of European Workshop on Periodontology. Peri-implant diseases: Consensus Report of the Sixth European Workshop on Periodontology. J Clin Periodontol. 2008;35(Suppl 8):282–5.
2. Lang NP, Berglundh T, Working Group 4 of Seventh European Workshop on Periodontology. Periimplant diseases: where are we now?–Consensus of the Seventh European Workshop on Periodontology. J Clin Periodontol. 2011; 38(Suppl 11):178–81.
3. Sanz M, Chapple IL, Working Group 4 of the Seventh European Workshop on Periodontology. Clinical research on peri-implant diseases: consensus report of Working Group 4. J Clin Periodontol. 2012;39(Suppl 12):202–6.
4. Klinge B, Meyle J, Working group 2 of the third EAO Consensus Conference 2012. Peri-implant tissue destruction. The Third EAO Consensus Conference 2012. Clin Oral Implants Res. 2012;23(Suppl 6):108–10.
5. Schwarz F, Becker K, Sager M. Efficacy of professionally-administered plaque removal in managing peri-implant mucositis. A systematic review and meta-analysis. J Clin Periodontol. 2015;42(Suppl 16):202–13.
6. Schwarz F, Schmucker A, Becker J. Efficacy of alternative or adjunctive measures to conventional treatment of peri-implant mucositis and peri-implantitis: a systematic review and meta-analysis. Int J Implant Dent. 2015; 1(1):22.
7. Schwarz F, Sahm N, Schwarz K, Becker J. Impact of defect configuration on the clinical outcome following surgical regenerative therapy of peri-implantitis. J Clin Periodontol. 2010;37(5):449–55.
8. Aghazadeh A, Rutger Persson G, Renvert S. A single-centre randomized controlled clinical trial on the adjunct treatment of intra-bony defects with autogenous bone or a xenograft: results after 12 months. J Clin Periodontol. 2012;39(7):666–73.
9. Schwarz F, Sahm N, Bieling K, Becker J. Surgical regenerative treatment of peri-implantitis lesions using a nanocrystalline hydroxyapatite or a natural bone mineral in combination with a collagen membrane: a four-year clinical follow-up report. J Clin Periodontol. 2009;36(9):807–14.
10. Roccuzzo M, Bonino F, Bonino L, Dalmasso P. Surgical therapy of peri-implantitis lesions by means of a bovine-derived xenograft: comparative results of a prospective study on two different implant surfaces. J Clin Periodontol. 2011;38(8):738–45.
11. Carcuac O, Derks J, Abrahamsson I, Wennström JL, Petzold M, Berglundh T. Surgical treatment of peri-implantitis. 3-year results from a randomized controlled clinical trial. J Clin Periodontol. 2017;44(12):1294–303.
12. Canullo L, Peñarrocha-Oltra D, Covani U, Botticelli D, Serino G, Penarrocha M. Clinical and microbiological findings in patients with peri-implantitis: a cross-sectional study. Clin Oral Implants Res. 2016;27(3):376–82.

comparable PD, marginal bone and plaque levels at both short-term (1–3 years) and long-term (> 3 years) follow-ups [19]. Moreover, the occurrence of peri-implant diseases or a progressive marginal bone loss was reported to be low and also comparable between different lateral hard tissue grafting protocols [20]. However, the data on whether former bone grafting procedures influence peri-implantitis treatment outcomes has not been reported in the literature.

Based on the findings of the current investigation, combined surgical treatment was associated with clinically important reduction in BOP and PD values and was not influenced by the presence or absence of the grafting procedure at the implant site. When interpreting these results, the relatively small number of patients in the group with grafted implant sites should be taken into consideration. Additionally, it should be noted that two different decontamination protocols (i.e., Er: YAG laser or debriding with plastic curettes and cotton pellets soaked in sterile saline) were applied. Nevertheless, according to the findings from the randomized clinical trial, the method used to decontaminate the implant surface had no impact on the clinical outcomes of the combined surgical therapy of peri-implantitis [16].

Conclusions

Within the limitations of the current study, it was concluded that the effectiveness of combined surgical therapy of peri-implantitis was comparable at both grafted and non-grafted implant sites and was not influenced by the initial bone-grafting procedures.

13. Schwarz F, Sahm N, Becker J. Impact of the outcome of guided bone regeneration in dehiscence-type defects on the long-term stability of peri-implant health: clinical observations at 4 years. Clin Oral Implants Res. 2012; 23(2):191–6.

14. Schwarz F, Sahm N, Iglhaut G, Becker J. Impact of the method of surface debridement and decontamination on the clinical outcome following combined surgical therapy of peri-implantitis: a randomized controlled clinical study. J Clin Periodontol. 2011;38(3):276–84.

15. Cohen J. Statistical power analysis for the behavioral sciences. 2nd ed. Hillsdale, NJ: Lawrence Erlbaum; 1988.

16. Schwarz F, John G, Schmucker A, Sahm N, Becker J. Combined surgical therapy of advanced peri-implantitis evaluating two methods of surface decontamination: a 7-year follow-up observation. J Clin Periodontol. 2017; 44(3):337–42.

17. Roccuzzo M, Pittoni D, Roccuzzo A, Charrier L, Dalmasso P. Surgical treatment of peri-implantitis intrabony lesions by means of deproteinized bovine bone mineral with 10% collagen: 7-year-results. Clin Oral Implants Res. 2017;28(12):1577–83.

18. Roos-Jansåker AM, Persson GR, Lindahl C, Renvert S. Surgical treatment of peri-implantitis using a bone substitute with or without a resorbable membrane: a 5-year follow-up. J Clin Periodontol. 2014;41(11):1108–14.

19. Sanz-Sánchez I, Carrillo de Albornoz A, Figuero E, Schwarz F, Jung R, Sanz M, Thoma D. Effects of lateral bone augmentation procedures on peri-implant health or disease: A systematic review and meta-analysis. Clin Oral Implants Res. 2018;29(Suppl 15):18–31.

20. Schwarz F, Giannobile WV, Jung R, Groups of the 2nd Osteology Foundation Consensus Meeting. Evidence-based knowledge on the aesthetics and maintenance of peri-implant soft tissues: Osteology Foundation Consensus Report Part 2-Effects of hard tissue augmentation procedures on the maintenance of peri-implant tissues. Clin Oral Implants Res. 2018;29(Suppl 15):11–3.

4

Comparative evaluation of the stability of two different dental implant designs and surgical protocols

David E. Simmons[1], Pooja Maney[1], Austin G. Teitelbaum[1], Susan Billiot[1], Lomesh J. Popat[2] and A. Archontia Palaiologou[1*]

Abstract

Background: The purpose of this study was to compare a parallel wall design implant to a tapered apex design implant when placed in the posterior maxilla using two different surgical protocols.

Methods: Twenty-seven patients (30 implants) were divided into three groups. All implants were 4 mm wide in diameter and 8 mm long.
Group A received 10 tapered implants (OSPTX) (Astra Tech OsseoSpeed TX™) using the soft bone surgical protocol (TXSoft).
Group B received 10 tapered implants (OSPTX) (AstraTech OsseoSpeedTX™) using the standard surgical protocol (TXStd).
Group C received 10 parallel wall implants (OSP) (AstraTech OsseoSpeed™) using the standard surgical protocol (OStd).
All implants were placed in the posterior maxilla in areas with a minimum of 8-mm crestal bone height.
Resonance frequency measurements (implant stability quotient (ISQ)) and torque values were recorded to determine initial implant stability. All implants were uncovered 6 weeks after placement and restored with a functionally loaded resin provisional screw-retained crown. Resonance frequency measurements were recorded at the time of implant placement, at 6 weeks and 6 and 12 months. Twelve months after implant placement, the stability of the implants was recorded and the final restorations were placed using custom CAD/CAM fabricated abutments and cement-retained PFM DSIGN porcelain crowns. After implant restoration, bone levels were measured at 6 and 12 months with standardized radiographs.

Results: Radiographic mean bone loss was less than 0.5 mm in all groups, with no statistically significant differences between the groups. Implant survival rate at 1 year was 93.3%, with 2/30 implants failing to integrate prior to functional loading at 6 weeks. No statistically significant difference was found between ISQ measurements between the three groups at all time intervals measured. Strong positive correlations were found between overall bone loss at 6 months and insertion torque at time of placement. A very weak correlation was found between insertion torque and ISQ values at time of implant placement.

Conclusions: Survival and stability of OSPTX and OSP implants is comparable. Osteotomy preparation by either standard or soft bone surgical protocol presented no significant effect on implant survival and stability for the specific implant designs.

Keywords: Dental implants, Implant stability, OsseoSpeed™, OsseoSpeed TX™, Resonance frequency analysis, Osstell™, Implant survival

* Correspondence: apalai@lsuhsc.edu
[1]Department of Periodontics, Louisiana State University Health Sciences Center School of Dentistry, 1100 Florida Avenue, New Orleans, LA 70119, USA
Full list of author information is available at the end of the article

Background

Dental implants are now a widely accepted treatment option for the replacement of missing teeth. The therapeutic goal of dental implants is to support restorations that replace single or multiple missing teeth so as to provide patient comfort, function, and esthetics as well as assist in the ongoing maintenance of remaining intraoral and perioral structures. However, anatomic limitations such as the maxillary sinus may limit the amount of bone available to place traditional length implants (>10 mm). To avoid invasive sinus elevation procedures, manufacturers have developed shorter implants (<10 mm). Multiple studies have proven that short implants are equally successful to longer implants [1–9]. Tapered implant design further enhances primary implant stability, especially in the posterior maxilla where bone quality is usually poor [10–12].

The purpose of this study was to evaluate the initial stability of the OsseoSpeed TX™1 tapered implant (OSPTX) and to compare it to the standard OsseoSpeed™1 parallel walled implant (OSP) as well as to compare the soft bone and standard surgical protocols. Both implants included in this study are manufactured from high-grade commercially pure titanium with surface roughness produced via a fluoride treatment process. The OSPTX and OSP implants are self-tapping implants. The implants used in this study were all of 4.0 mm in diameter and 8 mm in length. Microthreads™ characterize the coronal aspect of both implants. The OSPTX implant has the same features as OSP except the apex of the implant is tapered (Fig. 1).

Successful integration of dental implants is largely dependent on their primary stability [13]. Implants placed in the maxilla present more challenges due to the poor bone quality usually found in these areas. Another anatomic challenge in the posterior maxilla is the pneumatization of the maxillary sinus which can limit the length of implant that can be placed. To avoid invasive sinus augmentation procedures, implants have been designed in shorter lengths such as 8 mm. To further enhance short implant primary stability, a tapered design has been developed which has been proven to provide greater initial stability [10–12, 14]. Implant stability can be evaluated by different measures such as torque at the time of implant placement, resistance to reverse torque, and resonance frequency analysis (RFA). Multiple studies have established feasibility for validating implant stability in lab and animal models to justify using resonance frequency analysis in clinical trials [15, 16]. Limited literature exists on the OSPTX implant design, and to our knowledge, no clinical studies exist that compare OSP to OSPTX. A recent ex vivo comparison of two different designs of OSPTX implants in porcine mandibles demonstrated that a conical neck design presented higher primary stability (insertion torque and implant stability quotient (ISQ)) than a cylindrical neck design [17]. In our study, both the torque value and ISQ value were recorded at the time of placement. ISQ values were also recorded at implant uncovery at 6 weeks and also at 6 and 12 months when the final restoration was placed.

A recent systematic review by Stocchero et al. concluded that an undersized drilling protocol in soft bone is an effective way to enhance insertion torque but recommended that further clinical studies are needed to confirm these data [18]. Our study was designed to address this question, as it compared the standard drilling protocol to a soft bone protocol.

Our study hypothesis is that the stability of the OSPTX implant will be greater than that of the OSP implant due to the tapered design of the OSPTX implant.

The objectives of this study were the following:

1. To determine whether preparation of the osteotomy with a soft bone protocol (underpreparation of the osteotomy compared to the implant diameter by −0.5 mm at the body portion) results in greater primary implant stability
2. To investigate possible correlations between ISQ and torque values
3. To evaluate radiographic bone loss at 6 months and 1 year

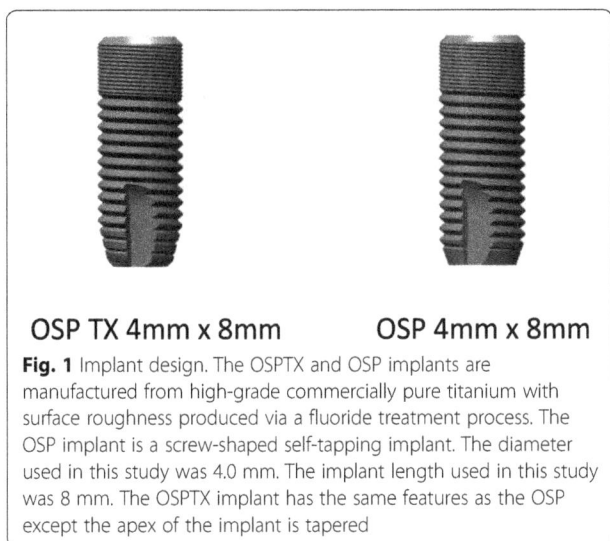

OSP TX 4mm x 8mm   OSP 4mm x 8mm

Fig. 1 Implant design. The OSPTX and OSP implants are manufactured from high-grade commercially pure titanium with surface roughness produced via a fluoride treatment process. The OSP implant is a screw-shaped self-tapping implant. The diameter used in this study was 4.0 mm. The implant length used in this study was 8 mm. The OSPTX implant has the same features as the OSP except the apex of the implant is tapered

Methods

Following proper approval by the LSUHSC Institution Review Board (LSUNO IRB#7438), 27 (30 implant sites) systemically healthy patients at least 18 years old were enrolled in the study and randomly divided into three groups as follows (inclusion and exclusion criteria are described in detail in Table 1):

Table 1 Patient selection criteria

Inclusion	Male or female
	At least 18 years old
	Healthy enough to undergo routine implant surgery and subsequent dental treatment
	Partially edentulous requiring single dental implants in the maxilla
	Adequate volume of native or grafted bone to accommodate dental implants at least 8 mm long
	No active infections
	Physically, emotionally, and financially able to undergo planned implant procedures
	Adequate compliance to meet study requirements and necessary appointments
Exclusion	Medical need for antibiotic premedication for infective endocarditis, artificial joints, or any other medication
	Uncontrolled hypertension
	Uncontrolled diabetes
	Serological human immunodeficiency virus (HIV) positive
	History of significant heart, stomach, liver, kidney, blood, immune system, or other organ impairment or systemic disease that would prevent undergoing the proposed treatment
	Smoke cigarettes or other tobacco products
	Use of investigational drugs during the previous month
	Unresolved dental conditions likely to require exiting the study for treatment, such as deep cavities, abscesses, or moderate to severe periodontal disease
	History of radiation therapy to the head and neck
	Unwilling or inability to sign the informed consent form
	Failure to demonstrate willingness to return for a required number of visits
	Need immediate dental implant placement following tooth extraction

Patient selection, inclusion, and exclusion criteria are presented

Group A received 10 OSPTX implants using the soft bone surgical protocol (OSPTXSoft).
Group B received 10 OSPTX implants using the standard surgical protocol (OSPTXStd).
Group C received 10 OSP implants using the standard surgical protocol (OSPStd).

To facilitate randomization, the manufacturer packaged each implant with a prescribed surgical protocol included. The surgeon was blinded to the implant type until the opening of the package when the patient was seated for the surgery.

The soft bone drilling protocol used for group A results in an underpreparation compared to the implant diameter by −0.5 mm at the body portion. Corresponding underpreparation at the apex is from the beginning of apex towards the tip of the implant −0.8, −0.4, and 0 mm, respectively. All implants were of 4 mm diameter and 8 mm length and were placed at sites coronal to the maxillary sinus where at least 8-mm bone height was available. Every patient received a cone beam computed tomography (CBCT) evaluation pre-operatively using an i-CAT[*2] unit. Bone quality was measured clinically by the surgeon during preparation of the osteotomy [19]. Implants were placed following a two-stage protocol. They were uncovered at 6 weeks at which time functionally loaded screw-retained provisional crown was delivered per a FDA approved protocol for this implant system. Implant stability was measured by insertion torque using a calibrated torque wrench[3] at the time of implant placement and by ISQ measurements using the Osstell[™4] unit at the time of implant placement and at 6 weeks and 6 and 12 months (Fig. 2). Standardized periapical radiographs were taken at the time of implant placement and at 6 and 12 months. Changes to the bone level heights were measured at 6 and 12 months by two blinded examiners using the ImageJ[®5] software. The final cement-retained PFM crown (DSIGN porcelain) was delivered at 12 months.

ANOVA was used to compare the mean implant stabilities between the three groups. Post hoc testing was done via Tukey's honestly significant differences test to calculate the differences between ISQ measurements at the time of implant placement, 6 weeks and 6 and 12 months (Fig. 2) as well as bone levels at 6 and 12 months (Fig. 3). The correlations of multiple parameters such as insertion torque, ISQ, and crestal bone level were calculated using the Pearson product-moment correlation coefficient.

Results

Overall implant survival rate was 93.3%. Two implants failed, one implant in group A (OSPTXSoft) and one in group B (OSPTXStd). Both implant failures occurred at the time of uncovery (at 6 weeks) and prior to loading of the implants and were attributed to lack of integration. With the exception of these two failed implants, there was 100% success for all remaining implants using the parameters described in Table 2. There are no statistically significant differences in mean crestal bone loss at 6 and 12 months (Fig. 3) or ISQ at insertion, 6 weeks and 6 and 12 months (Fig. 2) in between the three groups. Implant stability, as measured by ISQ, ranged between 83 and 84 at the 12-month time point in all groups (Fig. 2). Mean radiographic crestal bone loss at 6 and 12 months after implant placement was minimal (<0.5 mm) in all groups with no statistically significant difference between the groups (Fig. 3). Implant stability, as measured with ISQ, presented no

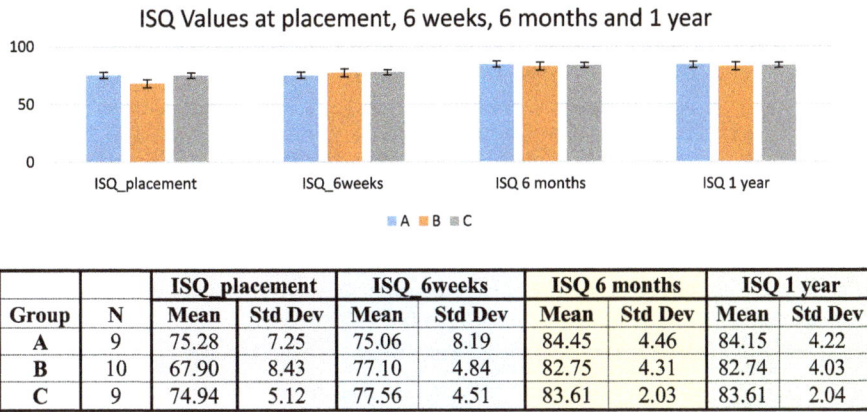

Fig. 2 ISQ values at placement, 6 weeks, 6 months, and 1 year. Mean and standard deviation of ISQ values taken at placement, 6 weeks, 6 months, and 1 year is presented. No statistical significant difference was determined between ISQ values at all time points. (*p* < 0.05)

ISQ Values at placement, 6 weeks, 6 months and 1 year

Group	N	ISQ_placement		ISQ_6weeks		ISQ 6 months		ISQ 1 year	
		Mean	Std Dev	Mean	Std Dev	Mean	Std Dev	Mean	Std Dev
A	9	75.28	7.25	75.06	8.19	84.45	4.46	84.15	4.22
B	10	67.90	8.43	77.10	4.84	82.75	4.31	82.74	4.03
C	9	74.94	5.12	77.56	4.51	83.61	2.03	83.61	2.04

statistically significant difference between the three groups at the time of insertion and at 6 and 12 months. Strong positive correlations were found between overall bone loss at 6 months and insertion torque at time of placement ($r = 0.7998$). When evaluating the correlation between torque values at the time of implant placement, a strong positive correlation was found with overall bone loss at 6 months ($r = 0.7995$) and with ISQ at 6 weeks ($r = 0.9078$). Insertion torque and ISQ at time of implant placement presented a very weak correlation ($r = 0.0509$).

Discussion

Augmentation of the maxillary sinus prior to dental implant placement is routinely performed in order to help patients restore their maxillary posterior dentition. Unfortunately, not all patients are candidates for this procedure due to either health, personal, or financial concerns. An alternative treatment without the need for a sinus elevation procedure is the use of a shorter implant. Research has shown that shorter implants (<10 mm) have comparable survival and success rates to

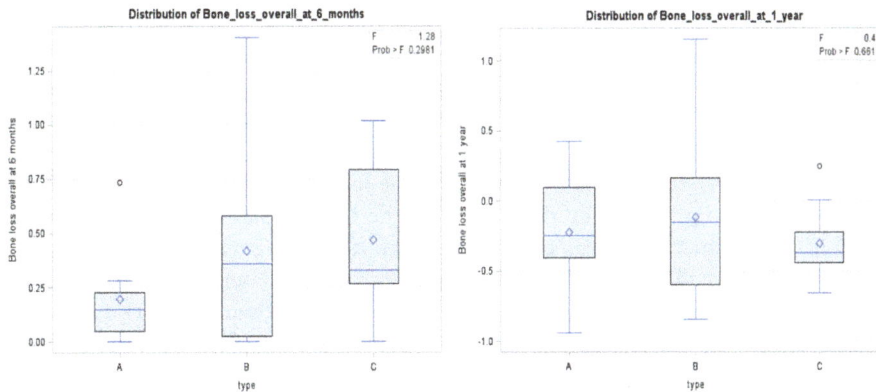

Mean Bone Loss						
		6 Months		1 Year		
Group	N	Mean	Std Dev	Mean	Std Dev	
A	9	0.1975	0.2357	-0.2201	0.4393	
B	10	0.4167	0.4766	-0.1132	0.5752	
C	9	0.4676	0.3444	-0.3033	0.2780	
		P-value= 0.2981		P-value= 0.6613		

Fig. 3 Mean bone loss at 6 months and 1 year. Mean bone loss distribution charts at 6 months and 1 year present no statistically significant difference. *p* value at 6 months was 0.2981 and at 1 year 0.6613

Table 2 Outcome success criteria

Implant success	Clinically immobile when tested manually and/or with RFA (minimum ISQ = 65)
	Absence of peri-implant radiolucency present on an undistorted radiograph
	Absence of unresolved pain, discomfort, infection or neuropathy, or peri-implant soft tissue complications attributable to the implant
	Implant placement that does not preclude delivery of a prosthetic crown with an appearance that is satisfactory to the patient and the dentist
	Crestal bone loss that is <1.5 mm after the first year of loading followed by not more than 0.2 mm of annual crestal bone loss thereafter
Prosthesis success	Absence of unresolved peri-implant soft-tissue complications, such as bleeding, swelling, suppuration or recession, attributable to the prosthetic restoration
	Absence of unresolved prosthetic complications, such as screw loosening or porcelain fracture
	Absence of esthetic complications, such as implant or abutment visibility, or compromised porcelain translucency or mismatched prosthetic tooth color
	Early loading success: a functional provisional crown placed ≥3 weeks and <3–6 months after implant placement, followed by delivery of a definitive crown after 12 months of function

Outcome success criteria are presented

longer implants (>10 mm) [1–4, 6–9]. Primary implant stability, as measured at the time of placement, is another important factor for both short and long implants. Tapered implant designs are considered to provide greater initial stability [12, 14]. Specifically, Lozano-Carrascal et al. in a prospective clinical study compared OSP implants to tapered MIS® implants placed in human mandibles. They reported the tapered implants achieved higher primary stability measured through ISQ and insertion torque [20]. Our study did not support these findings as we did not find a statistically significant difference in primary stability between the OSP and OSPTX implant designs. However, the OSPTX implants used in our study were tapered only at the apex as opposed to the MIS® implant which is tapered throughout the body of the implant. Furthermore, the mean insertion torque value observed in our study for the OSP group was lower (27.6 Ncm) than that observed by Lozano-Carrascal et al. in the maxilla for the same implant (35.8 Ncm) [20]. This difference may be attributed to the shorter implant length and wider diameter used in our study. The mean ISQ at insertion for the OSP implants in our study presented comparable values to an ex vivo study using the same implant placed in fresh porcine mandibles [17].

Surgical protocols have been developed to overcome the poor bone quality found in the posterior maxilla, so as to increase primary implant stability. Most surgical systems recommend a soft bone surgical protocol which requires a narrower diameter osteotomy than that of the implant being placed. This can involve underpreparing the complete length of the osteotomy or only underpreparing the apical ¾ of the osteotomy when the crestal bone is denser. In the posterior maxilla, the bone quality can vary greatly. By comparing the stability between the three groups, we found that implant stability was neither statistically significantly different between the two different implant designs or between the two different surgical protocols used. These findings are in agreement with Siera-Rebolledo et al., who also found no statistically significant differences between a soft bone drilling protocol and a standard drilling protocol [21].

Insertion torque presented a moderate to strong correlation with ISQ values at 6 weeks, 6 months, and 1 year but not at time of implant insertion. This finding is in agreement with Acil et al. who reported no statistically significant correlation between insertion torque and ISQ at time of implant placement [22].

Although a strong correlation was found between insertion torque and bone loss at all time points, the mean bone loss observed was minimal (<0.5 mm).

The OSP implant system has demonstrated high survival rates ranging from 94 up to 100% in previous long- and short-term studies [23–25]. Our findings are comparable with an overall 93.3% survival rate at 1 year, despite the fact that all implants were placed in the posterior maxilla.

Conclusions

Survival rates and stability of OSP and OSPTX implants was comparable.

Osteotomy preparation either by the standard or by the soft bone surgical protocol had no significant effect on implant survival, success, and stability.

Insertion torque presented a moderate to strong correlation with ISQ values at 6 weeks, 6 months, and 1 year.

Insertion torque presented a weak correlation to ISQ values at time of implant insertion.

Endnotes

[1]DENTSPLY International, Susquehanna Commerce Center, 221 West Philadelphia Street, York, PA 17401

[2]I-CAT 17 19; Imaging Services International LLC, 1910 North Penn Rd., Hatfield, PA 19440

[3]Intra-Lock International, 6560 S. West Rogers Circle, Suite 24, Boca Raton, FL 33487

[4]Osstell USA, 6700 Alexander Bell Drive, Suite 200, Columbia, MD 21046

[5]ImageJ 1.50i Wayne Rasband National Institutes of Health, USA; https://imagej.nih.gov/ij/; Java 1.8.0_77 (64bit)

Funding
This study was supported by Dentsply®. The company provided all Astra Dental implants and restorative parts needed for the completion of the study.

Authors' contributions
DES is a restorative dentist and Clinical Associate Professor of Periodontics who directs the Implant Restorative Fellowship Program at LSUHSC-SOD Department of Periodontics. He oversaw restoration of all implants placed. PM is an Associate Professor of Periodontics who teaches at both the undergraduate and postgraduate level. She assisted with IRB approval and oversight of surgical procedures. AGT was a Periodontics resident at the time. He assisted with data collection and analysis. SB was the study coordinator and assisted with all aspects of the study. LJP completed the statistical analysis of all data collected. AAP is an Associate Professor and Postgraduate Program Director who oversees all clinical activities at the postgraduate Periodontics clinic. She assisted with oversight of surgical procedures and manuscript preparation. All authors read and approved the final manuscript.

Competing interests
Dr. Simmons, Dr. Maney, Dr. Teitelbaum, Ms. Billiot, and Dr. Palaiologou state that they have no conflicts of interest.

Author details
[1]Department of Periodontics, Louisiana State University Health Sciences Center School of Dentistry, 1100 Florida Avenue, New Orleans, LA 70119, USA. [2]Tulane University SPHTM, 1440 Canal St, Suite 2001, New Orleans, LA 70130, USA.

References
1. Anitua E, Orive G. Short implants in maxillae and mandibles: a retrospective study with 1 to 8 years of follow-up. J Periodontol. 2010;81(6):819–26.
2. Feldman S, Boitel N, Weng D, Kohles SS, Stach RM. Five-year survival distributions of short-length (10 mm or less) machined-surfaced and Osseotite implants. Clin Implant Dent Relat Res. 2004;6(1):16–23.
3. Felice P, Cannizzaro G, Checchi V, Marchetti C, Pellegrino G, Censi P, et al. Vertical bone augmentation versus 7-mm-long implants in posterior atrophic mandibles. Results of a randomised controlled clinical trial of up to 4 months after loading. Eur J Oral Implantol. 2009;2(1):7–20.
4. Misch CE. Short dental implants: a literature review and rationale for use. Dent Today. 2005;24(8):64–6. 8.
5. Lee SA, Lee CT, Fu MM, Elmisalati W, Chuang SK. Systematic review and meta-analysis of randomized controlled trials for the management of limited vertical height in the posterior region: short implants (5 to 8 mm) vs longer implants (>8 mm) in vertically augmented sites. Int J Oral Maxillofac Implants. 2014;29(5):1085–97.
6. Mezzomo LA, Miller R, Triches D, Alonso F, Shinkai RS. Meta-analysis of single crowns supported by short (<10 mm) implants in the posterior region. J Clin Periodontol. 2014;41(2):191–213.
7. Monje A, Chan HL, Fu JH, Suarez F, Galindo-Moreno P, Wang HL. Are short dental implants (<10 mm) effective? A meta-analysis on prospective clinical trials. J Periodontol. 2013;84(7):895–904.
8. Monje A, Fu JH, Chan HL, Suarez F, Galindo-Moreno P, Catena A, et al. Do implant length and width matter for short dental implants (<10 mm)? A meta-analysis of prospective studies. J Periodontol. 2013;84(12):1783–91.
9. Nisand D, Renouard F. Short implant in limited bone volume. Periodontol 2000. 2014;66(1):72–96.
10. Abbou M. Primary stability and osseointegration: preliminary clinical results with a tapered diminishing-thread implant. Pract Proced Aesthet Dent. 2003;15(2):161–8. quiz 70.
11. Hall JA, Payne AG, Purton DG, Torr B. A randomized controlled clinical trial of conventional and immediately loaded tapered implants with screw-retained crowns. Int J Prosthodont. 2006;19(1):17–9.
12. O'Sullivan D, Sennerby L, Meredith N. Influence of implant taper on the primary and secondary stability of osseointegrated titanium implants. Clin Oral Implants Res. 2004;15(4):474–80.
13. Schwartz-Arad D, Herzberg R, Levin L. Evaluation of long-term implant success. J Periodontol. 2005;76(10):1623–8.
14. Alves CC, Neves M. Tapered implants: from indications to advantages. Int J Periodontics Restorative Dent. 2009;29(2):161–7.
15. Cawley P, Pavlakovic B, Alleyne DN, George R, Back T, Meredith N. The design of a vibration transducer to monitor the integrity of dental implants. Proc Inst Mech Eng H. 1998;212(4):265–72.
16. Meredith N, Shagaldi F, Alleyne D, Sennerby L, Cawley P. The application of resonance frequency measurements to study the stability of titanium implants during healing in the rabbit tibia. Clin Oral Implants Res. 1997;8(3):234–43.
17. Staedt H, Palarie V, Staedt A, Wolf JM, Lehmann KM, Ottl P, et al. Primary stability of cylindrical and conical dental implants in relation to insertion torque—a comparative ex vivo evaluation. Implant Dent. 2017;26(2):250–5.
18. Stocchero M, Toia M, Cecchinato D, Becktor JP, Coelho PG, Jimbo R. Biomechanical, biologic, and clinical outcomes of undersized implant surgical preparation: a systematic review. Int J Oral Maxillofac Implants. 2016;31(6):1247–63.
19. Misch CE. Contemporary implant dentistry. 3rd ed. St. Louis: Elsevier; 2008. p. 1102.
20. Lozano-Carrascal N, Salomo-Coll O, Gilabert-Cerda M, Farre-Pages N, Gargallo-Albiol J, Hernandez-Alfaro F. Effect of implant macro-design on primary stability: a prospective clinical study. Med Oral Patol Oral Cir Bucal. 2016;21(2):e214–21.
21. Sierra-Rebolledo A, Allais-Leon M, Maurette-O'Brien P, Gay-Escoda C. Primary apical stability of tapered implants through reduction of final drilling dimensions in different bone density models: a biomechanical study. Implant Dent. 2016;25(6):775–82.
22. Acil Y, Sievers J, Gulses A, Ayna M, Wiltfang J, Terheyden H. Correlation between resonance frequency, insertion torque and bone-implant contact in self-cutting threaded implants. Odontology. 2016. [Epub ahead of print]
23. Oxby G, Oxby F, Oxby J, Saltvik T, Nilsson P. Early loading of fluoridated implants placed in fresh extraction sockets and healed bone: a 3- to 5-year clinical and radiographic follow-up study of 39 consecutive patients. Clin Implant Dent Relat Res. 2015;17(5):898–907.
24. De Bruyn H, Raes F, Cooper LF, Reside G, Garriga JS, Tarrida LG, et al. Three-years clinical outcome of immediate provisionalization of single Osseospeed() implants in extraction sockets and healed ridges. Clin Oral Implants Res. 2013;24(2):217–23.
25. Ebler S, Ioannidis A, Jung RE, Hammerle CH, Thoma DS. Prospective randomized controlled clinical study comparing two types of two-piece dental implants supporting fixed reconstructions—results at 1 year of loading. Clin Oral Implants Res. 2016;27(9):1169–77.

Implant success and survival rates in daily dental practice: 5-year results of a non-interventional study using CAMLOG SCREW-LINE implants with or without platform-switching abutments

Sven Marcus Beschnidt[1], Claudio Cacaci[2], Kerem Dedeoglu[3], Detlef Hildebrand[4*] [iD], Helfried Hulla[5], Gerhard Iglhaut[6,7], Gerald Krennmair[8], Markus Schlee[9,10], Paul Sipos[11], Andres Stricker[12] and Karl-Ludwig Ackermann[13]

Abstract

Background: The performance of dental implants in controlled clinical studies is often investigated in homogenous populations. Observational studies are necessary to evaluate the outcome of implant restorations placed in real-life situations, according to standard practice, and to assess the needs of the patients. The aim of this non-interventional study was to reveal the survival, success, and general performance of CAMLOG SCREW-LINE implants and their restorations in daily dental practice.

Methods: Seventeen private practices across five countries participated in this prospective multicenter study. Patients received implants in the maxilla and mandible which were restored either with platform-matching or platform-switching abutments. Patients were followed-up for up to 5 years post-loading. Radiographs and clinical parameters were evaluated and patient satisfaction was evaluated.

Results: From a total of 196 patients planned, 185 patients with 271 implants were restored with abutments and fulfilled the follow-up inclusion criteria. Three implant failures were recorded, resulting in a cumulative survival rate of 98.6% after 5 years post-loading. One persistent complication of peri-implantitis occurred. The soft tissue health remained stable, and the papilla height improved after loading. At 5-year follow-up, the mean crestal bone loss was -0.28 ± 0.60 mm; over 99% of patients reported satisfaction with the restoration as excellent or good.

Conclusions: Implants placed and restored with both platform-matching and platform-switching abutments in daily dental private practice achieved excellent clinical outcomes with highly satisfied patients after 5 years of function, confirming the results obtained in well-controlled clinical trials.

Keywords: Implant success, Implant survival, Dental implants, Patient satisfaction, Daily dental practice, Non-interventional study, Platform switching, Hard tissue, Soft tissue

* Correspondence: hildebrand@dentalforum-berlin.de
[4]Private practice, Berlin, Germany
Full list of author information is available at the end of the article

Background

Success and survival rates of endosseous implants are well-documented in a number of controlled clinical trials and systematic reviews [1–3]. Generally, controlled trials evaluate endosseous implants in specific clinical situations; thus, the patient population is subjected to rigorous inclusion criteria and follow-up. Accordingly, controlled clinical trials do not reflect the real-life situation in private practice. Numerous factors including experienced clinicians, specialized clinics, restricted inclusion and exclusion criteria, specific indications, and increased time spent during follow-up, may affect or even bias the results, outcomes, or reported implant success and survival rates [4]. Consequently, there is an increasing trend in assimilating and reporting real-life data [4] allowing for the evaluation and assessment of dental implants in daily practice. An observational, non-interventional study in a non-homogeneous population better reflects daily practice than a controlled clinical study.

Various studies have reported on success and survival of endosseous implants in private practice settings. In a 5-year prospective observational study on 590 patients, Cochran et al. [5] evaluated 990 implants placed under routine private practice conditions. Very high cumulative survival and success rates were achieved after 3 years (> 99%) and 5 years (97%) of loading. These results were found to be comparable with the rates of survival and success of the same sand-blasted, large grit, acid-etched (SLA) implants achieved in a controlled, prospective, multicenter clinical study (Cochran et al. 2002 as cited in [5]).

Nevertheless, observational studies performed in private practice are not without their flaws; studies have shown that patients may be poorly motivated to attend follow-up appointments [6, 7], and results from various studies imply that, in non-controlled clinical settings, follow-up attendance may drop when patient satisfaction is high [6–8]. In contrast, regular follow-up appointment attendance is integral to the study design in controlled clinical trials; therefore, the patient's obligated attendance to follow-up appointments may mask their natural behavior when satisfied.

In the present study, CAMLOG SCREW-LINE implants with the Promote plus surface (sandblasted and acid-etched surface) were used. These implants in combination with platform-matching abutments have been shown to have high long-term success rates ranging from 97.8 to 100% at 5-year to 10-year follow-up [9–13]. They can be restored with either platform-matching or platform-switching abutments with the difference that platform-switching abutments have a narrower diameter than the implant, leading to an implant-abutment mismatch. The effects of platform switching on hard tissue outcomes are well-studied, with there being a tendency to better outcomes with respect to crestal bone loss with platform switching [14–23]. Regarding the CAMLOG SCREW-LINE implants, the effect of platform switching and platform matching was evaluated in a randomized controlled clinical trial (RCT) [21, 23]. At 1-year follow-up, implant success rates were 97.3% and 100%, and at 3 years, implant survival was 97.3% and 97.1%, for platform-switching and platform-matching implants respectively. Platform-switching implants showed a positive effect on marginal bone loss already at 1-year follow-up, and significantly less marginal bone loss was reported with the platform-switching versus platform-matching technique at 3 years (0.28 ± 0.56 mm vs. 0.68 ± 0.64, respectively; $p = 0.002$).

To understand the performance of the CAMLOG SCREW-LINE implants used with platform-switching and platform-matching abutments outside of a controlled clinical environment, we conducted a prospective, non-interventional study in private practice. The primary objective was to provide data for a life table analysis on the performance of the implants in private practice, to show the probability of survival and success of the dental implants after a follow-up time of 5 years post-loading. Secondary objectives were to evaluate patient satisfaction through the assessment of appearance, ability to chew, ability to taste, comfort, general satisfaction, and fit. The outcomes were also reported for platform-switching and platform-matching subgroups.

Methods
Study design

This was a prospective multicenter non-interventional study to assess implant success and survival rates in daily dental practices using the CAMLOG SCREW-LINE implants (CAMLOG Biotechnologies AG, Basel, Switzerland) used with or without platform-switching abutments. Patients were enrolled over a period of 2 years from October 2008 to September 2010 from 17 sites across five countries (Austria $n = 2$, Germany $n = 10$, Spain $n = 2$, the Netherlands $n = 2$, and Turkey $n = 1$). All patients gave their signed informed consent for participation in this study. The study was performed in accordance with the declaration of Helsinki, and institutional review board approval was obtained from the respective local review boards of the participating countries. The reporting of this study conforms to the STROBE statement [24].

The primary outcome of this study was the implant survival and success rates at 1, 3, and 5 years post-loading. The secondary outcomes were patient satisfaction as indicated by the assessment of the patient's ability to chew, ability to taste, comfort, appearance and fit of restoration, and general satisfaction.

Population

Male and female patients ≥ 18 years of age with sufficient bone at the implant site to achieve primary stability were included in this study. It was expected that the patients would return to the treatment center for prosthetic restoration and routine follow-up appointments at 1, 3, and 5 years post-loading. If socket preservation were to be performed, a minimum of 6 months must have elapsed before surgery. In such cases, this would be documented on the case report form. Patients were excluded if they had any contraindications to the package insert for the dental implant system, if primary stability at the implant insertion was not achieved, or if any bone graft and/or guided bone regeneration procedure was required. The treatment indications were single or multiple tooth replacement in the maxilla or mandible without the use of simultaneous augmentation or membrane, of which the implants were to be restored with either fixed single crown or fixed partial denture restorations.

Treatment procedure

Patients were to be treated according to standard practice for implant procedures applicable in the countries participating in the study. Implants used in this study were CAMLOG SCREW-LINE implants (K-Line) with diameters of 3.8 mm, 4.3 mm, 5.0 mm (or 6.0 mm), and lengths of 9 mm, 11 mm, and 13 mm. Both platform-matching and platform-switching abutments could be used. The protocol allowed freedom of choice, and the investigators selected the best option for the patients' indication. Implants were placed following normal treatment protocols of the participating site and were inserted following one-stage or two-stage surgery decided upon clinical need. Implants were restored after a healing period of at least 6 weeks post-surgery in bone class I–III and 12 weeks in bone class IV [25]. During surgery, the bone quality, crestal ridge width and height, and primary stability of the implant were documented.

Follow-up

The post-surgical examination took place between 1 and 2 weeks post-surgery according to the standard practice. At this time, patient complaints and adverse events were recorded. Patients underwent suture removal and were instructed in oral hygiene and plaque removal. Follow-up visits were scheduled according to standard practice and according to the surgical protocol. Patients undergoing two-stage surgery attended a re-entry surgery for placement of the healing abutment; otherwise, patients attended the clinic for abutment placement, provisional prosthesis placement, and definitive prosthesis placement as per individual treatment plan. Follow-up appointments then occurred at 6 months, 1, 2, 3,4, and

5 years post prosthetic installation. Standard maintenance care like check-ups for dental hygiene was performed as required.

Assessments

Throughout the study, only radiographs consistent with standard implant procedures were taken. Bone level changes were assessed based on available and evaluable standardized periapical radiographs with a film-holder using parallel-technique or panoramic radiographs (depending on the standard in the study centers). Baseline was defined as the time of the first prosthetic installation (loading). Each investigator performed their own measurements on either digital or analog radiographs, as available. In order to achieve standardized measurements, all analog radiographs were digitized and measurements were performed on all radiographs with the free-available software ImageJ 1.50i by an experienced independent person and subsequently validated by the investigators. All periapical and panoramic radiographs were individually calibrated (distance of three threads) to account for the distortion of the pictures. The distance from the implant shoulder to the first visible bone contact at the mesial and distal aspect of the implants was measured. The measurements at the mesial and distal site were averaged to obtain the bone level per implant. The changes in the bone level were calculated over several intervals: from loading to 5 years post-loading and at yearly intervals starting from 1 year post-loading to evaluate the success criteria. Bone quality [26] was assessed during the surgery (D1 to D4). Clinical parameters to assess the soft tissue health, including Modified Plaque Index (MPI), Papilla Index, Sulcus Bleeding Index (SBI), and pocket probing depth (PPD) (if measured), were recorded during abutment placement, during placement of the definitive prosthesis, and at each subsequent follow-up visit. The MPI and SBI were measured according to the criteria described by Mombelli [27]. The presence of the mesial and the distal papilla was evaluated according to the Jemt papilla score [28]. PPD, if routinely measured, was evaluated as a change in probing depths at 1, 3, and 5 years, compared with baseline. MPI, SBI, and PPD were determined on the buccal, lingual, distal, and mesial sites on each implant; the mean value of the scores was taken to provide the assessment of the implant.

The primary stability of the implant was assessed during surgery. Implant success and survival were evaluated in the group of implants restored with abutments [5, 29] at both placements of the provisional and definitive prostheses and at each follow-up visit thereafter. Implants were deemed successful in accordance with the criteria for implant success laid down by Albrektsson et al. [30]. Implants were successful if there was less than 0.2 mm bone loss annually after the first year of loading, if they were clinically immobile, if there was no peri-implant radiolucency, and if there was no persistent and/or irreversible pain, infection, neuropathies, or paresthesia. During the course of the study, the criterion of bone loss by Albrektsson et al. was scrutinized, and the scientific relevance was not considered to be suitable anymore [30, 31]; therefore, implant success was assessed post hoc, according to Buser et al. [29], that is, there was no persistent and/or irreversible signs or symptoms such as pain, infection, neuropathies, or paresthesia, no peri-implant infection with suppuration, no mobility, and no continuous radiolucency around the implant. Radiological evaluation for radiolucency and bone loss was measurable only with available evaluable radiographs; radiographs for some patients were missing or not evaluable. In the case that no complications were reported by the clinician, and the patients reported being satisfied according to the set criteria, then radiographs were not necessary and the implant was deemed successful.

The patients rated their satisfaction regarding the ability to chew, to taste, their comfort, appearance and fit of restoration, and general satisfaction on a categorical scale (very unsatisfied, unsatisfied, middle, satisfied, very satisfied) via a questionnaire at each visit beginning from loading [17, 22].

Safety

Adverse events were recorded on an adverse event form and reported as non-treatment associated or treatment-associated events.

Statistical methods

A minimum of 200 patients were planned to be included in the study. Analyses were performed on the per protocol population. In addition, to assess the correlation of implant success with anatomical and surgical parameters, analyses of the subgroups "platform matching" and "platform switching" (based on abutment type) were performed. Implant success and survival rates were calculated using a life table analysis 1 year after baseline and yearly thereafter. To test for significant differences for repeated measurements, the Wilcoxon signed-rank test was used, and to assess for significant differences between the subgroups, the Kruskal-Wallis test was used. p values of less than $p < 0.05$ were deemed significant. Changes in the crestal bone were quantitatively evaluated through the standardized measurements of the radiographs. Any non-standardized radiographs allowed for qualitative analysis only. Standardized measurements on radiographs for calculating bone level changes were done with the freely available software ImageJ 1.50i (https://imagej.nih.gov/ij/). Descriptive statistics were performed with IBM SPSS Statistics for Windows V24.0 (IBM Corp., Armonk, NY, USA).

Results

Patient demographics

In total, 196 patients from 17 centers met the inclusion criteria for this study and were included in the per-protocol analysis. In total, 285 implants were placed (Table 1). At the 5-year follow-up, data were available for the 137 patients who completed the study (Fig. 1). Patient demographic data is presented in Tables 2 and 3.

Implant success

Implant success was reported according to the criteria for implant success laid down by Albrektsson et al. [30], as well as that by Buser et al. [29]. According to Albrektsson et al., there were three implant failures post-loading and three implants which did not meet the success criteria due to bone loss ($n = 2$) and peri-implantitis ($n = 1$). According to Buser et al., there were three implant failures post-loading and one implant which did not meet the success criteria due to peri-implantitis ($n = 1$) (Table 4). The three implants which were late failures were lost at 2 years post-loading due to important bone loss and at 3.6 years and at 4.6 years post-loading (all platform switching). Additional five implants were lost before loading as a result of no osseointegration (early failures) and therefore were not considered for the analysis.

The cumulative success rates did not differ according to both criteria at 1-year follow-up or at 3-year follow-up, being 100% and 99.6%, respectively. However, at 5-year follow-up, the success rate according to Buser et al. was higher at 98.0% than that according to Albrektsson et al. at 97.1%. The sub-group analysis revealed that the success rate for platform-matching implants was 100% at 1-year and at 3-year and 96.2% at 5-year follow-up according to Albrektsson et al. and 100% at each follow-up according to Buser et al. Conversely, for platform-switching implants the success rate was 100% at 1-year follow-up, 99.4% at 3-year follow-up, and 97.4% at 5-year follow-up, according to both criteria.

Implant survival

The cumulative survival rate was 100% at 1-year follow-up, 99.6% at 3-year follow-up, and 98.6% at 5-year follow-up. All three late failures were in the platform-switching subgroup.

Clinical parameters/soft tissue parameters
Plaque index

Mean modified plaque indices were very low at below 0.5 for all but one measurement throughout the course

Table 1 Table of study centers

Investigator*	City/country	Number of patients included	Number of implants included
Dr. Helfried Hulla	Strass in Steiermark, Austria	10	15
Prof. DDr. Gerald Krennmair	Marchtrenk, Austria	10	20
Dr. S. Marcus Beschnidt (PI)	Baden-Baden, Germany	8	12
Dr. Karl-Ludwig Ackermann	Filderstadt, Germany	14	18
Dr. Thomas Barth	Leipzig, Germany	15	28
Dr. Claudio Cacaci	Munich, Germany	11	14
Dr. Christian Hammächer	Aachen, Germany	10	13
Dr. Detlef Hildebrand	Berlin, Germany	16	30
PD Dr. Gerhard Iglhaut	Memmingen, Germany	4	5
PD Dr. Dr. Markus Schlee	Forchheim, Germany	18	22
Dr. Dr. Manfred Wolf	Leinfelden-Echterdingen, Germany	14	17
PD Dr. Dr. Andres Stricker	Constance, Germany	11	18
Dr. Juan Manuel Vadillo	Madrid, Spain	12	17
Dr. Fernando Loscos Morató	Zaragoza, Spain	15	22
Dr. Gert de Lange / Dr. Paul Sipos	Amstelveen, Netherlands	15	18
Dr. Chris van Lith	Hoorn, Netherlands	4	4
Dr. Kerem Dedeoglu	Istanbul, Turkey	9	12

*All in private practice

of the study (Fig. 2a). At loading, the overall MPI was 0.27 ± 0.49 slightly increasing to 0.38 ± 0.52 at 5-year follow-up; the increase in MPI from loading to 5-year follow-up was statistically significant ($p < 0.001$). The MPI for the platform-switching subgroup was significantly lower than that for platform-matching subgroup at 3-year ($p = 0.025$), 4-year ($p = 0.001$), and 5-year ($p = 0.028$) follow-up.

Sulcus bleeding index
At loading, the overall SBI was 0.21 ± 0.47, remaining very low throughout the study and slightly increasing to 0.32 ± 0.49 at 5-year follow-up (Fig. 2b). The increase in SBI from loading to 5-year follow-up was statistically significant ($p < 0.001$). At 3-year follow-up, the SBI was significantly higher in the platform-matching subgroup than in the platform-switching subgroup (0.29 vs. 0.23; $p = 0.039$); this difference increased at 4-year and 5-year follow-up (0.41 vs. 0.20; $p = 0.001$ and 0.50 vs. 0.27; $p = 0.004$, respectively).

Pocket probing depth
At loading, the PPD was 2.16 ± 1.05 mm; it decreased to 1.89 ± 1.04 mm at 6 months post-loading, increasing to 2.12 ± 1.04 mm at 1-year follow-up (Fig. 2c). From this point onward, the PPD increased to 2.34 ± 1.18 mm at 5-year follow-up. The increase in mean PPD from loading to 5-year follow-up was statistically significant ($p = 0.032$). The mean PPD for the platform-switching

subgroup was significantly lower than that for the platform-matching subgroup at 4-year (2.20 mm vs. 2.77 mm; $p = 0.012$) and 5-year follow-up (2.23 mm vs. 2.70 mm; $p = 0.011$).

Jemt papilla score
At loading, the Jemt papilla score was 1.93 ± 1.01, significantly increasing to 2.14 ± 0.95 at 5-year follow-up ($p = 0.023$) (Fig. 2d). For the platform-switching subgroup, a significant difference was observed between baseline and 5-year follow-up ($p < 0.001$); however, no significant difference was observed for the platform-matching group over the same time period. Furthermore, at loading, the Jemt papilla score was significantly lower for the platform-switching subgroup than for the platform-matching subgroup (1.78 vs. 2.28; $p = 0.009$).

Bone level changes
Evaluable radiographs were available from 13 participating sites: eleven sites with periapical and two sites with orthopantographic radiographs. At loading and at 5-year follow-up, respectively, 148 and 119 evaluable radiographs were available. The mean bone level change from loading (baseline) to 5-year follow-up was (mean $\pm$ SD) -0.28 ± 0.60 mm. No significant differences in the mean bone level change from loading to 5-year follow-up were observed between the platform-switching and platform-matching subgroups (-0.32 ± 0.60 mm vs. -0.13 ± 0.29 mm). From

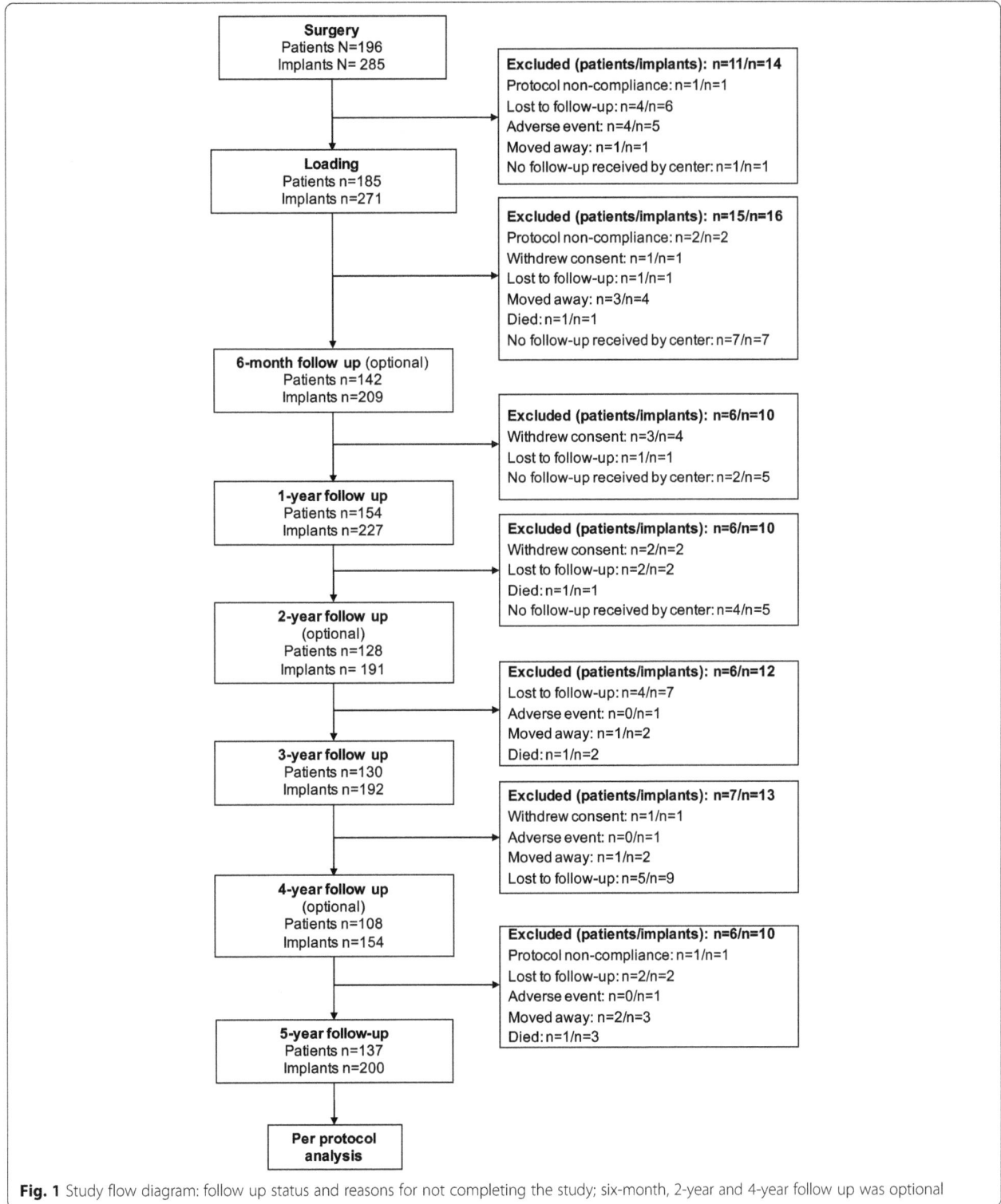

Fig. 1 Study flow diagram: follow up status and reasons for not completing the study; six-month, 2-year and 4-year follow up was optional

loading to 5-year follow-up, no bone loss or even bone gain was observed in 38% of evaluable implants. Figure 3 shows the frequency distribution of bone level changes from loading to 5-year follow-up for all implants.

Patient satisfaction

Patient satisfaction was reported as excellent by over 60% of all patients for each category at each time point during the course of the study, with almost all remaining

Table 2 Patient demographics

	Overall	Subgroup*	
		Platform switching	Platform matching
Patients, n (%)	196 (100)	144	41
Sex, n (%)			
Male	87 (44.4)	62 (43.1)	19 (46.3)
Female	109 (55.6)	82 (56.9)	22 (53.7)
Age, years			
Mean (SD)	51.5 (14.2)	53.1 (14.4)	47.4 (12.9)
Range	17.9–82.1	17.9–82.1	19.3–78.5
Pre-implant bone surgeries, n			
Autogenous bone grafting	31	n/a	n/a
Socket preservation	1	n/a	n/a
Others	16	n/a	n/a
Pre-implant soft tissue s urgeries, n			
Palatal soft tissue graft	15	n/a	n/a
Other	1	n/a	n/a
Bone quality, %			
D1: mainly homogenous bone	12.8	8.9	22.4
D2: compact bone thick	42.2	42.4	41.8
D3: compact thin/cancellous good density	42.2	45.3	35.8
D4: compact thin/cancellous low density	2.8	3.4	0.0
Reasons for tooth loss, n (%)			
Caries	53 (19.3)	36 (18.4)	13 (19.4)
Endodontic	96 (35.0)	67 (34.2)	24 (35.8)
Fracture	35 (12.8)	32 (16.3)	3 (4.5)
Periodontal	46 (16.8)	33 (16.8)	13 (19.4)
Endodontic and periodontal	3 (1.1)	3 (1.5)	0 (0.0)
Caries and periodontal	4 (1.5)	4 (2.0)	0 (0.0)
Endodontic and fracture	2 (0.7)	1 (0.5)	1 (1.5)
Others	35 (12.8)	20 (10.2)	13 (19.4)
Missing	11 (3.9)		
Smoking status, n (%)			
Non-smoker	166 (86.5)	121 (85.2)	37 (90.2)
Mild smoker (≤ 10/day)	18 (9.4)	13 (9.2)	4 (9.8)
Heavy smoker (> 10/day)	8 (4.2)	8 (5.6)	0 (0.0)
General health status, n (%)			
ASA P1	161 (85.6)	118 (85.5)	34 (82.9)
ASA P2	26 (13.8)	20 (14.5)	6 (14.6)
ASA P3	1 (0.5)	0 (0.0)	1 (2.4)

*Eleven patients with 14 implants were not loaded/restored with abutments due to early implant failures or because the patients were lost to follow-up (Fig. 1)

patients reporting good outcomes (Fig. 4). No more than three patients reported an outcome of fair for any category at any time point, and no patients reported an outcome of poor for any category at any time points. No differences were observed between the platform-switching and platform-matching subgroups for any category at any time point (data not shown).

Prosthetic complications

With regard to prosthetic complications, there were two cases of ceramic chipping in two patients; the restorations were corrected and no further complications were seen. There were three cases of crown loosening which resolved after re-cementing the crowns, and there were two cases of abutment screw loosening leading to crown mobility, which resolved after screw tightening.

Discussion and conclusions

This large, multicenter study provides real-life long-term data on 285 implants placed in 196 patients. The results show that the placement of CAMLOG SCREW-LINE implants with platform-matching or platform-switching abutments results in high survival and success in the long term. The overall success rate for implants was 97.1% at 5-year post-loading, and 97.4% and 96.2% for implants with platform-switching and platform-matching abutments, respectively, according to Albrektsson et al. [30]; the overall survival rate was 98.6%. For comparability to other studies, the success rates were assessed post hoc according to Buser et al. [29], revealing a 5-year overall success rate of 98.0%, and 100% and 97.4% for implants with platform-matching and platform-switching abutments, respectively.

These results compare positively with the results achieved for the CAMLOG SCREW-LINE implants in an RCT [23]. Here, the 3-year success rates—according to Buser et al. [29]—were 97.3% for platform-switching and 97.1% for platform-matching implants. In contrast, the present study achieved better 3-year success rates—according to Buser et al. [29]—for both platform-matching (100%) and platform-switching (99.4%) implants. Other private practice studies achieved similar results to our study, with success rates at 3 years of 93.5% for SLActive implants [4] and 99.12% and 97.58% at 3 and 5 years, respectively, for comparable SLA surface implants [5]. These studies [4, 5] also applied the success criteria, according to Buser et al. [29], namely absence of pain, infection, neuropathies or paresthesia, peri-implant infection with suppuration, mobility, and continuous radiolucency around the implant. Slight differences in success rates are seen with the two criteria [29, 30]. In our study, the success rates are lower at 5-year follow-up, according to Albrektsson et al., because bone level changes were measured to fulfill the first criterion (< 0.2 mm bone loss

Table 3 Patient demographics with respect to implants

	Overall	Subgroup*	
		Platform switching	Platform matching
Total Implants, n	285	203*	68*
Number of implants placed per patient, n (%)			
1	125 (63.8)	97 (67.4)	20 (48.8)
2	56 (28.6)	37 (25.7)	16 (39.0)
3	12 (6.1)	7 (4.9)	5 (12.2)
4	3 (1.5)	3 (2.1)	0 (0.0)
Implant position distribution, n			
Maxilla			
17	3	2	1
16	16	10	4
15	14	8	5
14	9	8	0
13	1	1	0
12	11	10	1
11	8	7	1
21	11	10	1
22	7	6	1
23	8	8	0
24	11	8	2
25	11	7	3
26	15	12	2
27	2	1	1
Mandible			
47	12	8	4
46	44	31	10
45	13	9	3
44	9	7	2
43	1	0	1
42	1	1	0
41	0	0	0
31	1	1	0
32	0	0	0
33	0	0	0
34	4	1	3
35	14	9	4
36	47	33	13
37	12	5	6

Diameter	Length of implant				Total	
	9 mm	11 mm	13 mm	16 mm	Total, n	Total, %
3.3 mm	0	1	0	0	1	0.4
3.8 mm	10	29	54	1	94	33.0
4.3 mm	15	43	50	2	110	38.6
5.0 mm	7	35	36	1	79	27.7

Table 3 Patient demographics with respect to implants (*Continued*)

	Overall		Subgroup*			
			Platform switching		Platform matching	
6.0 mm	0	1	0	0	1	0.4
Total n	32	109	140	4	285	100.0

*Eleven patients with 14 implants were not loaded/restored with abutments due to early implant failures or because the patients were lost to follow-up (Fig. 1)

annually after the first year of loading). At 3-year follow-up, bone loss was noted in one patient (reclassified as peri-implantitis at the 4-year follow-up) and an important bone loss (due to poor oral hygiene and bruxism; two implants) in a patient with psychosocial issues who could not be treated during the study. Such a patient would not have been included in an RCT. Consequently, three implants were lost based on the bone loss criterion. Being able to measure bone level changes is also dependent on the availability of evaluable radiographs. In our study, these were taken as per standard clinical protocol using the available equipment, which may differ to that available in a university clinic, a setting commonly found in controlled clinical studies. Thus, some radiographs were not digitized and were difficult to read. Also, if the protocol does not stipulate radiography, then the natural behaviors of patients in private practice are revealed. Some patients refused radiographs, other patients were followed up by referring dentists, and radiographs were not exchanged. Additionally, if radiographs are routinely acquired, the clinician is still reliant on follow-up attendance. Accordingly, the success rates measured in the present study should be assessed collectively. Other studies not assessing bone level changes may report higher success rates than those achieved if bone level changes were evaluated [4, 5].

Other factors need to be considered when reporting success [32]. Papaspyridakos et al. reported a relationship between the number of success criteria and the success rate: the higher the number of success criteria, the lower the reported success rate [32]. Also, the common criterion of bone loss being < 2.0 mm during the first year of function, followed by < 0.2 mm annually thereafter, may no longer be suitable, particularly with new implant systems, such as platform-switching implants, which lead to minimal crestal bone remodeling (Prosper et al. and Trammell et al. cited in [32]). Over the 5-year study period, we report < 2.0 mm bone level change for all implants, 0.1–0.5 mm for 40%, and no bone loss or bone gain for 38% of all implants. Additionally, bone loss was 0.32 ± 0.66 mm and 0.13 ± 0.29 mm for the platform-switching and platform-matching subgroups. Of note, in this study, the platform-matching and platform-switching groups were very unbalanced (67 vs. 206 implants) because the decision to choose abutment type was the clinician's choice according to the clinical situation. Furthermore, very few

Table 4 Life table analysis showing the cumulative success rate according to Albrektsson et al. and Buser et al.

Interval (months)	Implants in interval	According to Albrektsson et al.			According to Buser et al.		
		Implants withdrawn during interval	Failures during interval	Cumulative success rate (%)	Implants withdrawn during interval	Failures during interval	Cumulative success rate (%)
Loading – 12	271	27	0	100	27	0	100
12–24	244	6	0	100	6	0	100
24–36	238	17	1	99.6	17	1	99.6
36–48	220	11	3	98.2	13	1	99.1
48–60	206	50	2	97.1	50	2	98.0
60–72	154	94	0	97.1	94	0	98.0
72–84	60	48	0	97.1	48	0	98.0
> 84	12	12	0	97.1	12	0	98.0

radiographs were available for the platform-matching subgroup; thus, differences between the two subgroups are not conclusive. Nevertheless, the minimal crestal bone loss of 0.32 mm observed for platform-switching implants is comparable with the data reported in other studies on platform-switching implants [17, 23]. The bone gain of 0.12 ± 0.42 mm at 1-year follow-up [17] and of 0.16 ± 0.53 mm at 3 years follow-up [23] have been reported. In these studies, the outer geometry of the implant was comparable; however, Rocha et al. [23] used implants of the same kind while Moergel et al. [17] used implants with a conical connection.

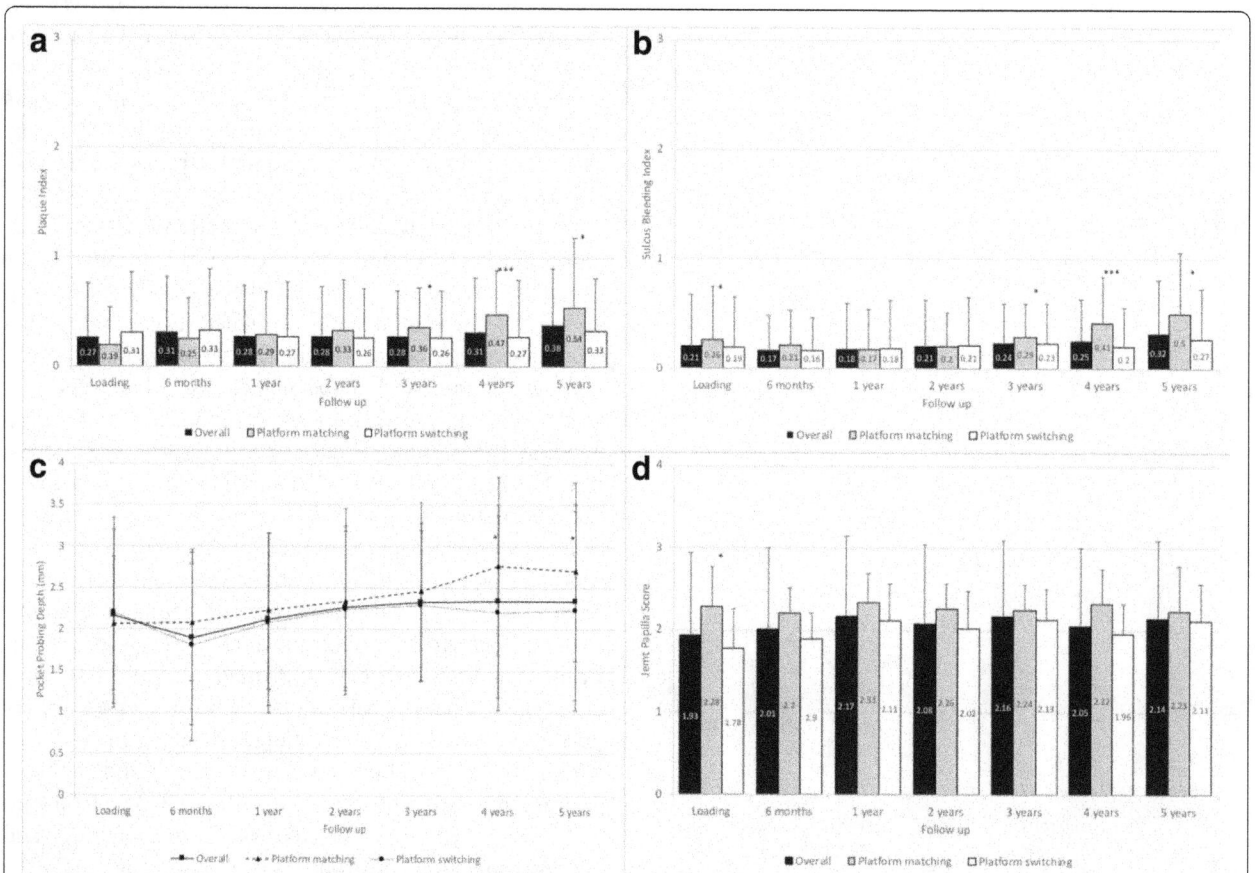

Fig. 2 Clinical parameters and soft tissue parameters. **a** Modified plaque index. Error bars indicate standard deviation. * = $p \leq 0.05$, *** = $p \leq 0.001$. **b** Sulcus bleeding index. Error bars indicate standard deviation. * = $p \leq 0.05$, *** = $p \leq 0.001$. **c** Pocket probing depth. The asterisk represents statistically significant differences (* = $p \leq 0.05$) observed between subgroups. **d** Jemt papilla score. The asterisk represents statistically significant differences (* = $p \leq 0.05$) observed between subgroups

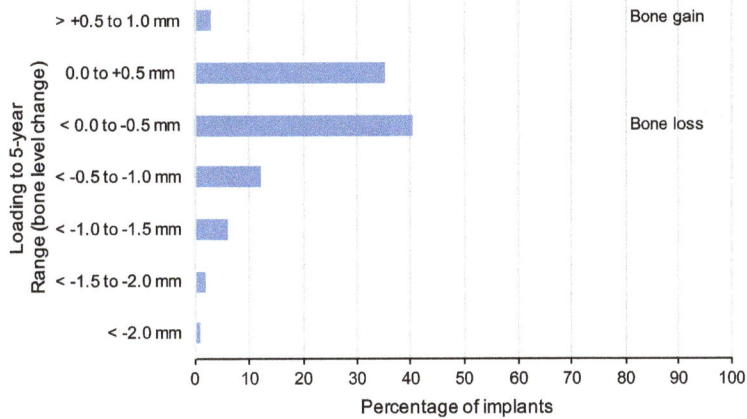

Fig. 3 Bone level changes from loading to 5-year follow up

The importance of the vertical soft tissue thickness has recently been reported [33, 34]. Platform-switching implants placed in thick tissues led to the preservation of the crestal bone level, while this was not observed in thin mucosal tissues. These studies were not yet published in the planning phase and initiation of the present study. Accordingly, pocket probing depth measurements were performed rather than vertical soft tissue thickness. These measurements may be biased; it is thought that the probe may stop at the horizontal shift instead of the pocket depth, yet, to our knowledge, there is no reference supporting this. In daily practice, probing was sometimes not performed if the implants showed no pathological findings. On the one hand, the variety of bone level changes in this study may be explained by different vertical soft tissue thicknesses, but cannot be validated due to these missing data. On the other hand, there are multiple confounding factors influencing the change in bone level, such as the size of the platform (mismatch), occlusal loading, and the microgap.

Additional to the standard success criteria, patient-reported outcomes are important factors when evaluating an implant system [32]. In our study, if the patient was satisfied, no further radiographs were taken, and the implant was deemed successful. Furthermore, in some success criteria, overall patient satisfaction should be good or excellent for the treatment to be successful (Levi et al. cited in Papaspyridakos et al. [32]). Our study reveals an exceptionally high level of patient satisfaction. The majority of patients reported excellent outcomes for all measured categories at each time point throughout the study, with most remaining patients reporting good outcomes (Fig. 4). No patient reported a poor outcome, and a maximum of three patients at any given time reported fair outcomes. The parameters assessed by patients are

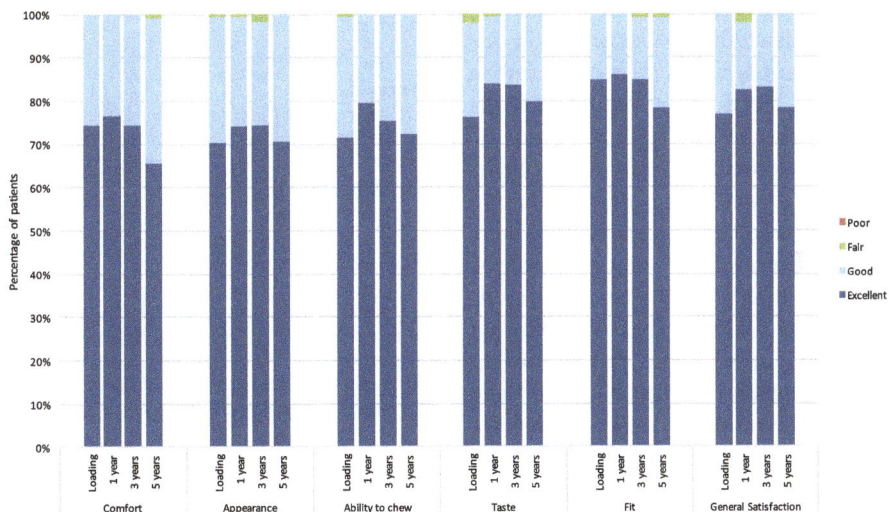

Fig. 4 Patient satisfaction throughout the study

closely related to soft tissue outcomes, which reflect oral hygiene and soft tissue health. The soft tissue parameters assessed in our study were MPI, SBI, PPD, and Jemt papilla score. For MPI, a statistically significant increase was observed from loading to the 5-year follow-up; however, the MPI at 5-year follow-up was, at 0.38 ± 0.52, still very low, with 0 equaling no detection of plaque and 1 equaling plaque only detectable after running a probe across the smooth marginal surface of the implant [27]. Similarly, the SBI remained very low throughout the study, despite a significant increase from loading to 5-year follow-up. At 5-year follow-up, the overall SBI was 0.32 ± 0.49, reflective of no bleeding given that 0 equals no bleeding and 1 equals isolated bleeding spots visible [27]. The PPD initially decreased within the first 6 months from which point it significantly increased to 2.34 ± 1.18 mm at 5-year follow-up. Nevertheless, the measured mean PPD still reflects the norm for conventionally placed implants, which at 2–4 mm is indicative of healthy tissues [35]. The same trend was observed for the Jemt papilla score [28], which significantly increased from loading to 5-year follow-up (2.14 ± 0.95). The ideal papilla score of 3 [28]corresponds to the optimal soft tissue contours; thus, the scores achieved in our study are close to the ideal. Although we observed some significant differences in these parameters between the platform-switching and platform-matching subgroups at 5 years, these are not clinically significant.

Our study should be particularly noted for its ability to recall patients for follow-up appointments. Patient attendance at follow-up appointments in trials performed in private practice can be troublesome [4, 6–8], and the inability to obtain full data from all patients at the later stages of a study may limit the interpretation of the final results. We obtained data for the 70% of patients completing the study at 5 years; this minimizes the limitations in the interpretation of results seen in comparable studies [5–8]. Although this study was performed in private practice, the investigators are very experienced in implantology and of good standing and understand the importance of follow-up and maintenance of good oral health. We observed a maximum of only five patients with poor oral hygiene at any given time (data not shown); additionally, the three late implant failures were in two patients with peri-implantitis or poor hygiene. The appearance of poorer oral hygiene later in the study also appears to correspond with the drop in follow-up attendance, which again supports the importance of follow-up. All other complications could be resolved and were not persisting. Furthermore, patients selected for inclusion in this study were optimal candidates for dental implants. Though the inclusion criteria predestinate the patient selection to some extent, the clinician's expertise likely influences selection of a "good" patient. The patients included in our study had good overall health; American Society of Anesthesiologists (ASA) scores of 1 were observed for 85.6% of patients, and 74% of patients had never smoked.

A limitation of this study was the imbalance in the use of platform-matching and platform-switching abutments. Platform-switching abutments are relatively new, and in practice, the "newer" method (platform switching) was likely chosen over the conventional method. Platform-switching implants have been shown to have better outcomes with regards to bone level changes, but overall patient satisfaction does not differ between the two types [23], also supported by the results of our study. Another limitation may be the non-homogeneous study population. There were no exclusion criteria apart from the standard contraindications for an implant treatment, and the patients descend from the standard pool of private practices. Nevertheless, the success and survival rates were very high and were comparable with clinical data obtained in well-controlled clinical trials with multiple inclusion and exclusion criteria.

Within the limitations of this study, we conclude that the CAMLOG SCREW-LINE implants placed with both platform-matching and platform-switching abutments in patients in a private practice setting seem to achieve clinical outcomes comparable with those achieved in controlled clinical trials. The crestal bone changes over a 5-year period were mainly limited to < 1 mm and could be interpreted as proper peri-implant tissue stability. We also draw attention to the importance of patient education and regular follow-up on clinical outcomes. The patients in our study were highly satisfied with their implants, soft tissue parameters were excellent, and bone level changes were minimal, leading to good overall success and survival of the implants.

Abbreviations

ASA: American Society of Anesthesiologists; MPI: Modified Plaque Index; PPD: Pocket probing depth; RCT: Randomized controlled clinical trial; SBI: Sulcus Bleeding Index; SD: Standard deviation; SLA: Sand-blasted, large grit, acid-etched

Acknowledgements

The authors thank Lyndsey Kostadinov BSc of Medicalwriters.com (Zurich, Switzerland) for providing medical writing support (writing and editing the manuscript) funded by OR Foundation (Basel, Switzerland). Thomas Barth, Christian Hammächer, Manfred Wolf, Juan Manuel Vadillo, Fernando Loscos Morató, Gert de Lange, and Chris van Lith and their practices were involved in the study in treating study patients and collecting study data.

Funding

The study was funded by an unrestricted grant of the Oral Reconstruction Foundation (former Camlog Foundation; ref. FTCAM 01/08).

Authors' contributions
SMB, CC, KD, DH, HH, GI, GK, MS, PS, AS, and KLA and their practices were involved in the study in treating study patients, collecting study data, discussing the results, and commenting on the manuscript. All authors read and approved the final manuscript.

Competing interests
All authors declare no specific conflict of interest regarding this study. The study centers of all authors received an unrestricted grant from the Oral Reconstruction Foundation. The following authors declare that they have received personal fees for lecturing from Camlog: SMB, CC, DH, GI, MS, PS, AS, and KLA.

Author details
[1]Private practice, Baden-Baden, Germany. [2]Private practice, Munich, Germany. [3]Private practice, Istanbul, Turkey. [4]Private practice, Berlin, Germany. [5]Private practice, Strass in Steiermark, Austria. [6]Private practice, Memmingen, Germany. [7]Department Oral and Maxillofacial Surgery/Plastic Surgery, University Hospital Freiburg, Center for Dental Medicine, Freiburg, Germany. [8]Private practice, Marchtrenk, Austria. [9]Private practice, Forchheim, Germany. [10]Department of Maxillofacial Surgery, Goethe University Frankfurt, Frankfurt, Germany. [11]Private practice, Amstelveen, Netherlands. [12]Private practice, Constance, Germany. [13]Private practice, Filderstadt, Germany.

References
1. Hjalmarsson L, Gheisarifar M, Jemt T. A systematic review of survival of single implants as presented in longitudinal studies with a follow-up of at least 10 years. Eur J Oral Implantol. 2016;9(Suppl 1):S155–62.
2. Jung RE, Zembic A, Pjetursson BE, Zwahlen M, Thoma DS. Systematic review of the survival rate and the incidence of biological, technical, and aesthetic complications of single crowns on implants reported in longitudinal studies with a mean follow-up of 5 years. Clin Oral Implants Res. 2012;23(Suppl 6):2–21.
3. Pjetursson BE, Thoma D, Jung R, Zwahlen M, Zembic A. A systematic review of the survival and complication rates of implant-supported fixed dental prostheses (FDPs) after a mean observation period of at least 5 years. Clin Oral Implants Res. 2012;23(Suppl 6):22–38.
4. Wallkamm B, Ciocco M, Ettlin D, Syfrig B, Abbott W, Listrom R, Levin BP, Rosen PS. Three-year outcomes of Straumann Bone Level SLActive dental implants in daily dental practice: a prospective non-interventional study. Quintessence Int. 2015;46:591–602.
5. Cochran D, Oates T, Morton D, Jones A, Buser D, Peters F. Clinical field trial examining an implant with a sand-blasted, acid-etched surface. J Periodontol. 2007;78:974–82.
6. Palmer RM, Smith BJ, Palmer PJ, Floyd PD. A prospective study of Astra single tooth implants. Clin Oral Implants Res. 1997;8:173–9.
7. Vermylen K, Collaert B, Linden U, Bjorn AL, De Bruyn H. Patient satisfaction and quality of single-tooth restorations. Clin Oral Implants Res. 2003;14:119–24.
8. Wilson TG Jr, Roccuzzo M, Ucer C, Beagle JR. Immediate placement of tapered effect (TE) implants: 5-year results of a prospective, multicenter study. Int J Oral Maxillofac Implants. 2013;28:261–9.
9. Franchini I, Capelli M, Fumagalli L, Parenti A, Testori T. Multicenter retrospective analysis of 201 consecutively placed camlog dental implants. Int J Periodontics Restorative Dent. 2011;31:255–63.
10. Nelson K, Semper W, Hildebrand D, Ozyuvaci H. A retrospective analysis of sandblasted, acid-etched implants with reduced healing times with an observation period of up to 5 years. Int J Oral Maxillofac Implants. 2008;23:726–32.
11. Krennmair G, Krainhöfner M, Piehslinger E. Retrospektive Vergleichsstudie zu implantatgetragenen Oberkieferdeckprothesen auf gefrästen Stegen. Frontaler Extensionssteg oder Seitenstege. Implantologie. 2008;16(3):287–98.
12. Semper W, Heberer S, Nelson K. Early loading of root form and conical implants with a sandblasted large-grit acid-etched surface: a 6-year clinical follow-up. Implants. 2008;2:14–19.
13. Vanlioglu B, Özkan Y, Kulak-Özkan Y. Clinical and radiographic outcome of Camlog implants in partially edentulous cases after an observation period of 10 years. Int Poster J Dent Oral Med. 2014;16:Poster 800.

14. Al-Nsour MM, Chan HL, Wang HL. Effect of the platform-switching technique on preservation of peri-implant marginal bone: a systematic review. Int J Oral Maxillofac Implants. 2012;27:138–45.
15. Becker J, Ferrari D, Mihatovic I, Sahm N, Schaer A, Schwarz F. Stability of crestal bone level at platform-switched non-submerged titanium implants: a histomorphometrical study in dogs. J Clin Periodontol. 2009;36:532–9.
16. Hsu YT, Lin GH, Wang HL. Effects of platform-switching on peri-implant soft and hard tissue outcomes: a systematic review and meta-analysis. Int J Oral Maxillofac Implants. 2017;32:e9–e24.
17. Moergel M, Rocha S, Messias A, Nicolau P, Guerra F, Wagner W. Radiographic evaluation of conical tapered platform-switched implants in the posterior mandible: 1-year results of a two-center prospective study. Clin Oral Implants Res. 2016;27:686–93.
18. Schwarz F, Alcoforado G, Nelson K, Schaer A, Taylor T, Beuer F, Strietzel FP. Impact of implant-abutment connection, positioning of the machined collar/microgap, and platform switching on crestal bone level changes. Camlog Foundation Consensus Report. Clin Oral Implants Res. 2014;25:1301–3.
19. Schwarz F, Hegewald A, Becker J. Impact of implant-abutment connection and positioning of the machined collar/microgap on crestal bone level changes: a systematic review. Clin Oral Implants Res. 2014;25:417–25.
20. Strietzel FP, Neumann K, Hertel M. Impact of platform switching on marginal peri-implant bone-level changes. A systematic review and meta-analysis. Clin Oral Implants Res. 2015;26:342–58.
21. Guerra F, Wagner W, Wiltfang J, Rocha S, Moergel M, Behrens E, Nicolau P. Platform switch versus platform match in the posterior mandible - 1-year results of a multicentre randomized clinical trial. J Clin Periodontol. 2014;41:521–9.
22. Molina A, Sanz-Sanchez I, Martin C, Blanco J, Sanz M. The effect of one-time abutment placement on interproximal bone levels and peri-implant soft tissues: a prospective randomized clinical trial. Clin Oral Implants Res. 2017;28:443–52.
23. Rocha S, Wagner W, Wiltfang J, Nicolau P, Moergel M, Messias A, Behrens E, Guerra F. Effect of platform switching on crestal bone levels around implants in the posterior mandible: 3 years results from a multicentre randomized clinical trial. J Clin Periodontol. 2016;43:374–82.
24. von Elm E, Altman DG, Egger M, Pocock SJ, Gotzsche PC, Vandenbroucke JP. The Strengthening the Reporting of Observational Studies in Epidemiology (STROBE) statement: guidelines for reporting observational studies. J Clin Epidemiol. 2008;61:344–9.
25. Lekholm U, Zarb G. Patient selection and preparation. In: GA BPZ, Albrektsson T, editors. Tissue integrated prostheses: osseointegration in clinical dentistry. Chicago: Quintessence Publishing Company; 1985. p. 199–209.
26. Misch CE. Density of bone: effect on treatment plans, surgical approach, healing, and progressive boen loading. Int J Oral Implantol. 1990;6:23–31.
27. Mombelli A, van Oosten MA, Schurch E Jr, Land NP. The microbiota associated with successful or failing osseointegrated titanium implants. Oral Microbiol Immunol. 1987;2:145–51.
28. Jemt T. Regeneration of gingival papillae after single-implant treatment. Int J Periodontics Restorative Dent. 1997;17:326–33.
29. Buser D, Ingimarsson S, Dula K, Lussi A, Hirt HP, Belser UC. Long-term stability of osseointegrated implants in augmented bone: a 5-year prospective study in partially edentulous patients. Int J Periodontics Restorative Dent. 2002;22:109–17.
30. Albrektsson T, Zarb G, Worthington P, Eriksson AR. The long-term efficacy of currently used dental implants: a review and proposed criteria of success. Int J Oral Maxillofac Implants. 1986;1:11–25.
31. Geraets W, Zhang L, Liu Y, Wismeijer D. Annual bone loss and success rates of dental implants based on radiographic measurements. Dentomaxillofac Radiol. 2014;43:20140007.
32. Papaspyridakos P, Chen CJ, Singh M, Weber HP, Gallucci GO. Success criteria in implant dentistry: a systematic review. J Dent Res. 2012;91:242–8.
33. Linkevicius T, Apse P, Grybauskas S, Puisys A. Influence of thin mucosal tissues on crestal bone stability around implants with platform switching: a 1-year pilot study. J Oral Maxillofac Surg. 2010;68:2272–7.
34. Linkevicius T, Puisys A, Steigmann M, Vindasiute E, Linkeviciene L. Influence of vertical soft tissue thickness on crestal bone changes around implants with platform switching: a comparative clinical study. Clin Implant Dent Relat Res. 2015;17:1228–36.
35. Lang NP, Berglundh T, Heitz-Mayfield LJ, Pjetursson BE, Salvi GE, Sanz M. Consensus statements and recommended clinical procedures regarding implant survival and complications. Int J Oral Maxillofac Implants. 2004;19(Suppl):150–4.

6

Reusing dental implants?: an experimental study for detecting the success rates of re-osseointegration

Murat Ulu[1*], Erdem Kılıç[2], Emrah Soylu[3*] (iD), Mehmet Kürkçü[4] and Alper Alkan[2]

Abstract

Background: The aim of this study was to histomorphometrically compare the implant-host integration between retrieved implants and new implants.

Methods: Jaws in 10 male beagle dogs were divided into four groups, and 36 dental implants were inserted into the jaws. In groups 1 and 2, experimental peri-implantitis was induced within 2 months after implant insertion. In group 1, surface decontamination of implants was achieved using air-flow and citric acid. In group 2, implants were sterilized with autoclave after air-flow and citric acid surface decontamination. Subsequently, these implants were inserted in contralateral jaws of the same dogs and a 3-month period was allowed for osseointegration. In group 3, the implants were removed from human jaws due to peri-implantitis and were inserted into dog jaws following surface cleaning protocol and sterilization with autoclave and a 3-month period was allowed for osseointegration. Group 4 was set as the control group. After the osseointegration period, all the animals were sacrificed. The degree of osseointegration in all groups was evaluated by evaluating the ISQ values and by using histomorphometric measurements.

Results: Histological findings showed that bone-implant contact (BIC) percentage (mean ± SD) was 83.39% ± 6.37 in group 1, 79.93% ± 11.83 in group 2, 75.45% ± 9.09 in group 3, and 80.53 ± 5.22 in group 4. Moreover, the resonance frequency analysis (RFA) and ISQ values were similar in all four groups both before and after the implantation.

Conclusions: The results of this experimental study indicated that there is no significant difference between new dental implants and re-used dental implants with regards to osseointegration around the implant.

Keywords: Dental implant, Osseointegration, Peri-implantitis, Surface characteristics

Background

Branemark et al. conducted the first experimental trial with titanium dental implants and created a new vision by defining the term "osseointegration" in the 1960s [1]. Despite the advances in implant technology and protocols and the accumulating evidence in the literature, implant failure/loss may still occur due to several reasons [2]. On the other hand, although dental implant therapy is a successful treatment option for edentulous patients, it may lead to undesired complications after the insertion of the implant such as implant mobility, radiolucency around the implant, and inflammation of peri-implant tissues, or subjective complaints from the patients [3]. Peri-implantitis is a major complication of implant treatment characterized by inflammation of the soft tissues surrounding implants combined with loss of bone [4]. If this complication is not treated appropriately, implant retrieval may be necessary. On the other hand, the primary reasons for an unsuccessful implant treatment include anatomical complexity, inexperience of the surgeon, poor oral hygiene, and smoking [5].

The most undesired complication in implant therapy is peri-implantitis which leads to retrieval of a dental implant. Similar to gingivitis and periodontitis, the main etiologic factor for peri-implant mucositis and peri-implantitis

---

* Correspondence: muratulu81@hotmail.com; dtemrahsoylu@hotmail.com
[1]Faculty of Dentistry, Oral and Maxillofacial Department, İzmir Katip Celebi University, İzmir, Turkey
[3]Faculty of Dentistry, Oral and Maxillofacial Department, Erciyes University, Kayseri, Turkey

is microbial dental plaque. Once an implant is inserted, bacterial colonization begins to occur on its surface [6]. The primary goal in nonsurgical treatment of peri-implant mucositis and peri-implantitis is to eliminate or reduce the bacteria levels in the peri-implant area and, ultimately, to re-establish a clinically healthy environment. However, with conventional treatment modalities, it is often difficult to eradicate microorganisms from threads and rough surfaces [7]. Instead, a number of techniques including laser treatment, air abrasion, citric acid application and conventional mechanical therapy have been used in peri--implantitis therapy. Nevertheless, despite the use of different techniques, complete elimination of pathogens around the implants may not always be possible. In particular, adequate decontamination may not be achieved due to the difficulty of attaining sufficient access to all the dental implant surfaces.

In the present study, a novel approach for peri-implantitis treatment is described, in which the infected implants are removed and the surface treatment is performed extra-orally due to the difficulty of implant surface decontamination inside the bone, and the implants are inserted into the bone for a second time after decontamination.

The aim of this study was to evaluate the implant-bone integration after the removal of an infected implant from the bone and to compare the success rate of this approach with that of new implants by using resonance frequency analysis and histomorphometry.

Methods

Research design

This in vivo study had a comparative, randomized, prospective research design, and each group consisted of 10 male beagle dogs that were veterinarian-controlled, healthy, and of similar weight. Animal Research Reporting in Vivo Experiment (ARRIVE) guidelines were used, and surgical procedure was approved by the Local Animal Experiments Ethical Committee of Erciyes University. Adequate measures were taken to minimize the pain or discomfort in the animals. A total of 36 dental implants (tissue level, 3.3 × 10 mm, Straumann AG, Basel, Switzerland) were inserted in the animals according to the non-submerged healing protocol. Figure 1 presents the flowchart of the research design employed in the study.

Sedation, anesthesia, animal care, and sacrifice

All the interventions were performed under general anesthesia. Enteral nutrition was stopped 12 h before the surgical procedure. General anesthesia was achieved with 2 mg/kg xylazine hydrochloride (i.m.) (Rompun, Bayer, Istanbul, Turkey) and 5 mg/kg ketamine hydrochloride (i.m.) (Alfamyne, Egevet, Izmir, Turkey). After

the surgery, a 3-day antibiotic therapy with Streptomycin 0.5 g/day (I.E. Ulagay, Istanbul, Turkey) was administered in each dog. Postoperative care included daily observations regarding appetite and the documentation of adverse events such as bleeding, pain, swelling, and discomfort. At the end of the experiment, all the animals were sacrificed with a large dose of pentobarbital (i.v.). The animals in groups 3 and 4 were sacrificed at month 6 and the animals in groups 1 and 2 were sacrificed at month 8 after the extraction surgery.

Surgical procedure

The surgical procedure was commenced by the extraction of the mandibular second, third, fourth pre-molars, and the first molar bilaterally. The pupillary reflex was controlled after the administration of anesthetic drugs. Peri- and intra-oral tissues were disinfected with 10% povidone-iodine solution, and the surgical area was covered with sterile covering. Infiltration anesthesia with 2% articaine (Ultracaine DS, Sanofi Aventis Drugs, Istanbul, Turkey) was applied to the premolar area for hemostasis and for post-operative pain control. A full-thickness vestibular flap was elevated gently, and surgical tooth extraction was performed using surgical burs with straight elevators. Surgical wounds were closed with 3/0 vicryl sutures and streptomycin 0.5 g/day was administered for 3 days postoperatively. After the extraction, a 3-month period was allowed for healing of the alveolar bone and soft tissue (Fig. 2).

After the 3 month healing period, a second surgery was performed for implant insertion. Pre-surgical procedures were the same as those described above. In addition, a horizontal incision was made along the edentulous premolar area. A mucoperiosteal flap was gently elevated to expose the recipient bone and the implant sockets were prepared using a commercially available surgical set (Straumann® instruments, Straumann AG, Waldenburg, Sweden) under sterile saline irrigation. All the implants had a sandblasted and acid-etched (SLA) surface and were of the same size and length (3.3 × 10 mm, tissue level). All implants were inserted to the level of the machined surface left below the bone. Non-submerged healing protocol was performed in all the groups and the flaps were closed with 3/0 vicryl sutures.

In group 1, after the insertion of the implants, 3/0 silk sutures (Doğsan, Trabzon, Turkey) were placed below the free gingival/mucosal margin around the implants and plaque control was terminated for 2 months (Fig. 3). To promote plaque retention and peri-implantitis, the animals were fed a soft diet. The implants were removed with reverse torque after the induction of peri-implantitis (Fig. 4). After the removal, all the implant surfaces were cleaned by air-flow with bi-carbonate granules for 1 min prior to the treatment with citric acid

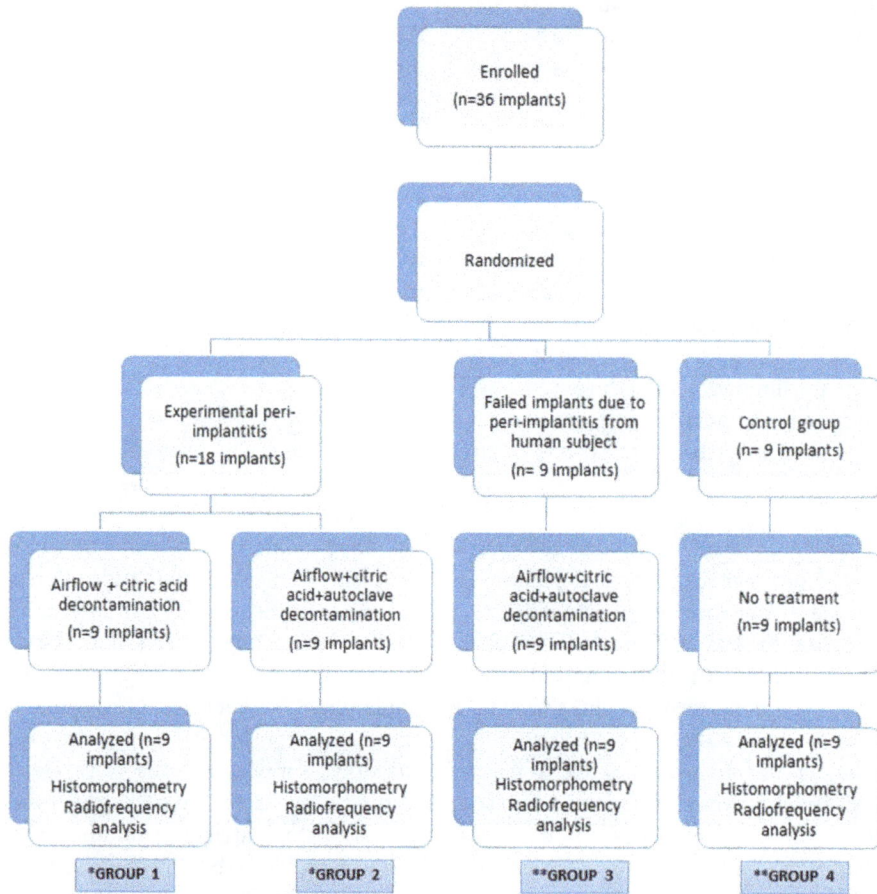

Fig. 1 Flowchart of the research design employed in the study. *Three dogs were used in each group 1 and 2. Three implants were inserted right side of the mandibles. After peri-implantitis period, extracted implants were inserted into the left side of the mandibles. **Two dogs were used in each group 3 and 4. Six failed implants from human inserted into the one dog's mandible bilaterally and three implants inserted into the other dog's mandible unilaterally in group 3. Six implants inserted into the one dog's mandible bilaterally and three implants inserted into the other dog's mandible unilaterally in group 4 (control group)

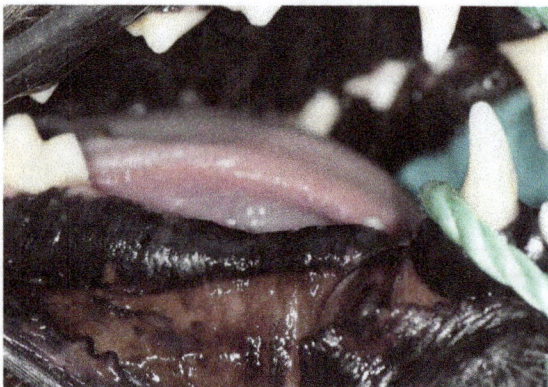

Fig. 2 Edentulous posterior mandible of the dog at 3 months after tooth extraction

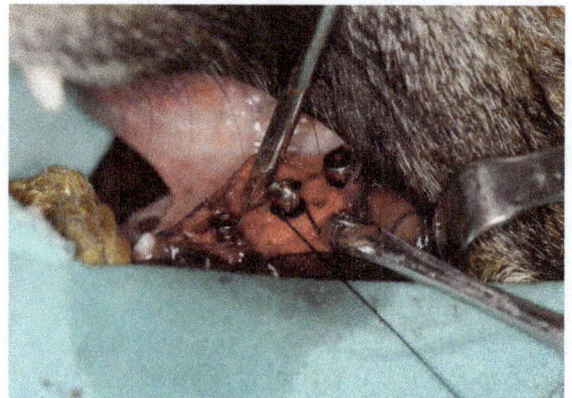

Fig. 3 Silk ligatures placed in a submarginal position around the implants

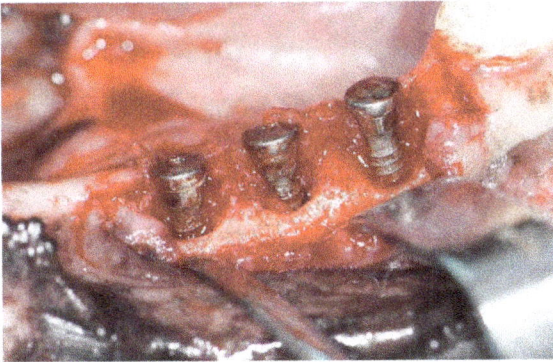

Fig. 4 A 2-month period was allowed for plaque retention and peri-implantitis

(pH: 1). Subsequently, the implant surfaces were rinsed with sterile saline solution and then all the implants were inserted in the contralateral side of the mandible of the same dog. After a 3-month osseointegration period, the animals were sacrificed with a high dose of pentobarbital (i.v.).

In group 2, the same procedures were applied as in group 1. However, unlike the implants in group 1, the implants in group 2 were sterilized by autoclave treatment at 121 °C for 30 min. Afterwards, the sterilized implants were inserted in the contralateral side of the mandible of the same dog from which the implants were retrieved. After a 3-month osseointegration period, the animals were sacrificed with a high dose of pentobarbital (i.v.).

In group 3, failed implants due to peri-implantitis were obtained from human subjects. The surface of the implants were cleaned and sterilized with autoclave and then the implants were inserted into the mandibles of the dogs. After a 3-month osseointegration period, the animals were sacrificed with a large dose of pentobarbital (i.v.).

In group 4 (control group), no implant insertion was performed and after a 3-month osseointegration period, the animals were sacrificed with a large dose of pentobarbital (i.v.). The preparation times, surgeries, and observation time points of all four groups were summarized on the time arrow (Fig. 5).

Experimental design

Resonance frequency analysis (RFA) measurements

Implant stability was measured using resonance frequency analysis (RFA) with an Osstell® device (Osstell AB, Goteborg, Sweden). All implants were placed with non-submerged healing protocol and the Osstell® sensor was positioned perpendicular to the long axis of the implant in accordance with the guidelines provided by the manufacturer. The results were calculated in the form of objective ISQ values (ranging from 1 to 100). The RFA measurements were performed from four different directions (mesial, distal, lingual, and vestibule), and the mean ISQ was recorded as the final value.

Removal and preparation of the implant-bone specimens

The implants with a neighboring bone were removed en bloc, and the adhesive soft tissues were dissected to investigate the healing status and the bone-implant contact (BIC) percentage. The specimens were fixed in 10% neutral buffered formalin for 48 h and dehydrated in subsequent concentrations of 70–99.9% ethanol. After dehydration, the specimens were embedded in methyl methacrylate (Technovit 7200 VLC, Heraeus Kulzer GmbH & Co. KG, Wehrheim, Germany) without decalcification. 200-μm-thick slides were cut from the blocks using a band saw (Exakt 300 CL, Exakt Apparatebau, Norderstad, Germany).

Histologic and histomorphometric analysis

The 50-μm-thick final histological slides were prepared by grinding with 320–4000 grit sandpapers (Hermes Schleifmittel GmbH & Co. KG, Hamburg, Germany). The final sections were mounted and stained with toluidine blue for histologic and histomorphometric analysis. In order to measure the BIC percentage, digital images of the sections were obtained by a digital camera (Olympus DP 70, Olympus, Tokyo, Japan) attached to a microscope (Olympus BX50). The obtained images were transferred to a computer and were histomorphometrically analyzed using ImageJ analysis software (ImageJ, National Institutes of Health, Bethesda, Maryland, USA) (Fig. 6). The BIC percentage was calculated by an experienced researcher blinded to the study protocol.

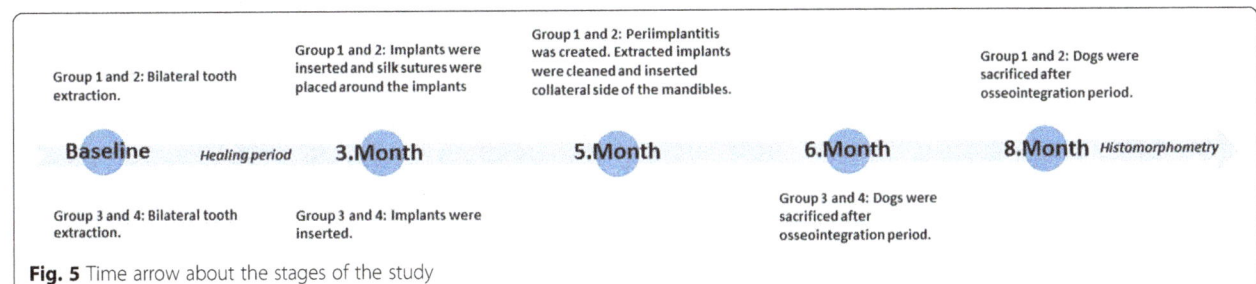

Group 1 and 2: Bilateral tooth extraction.	Group 1 and 2: Implants were inserted and silk sutures were placed around the implants	Group 1 and 2: Perimplantitis was created. Extracted implants were cleaned and inserted collateral side of the mandibles.		Group 1 and 2: Dogs were sacrificed after osseointegration period.
Baseline *Healing period*	**3.Month**	**5.Month**	**6.Month**	**8.Month** *Histomorphometry*
Group 3 and 4: Bilateral tooth extraction.	Group 3 and 4: Implants were inserted.		Group 3 and 4: Dogs were sacrificed after osseointegration period.	

Fig. 5 Time arrow about the stages of the study

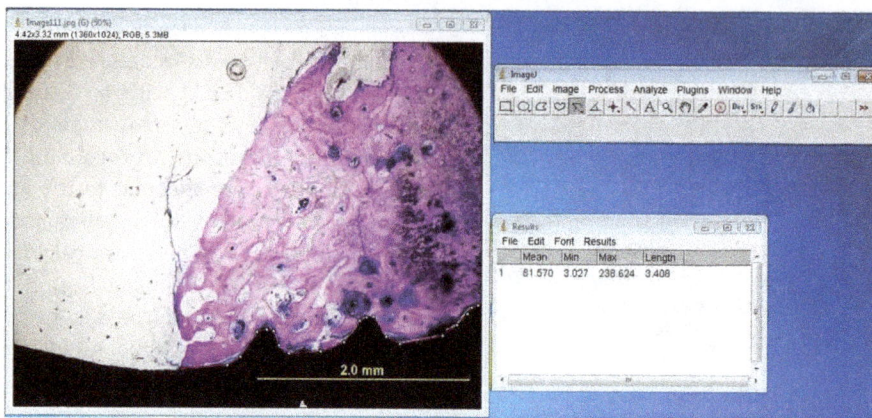

Fig. 6 BIC percentage measured with ImageJ analysis software

Statistical analysis

Statistical analyses were performed using SPSS v.20.0 (IBM, Chicago, IL, USA). The Shapiro-Wilks normality test was used to verify the normality of the data. All variables were normally distributed and thus parametric tests were used for intra-group (paired sample t test) and inter-group (one-way ANOVA/ Tukey's test) comparisons. A p value of < 0.05 was considered significant.

Results

The experimental period and the laboratory workup of the study were unremarkable. Surgical operations were uneventful and the post-operative healing periods were completed with no complications. Histologic analysis and the ISQ values indicated that osseointegration was achieved in all the implants.

Histomorphometric analysis

Histomorphometric analysis demonstrated that adequate bone formation in neighboring tissues was achieved in all four groups. In the histomorphometric analysis of the sections, the highest BIC percentage was seen in group 1 (83.39 ± 6.37) and the lowest BIC percentage was seen in group 3 (75.45 ± 9.09). However, no significant difference was found among the groups and all four groups were statistically similar with regards to BIC percentage. Tables 1 and 2 presents the histomorphometric measurements of the groups.

RFA measurements

Table 3 presents the RFA measurements of the groups. In all four groups, the RFA measurements were performed after the insertion and before the removal of the implants. The highest RFA values after the insertion were observed in groups 3 (71.77 ± 5.71) and 4 (70.44 ± 5.15), whereas the highest RFA values before the insertion were observed in groups 2 (79.44 ± 2.55) and 4 (79.12 ± 4.61). No significant difference was established between the groups. Nevertheless, the only significant difference between the initial and final ISQ values was found in group 2.

Discussion

Approximately two million new dental implants are inserted per year around the world and tens of millions of implants are still in use. Moreover, it is estimated that approximately 200,000–250,000 implants are removed every year [8]. Peri-implantitis is the major cause of the implant retrieval and also the most common complication caused by implant surgery. Mombelli et al. reported that plaque formation can occur on dental implant surfaces similar to that of tooth surfaces [9].

The mainstay treatment for peri-implantitis includes the elimination of etiologic factors and the mechanical removal of calculus, cement, and plaque followed by subgingival irrigation with tetracycline and chlorhexidine base mouthwash. Lang et al. first described a treatment protocol for peri-implantitis including mechanical cleaning, decontamination of the implant surface, antibiotic regimen, and regenerative surgery (if required) in 1997 [10]. However, literate indicates that the use of air-

Table 1 Comparison of BIC percentages of over the entire implant length at 3-month follow-up

Group 1 [Mean ± SD]	Group 2 [Mean ± SD]	Group3 [Mean ± SD]	Group 4 [Mean± SD]	p
83.39 ± 6.37	79.93 ± 11.83	75.45 ± 9.09	80.53 ± 5.22	290[*]

*Statistically not significant

Table 2 Comparison of BIC percentages of 3 mm crestal area of the implants at 3-month follow-up

Group 1 [Mean ± SD]	Group 2 [Mean ± SD]	Group3 [Mean ± SD]	Group 4 [Mean ± SD]	p
77.67 ± 5.03	75.28 ± 10.65	71.86 ± 8.34	80.63 ± 5.58	.144[*]

*Statistically not significant

Table 3 Inter- and intra-group ISQ analysis and measurements on day of surgery and at 3-month follow-up

	Mean ± SD ISQ day 0	Mean ± SD ISQ at 3 month	p
Group 1	69.33 ± 8.48	77.77 ± 1.78	.019
Group 2	68.88 ± 5.90	79.44 ± 2.55	.001*
Group 3	71.77 ± 5.71	75.11 ± 5.84	.366
Group 4	70.44 ± 5.15	79.12 ± 4.61	.022
p	.782	.115	

*Statistically significant

powder abrasive (APA) treatment for the decontamination of the implant surface remains controversial. Although some reports advocate that the in vivo usage of APA systems pose a potential risk of emphysema and may have limited clinical applications [11, 12], some other studies, such as the study reported by Duarte et al. found that APA is more effective in the decontamination of dental implants than lasers, metal curettes, and plastic curettes [13]. On the other hand, Renvert et al. compared the use of APA and Er:YAG laser application on dental implant surfaces and found that the two methods produced similar outcomes with regards to the decontamination of implant surfaces. In the present study, we used a combination of APA and citric acid for the decontamination of the surfaces of the retrieved implants, mainly because both methods are easily available, have minimal cost, and are easy to use when compared to laser treatment [14].

Another controversy reported in the literature is concerned with the re-healing process around the contaminated implant surface. Although some studies contend that re-healing is possible around the dental implants affected by peri-implantitis depending on the implant surface treatment modalities employed prior to re-insertion [15, 16], some other studies, such as the study reported by Persson et al. showed that they did not detect any re-osseointegration around the contaminated non-modified surface of the dental implants after the treatment of the implant surfaces affected by peri-implantitis [17]. On the other hand, Hürzeler et al. detected re-osseointegration with guided bone regeneration [18], Persson et al. found re-osseointegration in 84% of SLA implants [19], and Alhag et al. showed re-osseointegration on plaque-covered implant surfaces after the removal of the plaque by means of citric acid, tooth brush, and hydrogen peroxide [20].

Levin et al. conducted a similar study and investigated the success rate of retrieved dental implants that were re-implanted into dogs. The infected implants were re-implanted into dog jaws without any chemical or mechanical cleaning and the authors reported that there was no difference in terms of BIC percentage between the infected/reinserted and new dental implants after an appropriate healing period [21]. In our study, the experimental groups were formed in line with the literature; in group 1, a highly effective decontamination method (APA and citric acid) was used [22], whereas in groups 2 and 3, autoclave sterilization was used for the decontamination of implant surfaces since autoclave is the most common method for the sterilization of surgical instruments and is widely used in dental implant laboratory studies [23]. After the experiment, it was revealed that autoclave sterilization does not interfere with osseointegration, which implicates that autoclave sterilization is a useful method to be used in re-implantation procedures.

The main purpose of the current study was to evaluate the degree of osseointegration in the dental implants inserted for a second time following the treatment of the implant surfaces with peri-implantitis therapy. Unlike other peri-implantitis therapy approaches, the approach developed in this experiment allowed all the treatment procedures to be performed outside the mouth, thereby enabling the decontamination methods to be applied easily and uniformly to all the regions of the implants in a more standardized manner than would be possible intra-orally.

Conclusions

In conclusion, the results of this study indicated that there was no significant difference in the BIC percentages and the RFA measures between the implants retrieved due to peri-implantitis and re-implanted in the dog jaws and the new dental implants inserted for the first time. Moreover, the results also suggested that a dental implant retrieved due to peri-implantitis may be re-used in the same patient after decontamination of the implant surface. Nevertheless, despite the encouraging findings presented by this study, further studies including a larger number of implants are needed to substantiate the findings of our study.

Abbreviations
APA: Air powder abrasive; ARRIVE: Animal Research Reporting in Vivo Experiment; BIC: Bone-implant contact; IM: Intramuscular; IV: Intravenous; RFA: Resonance frequency analysis; SLA: Sandblasted and acid-etched

Funding
The Scientific and Technological Research Council of Turkey - Health Sciences Research Group (TUBITAK-SBAG) (Project Number: 109S346).

Availability of data and materials
In terms of the agreement between the authors and the funding source (The Scientific and Technological Research Council of Turkey - Health Sciences Research Group (TUBITAK-SBAG), sharing the data is forbidden. Hence, we cannot share the data.

Authors' contributions
Asst. Prof. Dr. MU and Asst. Prof. Dr. ES contributed in this study with the following processes: study design, Surgical operations of the animals, animal follow-up, data collection and analysis of the results, article drafting and proofreading, and approval of the article. Assoc. Prof. Dr. EK and Prof. Dr. AA are the mentors of this study and also contributed in this study with the

following processes: study design, surgical operations of the animals, analysis of the results, article drafting and proofreading, approval of the article. Prof. Dr. MK contributed in this study with the following processes: preparation of the histological samples, histological and histomorphometric analysis of the samples. All authors read and approved the final manuscript.

Competing interests

Murat Ulu, Erdem Kılıç, Emrah Soylu, Mehmet Kürkçü, and Alper Alkan declare that they have no competing interests.

Author details

[1]Faculty of Dentistry, Oral and Maxillofacial Department, İzmir Katip Celebi University, İzmir, Turkey. [2]Faculty of Dentistry, Oral and Maxillofacial Department, Bezmialem University, İstanbul, Turkey. [3]Faculty of Dentistry, Oral and Maxillofacial Department, Erciyes University, Kayseri, Turkey. [4]Faculty of Dentistry, Oral and Maxillofacial Department, Cukurova University, Adana, Turkey.

References

1. Branemark PI, Hansson BO, Adell R, et al. Osseointegrated implants in the treatment of the edentulous jaw. Experience from a 10-year period. Scand J Plast Reconstr Surg Suppl. 1977;16:1–132.
2. Esposito M, Hirsch JM, Lekholm U, et al. Biological factors contributing to failures of osseointegrated oral implants. (II). Etiopathogenesis. Eur J Oral Sci. 1998;106:721–64.
3. Manzano G, Montero J, Martin-Vallejo J, et al. Risk factors in early implant failure: a meta-analysis. Implant Dent. 2016;25:272–80.
4. Lindhe J, Meyle J, Group D of European Workshop on Periodontology. Peri-implant diseases: consensus report of the sixth European workshop on periodontology. J Clin Periodontol. 2008;35:282–5.
5. Chrcanovic BR, Albrektsson T, Wennerberg A. Reasons for failures of oral implants. J Oral Rehabil. 2014;41:443–76.
6. Salvi GE, Fürst MM, Lang NP, et al. One-year bacterial colonization patterns of Staphylococcus aureus and other bacteria at implants and adjacent teeth. Clin Oral Implan Res. 2008;19:242–8.
7. Lamont RJ, Jenkinson HF. Subgingival colonization by porphyromonas gingivalis. Oral Microbiol Immun. 2000;15:341–9.
8. Machtei EE, Mahler D, Oettinger-Barak O, et al. Dental implants placed in previously failed sites: survival rate and factors affecting the outcome. Clin Oral Implants Res. 2008;19:259–64.
9. Mombelli A, Lang NP. Microbial aspects of implant dentistry. Periodontol. 1994;4:74–80.
10. Lang NP, Mombelli A, Tonetti MS, et al. Clinical trials on therapies for peri-implant infections. Ann Periodontol. 1997;2:343–56.
11. Rasmusson L, Meredith N, Kahnberg KE, et al. Effects of barrier membranes on bone resorption and implant stability in onlay bone grafts. An experimental study. Clin Oral Implants Res. 1999;10:267–77.
12. Glauser R, Sennerby L, Meredith N, et al. Resonance frequency analysis of implants subjected to immediate or early functional occlusal loading. Successful vs. failing implants. Clin Oral Implants Res. 2004;15:428–34.
13. Duarte PM, Reis AF, de Freitas PM, et al. Bacterial adhesion on smooth and rough titanium surfaces after treatment with different instruments. J Periodontol. 2009;80:1824–32.
14. Renvert S, Lindahl C, Roos Jansaker AM, et al. Treatment of peri-implantitis using an Er:YAG laser or an air-abrasive device: a randomized clinical trial. J Clin Periodontol. 2011;38:65–73.
15. You TM, Choi BH, Zhu SJ, et al. Treatment of experimental peri-implantitis using autogenous bone grafts and platelet-enriched fibrin glue in dogs. Oral Surg Oral Med Oral Pathol Oral Radiol Endod. 2007;103:34–7.
16. Shibli JA, Martins MC, Ribeiro FS, et al. Lethal photosensitization and guided bone regeneration in treatment of peri-implantitis: an experimental study in dogs. Clin Oral Implants Res. 2006;17:273–81.
17. Persson LG, Ericsson I, Berglundh T, et al. Osseintegration following treatment of peri-implantitis and replacement of implant components. An experimental study in the dog. J Clin Periodontol. 2001;28:258–63.
18. Hurzeler MB, Quinones CR, Schupback P, et al. Treatment of peri-implantitis using guided bone regeneration and bone grafts, alone or in combination, in beagle dogs. Part 2: histologic findings. Int J Oral Max Impl. 1997;12:168–75.
19. Persson LG, Berglundh T, Lindhe J, et al. Re-osseointegration after treatment of peri-implantitis at different implant surfaces. An experimental study in the dog. Clin Oral Implants Res. 2001;12:595–603.
20. Alhag M, Renvert S, Polyzois I, et al. Re-osseointegration on rough implant surfaces previously coated with bacterial biofilm: an experimental study in the dog. Clin Oral Implants Res. 2008;19:182–7.
21. Levin L, Zigdon H, Coelho PG, et al. Reimplantation of dental implants following ligature-induced peri-implantitis: a pilot study in dogs. Clin Implant Dent Relat Res. 2013;15:1–6.
22. Sanchez-Garces MA, Gay-Escoda C. Periimplantitis. Med Oral Patol Oral Cir Bucal. 2004;9 Suppl:69–74. 63–9
23. Martin JY, Dean DD, Cochran DL, et al. Proliferation, differentiation, and protein synthesis of human osteoblast-like cells (MG63) cultured on previously used titanium surfaces. Clin Oral Implants Res. 1996;7:27–37.

7

A 1–7 year retrospective follow-up on consecutively placed 7-mm-long dental implants with an electrowetted surface

Paul S. Rosen[1,2]* ⓘ, Herman Sahlin[3], Rudolf Seemann[4] and Ari S. Rosen[5]

Abstract

Background: This retrospective consecutive case series study was performed to determinate the survival rate and implant stability of short (7 mm length) dental implants with an electrowetted hydrophilic surface that were in function from 1 to 7 years.

Methods: A retrospective chart review identified and evaluated 86 consecutively placed 7-mm-long dental implants (ProActive, Neoss Ltd., Harrogate, England) in 75 patients. Analysis was performed for implant survival as well as implant stability, as measured by insertion torque (IT) and resonance frequency analysis (RFA).

Results: Clinical follow-ups were performed from 1.0 to 7.0 years after implant placement (mean 4.0 ± 2.1 years). Two implants failed prior to loading resulting in a 5-year cumulative survival rate (CSR) of 97.7%. An additional late failure occurred at 60 months post-loading for a 7-year CSR of 94.8%. Mean insertion torque was 30.1 ± 7.4 Ncm and mean RFA at insertion was 73.6 ± 8.1 ISQ. Follow-up RFA measurements suggested that the achieved primary stability was maintained throughout the healing phase.

Conclusion: The present study demonstrates that treatment with short implants can be a predictable treatment option with high survival rate in sites with limited available bone.

Keywords: Short implants, Cumulative survival rate, Implant stability, Electrowetted surface

Background

In the past decades, the osseointegration rate of dental implants has dramatically increased, particularly in sites of softer dental bone, which may be attributed to the introduction of moderately roughened surfaces [1, 2]. Moreover, because of this increase in success, clinicians have attempted to push the envelope and place implants into sites that may provide a greater challenge as they wish to meet their patients' oral health needs. Short dental implants have been explored in various indications such as close proximity to the inferior alveolar nerve or at an area where there is a highly pneumatized sinus floor to potentially reduce the time associated with the surgery and the prolonged healing period attendant with complex grafting/surgical procedures

that would be needed for placing longer dental implants. Moreover, these grafting procedures may introduce certain post-operative morbidities not seen with standard dental implant placements. Three randomized controlled studies comparing short to longer dental implants that were placed into augmented sites found no significant differences in implant survival between the groups [3–5], suggesting comparable clinical outcomes for short and longer implants up to 3 years after implant surgery. Several systematic reviews/meta-analyses on the use of short implants have also demonstrated similar results [2, 6–8]. Esposito et al. performed a meta-analysis that demonstrated a non-significant trend of more implant failures (OR = 5.74) and more complications (OR = 4.97) in the group of implants placed into vertically augmented sites versus the short dental implant group [6]. Pommer et al. performed a systematic review and found that short implants with a machined surface had a higher early failure rate than longer implants with a machined surface (OR = 2.2) [2]. However, with rougher surfaces, no

* Correspondence: paul@psrperioimplant.com; psr907@gmail.com
[1]Clinical Professor of Periodontics, Baltimore College of Dental Surgery, University of Maryland Dental School, Baltimore, MD, USA
[2]Private Practice limited to Periodontics and Dental Implants, 907 Floral Vale Boulevard, Yardley, PA 19067, USA

difference was seen (OR = 1.1). Another systematic review and meta-analysis comparing short and long implants found that short implants are as predictable as long implants (CSR 88.1 vs. 86.7%), but the failures tend to occur at an earlier time point [8]. A recent systematic review by Lemos et al. found that short implants (8 mm and shorter) were as predictable as standard implants (> 8 mm). However, implants shorter than 8 mm showed lower survival rates than standard implants (RR = 2.05) [7].

The aim of this retrospective consecutive case series study was to investigate implant survival rate and analyze possible factors affecting the survival of short implants placed in one surgical practice focused on implantology and periodontology in a temporal cohort.

Methods

A retrospective study on short 7 mm hydrophilic implants from a single center was conducted in a private practice limited to periodontics and surgical dental implant placements from one of the authors, PSR (Yardley, Pennsylvania, USA). An exhaustive chart review identified 75 patients for analysis that were treated with 86 short (7 mm) implants during a 5-year period (September 1, 2009, to November 1, 2014). The study was performed in compliance with the Declaration of Helsinki. Data collection was performed in such a manner that subjects could not be identified, and therefore, it was exempt from IRB review according to Federal Regulation 45 CFR 46.101(b).

All implants had a hydrophilic electrowetted surface (ProActive™, Neoss Ltd., Harrogate, UK) and were placed according to the manufacturer's instructions using either a one-stage protocol with a transgingival healing abutment or a two-stage submerged healing for 5–8 weeks. Implants were loaded after 2 to 6 months (Figs. 1 and 2).

Postoperative management included the use of amoxicillin 875 mg twice daily for 7 days along with the use of 0.12% chlorhexidine gluconate mouthrinse topically applied twice daily for at least the first 28 days. If the patient was allergic to amoxicillin, then either clindamycin 150 mg taken four times daily for 7 days or azithromycin 500 mg taken on the first day followed by 250 mg per day for the next 4 days was substituted. For pain management, patients used ibuprofen 600–800 mg up to four times per day or acetaminophen with codeine # 3 taken every 4–6 hours if non-steroidal anti-inflammatory agents could not be taken.

Suture removal took place at 14 ± 3 days post-implant insertion. RFA was repeated at varying time points depending upon the data recorded at initial placement. Due to the study design (retrospective analysis of patient records compiled in a private practice setting), standardized annual radiographs were not taken. Timing and frequency of radiographic examination varied depending upon when the patients returned back to the surgeon's clinic and thus did not allow for a systematic analysis as part of the study.

Baseline parameters, both patient- and implant-related, as well as follow-up parameters (implant survival, follow-up time, and resonance frequency analysis) were collected from a review of the patient records.

Statistics

The main study parameters (principal outcome parameters) were defined to be implant loss and follow-up time.

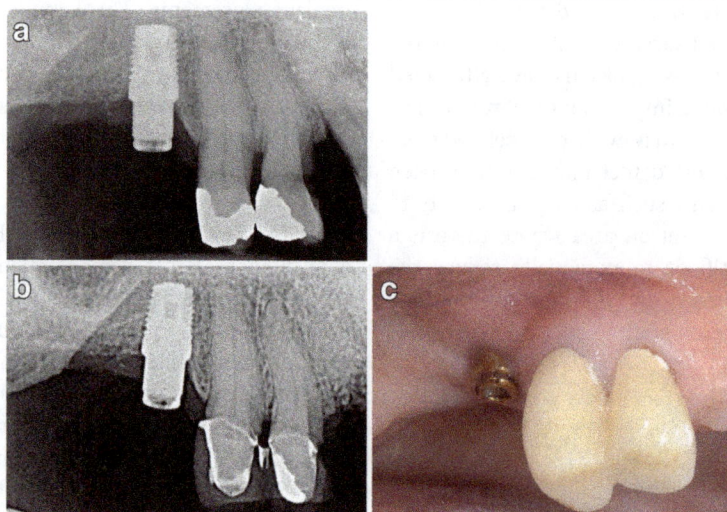

Fig. 1 a Initial radiograph exposed at abutment installation on a 5-mm-wide by 7-mm-length dental implant used to help support a removable partial denture for a 71-year-old Caucasian male. **b** Radiograph of the area taken at 82 months demonstrates good bone stability. **c** Clinical image of the area 82 months later. Soft tissue remains healthy. The two teeth anterior are in the process of receiving a two-unit fixed splint

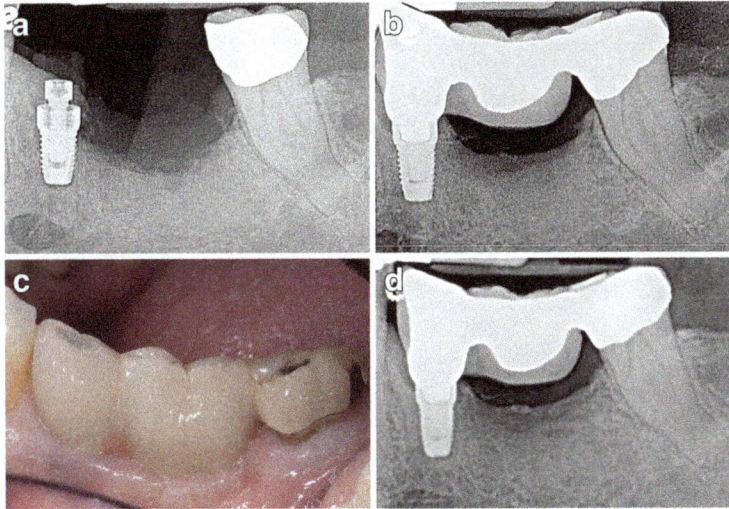

Fig. 2 a Radiographic image of a 3.5-mm-wide by 7-mm-length dental implant at the time of its placement at the mandibular left second premolar in a 63-year-old Caucasian female. **b** Radiographic image of a three-unit fixed partial denture upon its initial placement. The dental implant is the anterior abutment with the prosthesis screw retained to it. The distal abutment is the mandibular left second molar. A coping has been placed in the event of intrusion. **c** Clinical image of the three-unit fixed partial denture at 58 months post-loading. Soft tissue health has been maintained around both the tooth and the dental implant. **d** Radiograph exposed at 58 months demonstrating the steady state of bone on both the dental implant and the natural tooth abutments. There is no suggestion of any intrusion occurring with the mandibular left second molar

The cumulative survival rate was estimated. The influence of several factors on survival was tested in Cox proportional hazard models: age, sex, smoking, diabetes, osteoporosis, jaw, implant position, bone type, implant diameter, insertion torque, RFA at insertion, healing protocol, and prosthetic restoration. In case of continuous variables (age, torque, and RFA), an optimal cutoff value for implant failure prediction was computed based on the Youden's index [9]. Finally, all factors were added to a multivariate Cox proportional hazard model to correct for multiple testing.

Results

The chart review identified 86 placed implants in 75 patients. Table 1 summarizes the patient demographics of the 75 patients. Patients ranged in age from 29 to 88 years with a mean of 61.0 ± 12.5 years. Twenty-seven of the patients were males and 48 were females. Table 2 summarizes the implant and site-related information of the 86 placed implants. Mean insertion torque was 30.1 ± 7.4 Ncm (range 10–50), and mean RFA at the time of implant placements was 73.6 ± 8.1 ISQ (range 35–87).

Of the 86 implants, 84 (97.7%) successfully osseointegrated and were restored. Clinical follow-ups were recorded up to 7.0 years after implant placement with a mean follow-up time of 4.0 ± 2.1 years. There were three (3.5%) failed implants recorded in three (4.0%) different patients. Specifications on the failures are given in Table 3. The implant-based cumulative survival rate was 97.7% after 1 year, 97.7% after 5 years, and 94.8% after 7 years (Table 4).

Subgroup analysis was performed to identify if any factors had an effect on implant survival, i.e., if they were risk factors. The analysis failed to reveal any significant differences between subgroups, i.e., $p > 0.05$ for all tested parameters. Hence, none of the factors were identified as a risk factor. The mean insertion torque was 30.1 ±

Table 1 Patient demographics

		Number	Percent
Age (years)	20–29	1	1.3
	30–39	4	5.3
	40–49	6	8.0
	50–59	19	25.3
	60–69	27	36.0
	70–79	12	16.0
	80–89	6	8.0
Sex	Female	48	64.0
	Male	27	26.0
Smoker	No	69	92.0
	Yes	6	8.0
Diabetes	No	71	94.7
	Yes	4	5.3
Osteoporosis	No	66	88.0
	Osteopenia	5	6.7
	Osteoporosis	4	5.3
Penicillin-VK allergy	No	65	86.7
	Yes	10	13.3

Table 2 Implant and site-related specifications

		Number	Percent
Jaw	Maxilla	60	69.8
	Mandible	26	30.2
Position	Anterior	2	2.3
	Posterior	84	87.7
Implant diameter	3.5 mm	4	4.7
	4.0 mm	14	16.3
	4.5 mm	13	15.1
	5.0 mm	21	24.4
	5.5 mm	32	37.2
	6.0 mm	2	2.3
Site type	Healed site	48	55.8
	Immediate extraction	31	36.0
	Implant replacement	1	1.2
	Sinus	6	7.0
Bone quality (Lekholm/Zarb)	Type 1	4	4.7
	Type 2	54	62.8
	Type 3	26	30.2
	Type 4	2	2.3
Insertion torque (Ncm)	10–19	6	7.0
	20–29	14	16.3
	30–39	59	68.6
	40–49	4	4.7
	50	3	3.5
Implant stability at placement (ISQ)	30–39	1	1.2
	40–49	1	1.2
	50–59	1	1.2
	60–69	17	19.8
	70–79	44	51.2
	80–89	22	25.6
Surgery	One-stage	44	51.2
	Two-stage	42	48.8
Type of restoration	Crown	48	55.8
	Bridge	35	40.7
	Locator	3	3.5

Table 3 Specification of failed implants (three implants in three patients)

Sex	Age	Smoker	Risk factors	Position	Implant diameter	Insert. torque	ISQ at insert.	Time of failure
Male	75	No	Diabetes	Maxillary premolar	5.5 mm	20	75	0 months
Male	73	No	No	Maxillary premolar	4.5 mm	32	80	60 months
Female	77	No	Osteoporosis	Mandibular molar	5.0 mm	32	70	0 months

Table 4 Implant survival, life table analysis

Interval	Implants	Failed	Not followed	CSR (%)
Insertion to 1 year	86	2	3	97.7
1 to 2 years	81	0	19	97.7
2 to 3 years	62	0	6	97.7
3 to 4 years	56	0	6	97.7
4 to 5 years	50	0	16	97.7
5 to 6 years	34	1	16	94.8
6 to 7 years	17	0	15	94.8
7 years	2	–	–	–

7.5 Ncm in successful implants and 28.0 ± 6.9 Ncm in the three that failed. The mean ISQ value was 73.6 ± 8.2 in the successful implant group and 75.0 ± 5.0 in the failed implants group.

RFA measurements during the healing phase, i.e., up to 16 weeks, are presented in Table 5. The high mean RFA value at insertion (73.6 ± 8.1 ISQ) was well maintained up until 16 weeks, indicating maintained implant stability at a high level throughout the healing period.

Discussion

This retrospective study is the first to look at short dental implants with a hydrophilic electrowetted surface. The survival data suggest that this treatment is a viable option to care. In a systematic review that identified 13 studies on implants shorter than 10 mm, the CSR from the individual studies ranged from 80 to 100% with a combined CSR of 98.3% after 5 years, 94.8% after 6 years, and 88.1% after 14 years [8]. It should be noted that the CSR of the current study is comparable to the combined CSR for the identified 13 studies although the majority (56%) of the reported short implants in the reviews were 8–9 mm, i.e., longer than the implants followed in the current study. Another systematic review that looked only at comparative studies between short and long implants found a combined failure rate of 4.6% (32 of 700) for implants shorter than 8 mm after an average of 1.8 years (range 0.25–5 years) [7]. The present study demonstrated a slightly lower failure rate of 3.5% (3 of 86) after an average of 4.0 years. The cumulative survival rate for the current study (97.7% after 5 years, 94.8% after 7 years) was in the upper end of the range reported in these other studies on

Table 5 Resonance frequency analysis

Time	ISQ	n
Implant insertion	73.6 ± 8.1	86
1–4 weeks	79.4 ± 4.1	28
5–8 weeks	77.3 ± 5.0	34
9–12 weeks	74.9 ± 5.6	20
13–16 weeks	73.3 ± 4.4	11

short implants, indicating treatment outcomes well in line with or even better than the majority of short implant studies reported in the literature. In current scientific literature, a 13.4-year CSR of long implants was reported to be 94.6% [10]. This CSR for standard dental implants is at the same level as the 7-year survival rate for the 7-mm implants in the current study.

Since the treatment protocol is kept simple, it might be preferred by both patients and clinicians to treatments that involve more invasive techniques such as nerve transposition, guided bone regeneration, and sinus elevation procedures. The success of the reported treatment approach might in part be due to the use of implants with a diameter wider than 4 mm (68 of 86 implants). The wider implants were placed into sites with significant lateral bony dimensions to allow for their placement without over-preparing the sites and compromising residual bone width. This helped to maximize the implant surface and hence the implant-bone interface needed for successful osseointegration.

A wide distribution in implant insertion torque (10–50 Ncm) was seen in the study. This reflects the variety of clinical situations in which the implants were placed. Assessments were made by using both the RFA value and the insertion torque as to first whether an implant should have been left to heal in the first place and if so, how this would be best accomplished, i.e., through its submergence with a cover screw or by transgingival exposure with a healing abutment.

The study aimed at identifying factors affecting survival of 7-mm electrowetted-surfaced implants. In the temporal cohort of this study, none of the tested parameters showed any significance. This means that none of the factors were identified as risk factors for short implants. However, in a study cohort with only three implant failures in total, the possibility of missing a true risk factor is high for pure mathematical reasons. Therefore, larger patient populations are needed to properly identify the risk factors.

In the current study, two early losses occurred within 1 year. This is in line with a systematic review on 690 short (6 mm) implants, which reported that 76% of all losses were early [11]. Two of the three patients that lost implants had comorbidities such as diabetes (type 2) and osteoporosis. Diabetes, although known as a risk factor for periodontitis, has not been confirmed to affect implant survival [12]. Osteoporosis is also not confirmed as a risk factor, but at least has demonstrated a trend [13]. Diabetes and osteoporosis were not significant factors in this study. This may well be related to the small number of patients who had these systemic diseases thus providing a small overall effect.

The maxilla is commonly seen as having less favorable bone quality than the mandible [14]. Therefore, one concern would be that 7-mm-long implants placed in the maxillary arch might be at higher risk for failure than those placed in the mandible. In the current retrospective, the survival rate was similar between the two arches. Hence, the notion that one arch versus the other would be at greater risk with this particular short dental implant appears to hold no validity. A larger prospective study would need to be undertaken with more sites/clinicians placing the implants to determine if this finding is generalizable.

Thirty-six percent of the implants in the study were placed in extraction sockets. Provided that sufficient initial implant stability is achieved, there should be no additional risk factors compared to implants in healed sites. Studies have shown no difference in marginal bone remodeling between immediately placed and delayed implants [15].

The biggest limitation of the current study is its very nature as retrospective single-center study with a limited sample size. The included patients received 7-mm-long implants. There is no control group with longer dental implants of the same surface to allow for direct comparisons to be made.

Conclusion

The current retrospective consecutive case series study provides preliminary data that treatment with 7-mm-length short implants with a hydrophilic electrowetted surface is a reasonable approach in sites with limited vertical bone dimension. It adds to the body of evidence supporting short implant use for compromised sites. The success seen might be attributed to the larger implant diameters that were used to increase surface area. Further prospective studies need to be performed in larger patient population and with multiple centers to determine the generalizability of this approach.

Abbreviations
CSR: Cumulative survival rate; ISQ: Implant stability quotient; IT: Insertion torque; OR: Odds ratio; RFA: Resonance frequency analysis; RR: Relative risk

Authors' contributions
PSR was responsible for the preparation of the study protocol, clinical treatment, data acquisition, and approval of the final manuscript. HS was responsible for the data management, interpretation of the data, and preparation of the manuscript. RS was responsible for the statistics, interpretation of the data, and preparation of the manuscript. ASR was responsible for data acquisition and data management. All authors read and approved the final manuscript.

Competing interests
Herman Sahlin is an employee of Neoss Ltd. Authors Paul S. Rosen, Rudolf Seemann, and Ari S. Rosen declare no competing interests.

Author details
[1]Clinical Professor of Periodontics, Baltimore College of Dental Surgery, University of Maryland Dental School, Baltimore, MD, USA. [2]Private Practice limited to Periodontics and Dental Implants, 907 Floral Vale Boulevard, Yardley, PA 19067, USA. [3]Neoss Ltd, Gothenburg, Sweden. [4]University Clinic of Craniofacial, Maxillofacial and Oral Surgery, Vienna, Austria. [5]University of Delaware Newark, Delaware, USA.

References
1. Jemt T, Olsson M, Franke SV. Incidence of first implant failure: a retroprospective study of 27 years of implant operations at one specialist clinic. Clin Implant Dent Relat Res. 2015;17(Suppl 2):e501–10.
2. Pommer B, Frantal S, Willer J, Posch M, Watzek G, Tepper G. Impact of dental implant length on early failure rates: a meta-analysis of observational studies. J Clin Periodontol. 2011;38(9):856–63.
3. Esposito M, Pistilli R, Barausse C, Felice P. Three-year results from a randomised controlled trial comparing prostheses supported by 5-mm long implants or by longer implants in augmented bone in posterior atrophic edentulous jaws. Eur J Oral Implantol. 2014;7(4):383–95.
4. Gulje F, Abrahamsson I, Chen S, Stanford C, Zadeh H, Palmer R. Implants of 6 mm vs. 11 mm lengths in the posterior maxilla and mandible: a 1-year multicenter randomized controlled trial. Clin Oral Implants Res. 2013;24(12):1325–31.
5. Pohl V, Thoma DS, Sporniak-Tutak K, Garcia-Garcia A, Taylor TD, Haas R, Hammerle CH. Short dental implants (6 mm) versus long dental implants (11-15 mm) in combination with sinus floor elevation procedures: 3-year results from a multicentre, randomized, controlled clinical trial. J Clin Periodontol. 2017;44(4):438–45.
6. Esposito M, Grusovin MG, Felice P, Karatzopoulos G, Worthington HV, Coulthard P. Interventions for replacing missing teeth: horizontal and vertical bone augmentation techniques for dental implant treatment. Cochrane Database Syst Rev. 2009;4:CD003607.
7. Lemos CA, Ferro-Alves ML, Okamoto R, Mendonca MR, Pellizzer EP. Short dental implants versus standard dental implants placed in the posterior jaws: a systematic review and meta-analysis. J Dent. 2016;47:8–17.
8. Monje A, Chan HL, Fu JH, Suarez F, Galindo-Moreno P, Wang HL. Are short dental implants (<10 mm) effective? A meta-analysis on prospective clinical trials. J Periodontol. 2013;84(7):895–904.
9. Youden WJ. Index for rating diagnostic tests. Cancer. 1950;3(1):32–5.
10. Moraschini V, Poubel LA, Ferreira VF, Barboza ES. Evaluation of survival and success rates of dental implants reported in longitudinal studies with a follow-up period of at least 10 years: a systematic review. Int J Oral Maxillofac Surg. 2015;44(3):377–88.
11. Srinivasan M, Vazquez L, Rieder P, Moraguez O, Bernard JP, Belser UC. Survival rates of short (6 mm) micro-rough surface implants: a review of literature and meta-analysis. Clin Oral Implants Res. 2014;25(5):539–45.
12. Chrcanovic BR, Albrektsson T, Wennerberg A. Diabetes and oral implant failure: a systematic review. J Dent Res. 2014;93(9):859–67.
13. Giro G, Chambrone L, Goldstein A, Rodrigues JA, Zenobio E, Feres M, Figueiredo LC, Cassoni A, Shibli JA. Impact of osteoporosis in dental implants: a systematic review. World J Orthop. 2015;6(2):311–5.
14. Chrcanovic BR, Albrektsson T, Wennerberg A. Reasons for failures of oral implants. J Oral Rehabil. 2014;41(6):443–76.
15. Kinaia BM, Shah M, Neely AL, Goodis HE. Crestal bone level changes around immediately placed implants: a systematic review and meta-analyses with at least 12 months' follow-up after functional loading. J Periodontol. 2014;85(11):1537–48.

8

Direct activation of platelets by addition of CaCl$_2$ leads coagulation of platelet-rich plasma

Toshihisa Toyoda[1], Kazushige Isobe[1], Tetsuhiro Tsujino[1], Yasuo Koyata[1], Fumitaka Ohyagi[1], Taisuke Watanabe[1], Masayuki Nakamura[1], Yutaka Kitamura[1], Hajime Okudera[1], Koh Nakata[2] and Tomoyuki Kawase[3]* (iD)

Abstract

Background: Based on the notion that full activation of platelets is required for a growth factor release, in regenerative dentistry, platelet-rich plasma (PRP) in liquid form is usually clotted by addition of CaCl$_2$ in glassware before topical implantation. However, there has been no evidence as to which is better, full or partial activation of platelets, for minimizing the loss of growth factors and improving the controlled release of growth factors from coagulated PRP. To address this matter, here, we primarily examined direct effects of CaCl$_2$ on platelets in PBS and on coagulation in citrated PRP.

Methods: PRP was prepared from healthy volunteers' blood. Platelets' actions were monitored by scanning electron microscopy, flow cytometry, digital holographic microscopy, and immunofluorescent staining. Clot formation was examined in plasma.

Results: In plasma-free PBS, 0.1% CaCl$_2$ immediately upregulated CD62P and CD63, causing a release of microparticles and fibrinogen/fibrin; consequently, platelets aggregated and adhered to polystyrene culture dishes with enlargement of their attachment area. In a clot formation assay in plasma, CaCl$_2$ initially induced platelet aggregation, which triggered loop-like matrix formation and subsequently induced coagulation on a watch glass. Such changes were not clearly observed either with PRP in a plastic dish or in platelet-poor plasma on a watch glass: coagulation was delayed in both conditions.

Conclusions: These findings indicate that besides the well-known coagulation pathway, which activates platelets via thrombin conversion in a coagulation cascade, CaCl$_2$ directly activates platelets, which then facilitate clot formation independently and in cooperation with the coagulation pathway.

Keywords: Platelet, Activation, Coagulation, Fibrin, Flow cytometry, Calcium

Background

Since Marx's report [1], platelet-rich plasma (PRP) and subsequently modified PRP derivatives have been widely applied in regenerative dentistry. Unlike self-clotted platelet-rich fibrin (PRF), for better handling efficiency and minimizing the loss of growth factors to diffusion, PRP and some other derivatives in liquid form are usually clotted by addition of exogenous coagulation factors, such as thrombin and/or CaCl$_2$. For example, in the case of

plasma-rich in growth factors (PRGF) (the most successful PRP derivative) [2], venipuncture is performed with anti-coagulants, usually citrate or acid citrate dextrose (ACD), to chelate plasma Ca^{2+} [3]. Somewhat excessive amounts of Ca^{2+} are recommended for addition to citrated PRGF preparations to reconstitute plasma by recovering free Ca^{2+} levels on a watch glass at 37 °C [4, 5].

Behind this clot formation, there is the intrinsic coagulation pathway, which is activated at the level of factor XII by the glass surface and proceeds in the presence of Ca^{2+} to convert prothrombin to thrombin, subsequently fibrinogen to fibrin, and consequently facilitates fibrin polymerization and cross-linking [6]. In this process,

* Correspondence: kawase@dent.niigata-u.ac.jp
[3]Division of Oral Bioengineering, Institute of Medicine and Dentistry, Niigata University, Niigata, Japan
Full list of author information is available at the end of the article

thrombin converted from prothrombin is known to activate platelets via specific subtypes of protease-activated receptors [7, 8]. Therefore, it is likely that added $CaCl_2$ indirectly activates platelets through activation of a coagulation pathway in citrated PRP in glassware. The resulting fibrin fibers are thick and well cross-linked and are almost identical to those formed in a preparation of PRF [9].

In contrast to Ca^{2+}, when an alternative coagulation factor, e.g., thrombin, is added to citrated PRP, the resulting fibrin fibers are thin and often fused together turning into a sheet-like matrix. Because this thrombin-induced fibrin matrix is relatively easily degradable [9], to stabilize its existence at an implantation site and to retain its growth factors longer, it is better to use Ca^{2+} as a coagulation factor and to employ glassware for activation of the intrinsic coagulation pathway. This approach is not limited to PRP and PRGF and can be extended to PRF preparation from stored whole-blood samples. Nonetheless, direct effects of exogenously added Ca^{2+} on platelets in vitro have been poorly investigated and understood.

In this study, we attempted to dissociate platelets from the coagulation pathway and to evaluate possible direct action of Ca^{2+} on platelet functions in citrated whole-blood samples. In addition, in response to recent increasingly frequent requests for scheduled or outsourced, but not immediate on-site, preparation of various platelet concentrate types [4, 5], we examined time course changes in platelet responsiveness to added $CaCl_2$ along with coagulation time in stored whole-blood samples.

Methods
Preparation of the PRP fraction and clotting
Blood samples were collected from eight nonsmoking healthy male volunteers at ages from 32 to 68 years. The study design and consent forms of all the procedures performed were approved by the ethics committee for human participants of the Niigata University School of Medicine (Niigata, Japan) in accordance with the Helsinki Declaration of 1964 as revised in 2013.

Peripheral blood (~ 9 mL) was collected into plastic vacuum plain blood collection tubes (Neotube; NIPRO, Osaka, Japan) containing 1 mL of the A-formulation of ACD (ACD-A; Terumo, Tokyo, Japan) and was immediately centrifuged at $530 \times g$ for 10 min. The upper plasma fraction was collected, transferred to fresh tubes, and served as a PRP fraction [10]. The numbers of platelets and other blood cells in whole-blood samples and PRP preparations were determined on an automated hematology analyzer (pocH 100iV, Sysmex, Kobe, Japan).

Evaluation of platelet surface antigen expression by immunofluorescence (IT) staining

Platelet concentrates were prepared from citrated whole-blood samples, pretreated with 5 µg/mL prostaglandin E_1 (PGE$_1$; Cayman Chemical Co., Ann Arbor, MI, USA)

for 5 min, rinsed, and resuspended in PBS in sample tubes. Washed platelets were then treated with $CaCl_2$ at a final concentration of 0.1% and incubated in polystyrene culture dishes for up to 30 min at ambient temperature. At the end of the incubation, the reaction was stopped by adding 10% of neutralized formaldehyde. Platelets were washed twice, blocked with 0.1% Block-Ace (Sumitomo Dainippon Pharma Co., Ltd., Osaka, Japan) in 0.1% Tween 20-containing Tris-buffered saline (TBS) (T-TBS) for 1 h, and treated with a mouse monoclonal anti-human CD41, anti-CD62P, or anti-CD63 antibody (1:20 dilution; BioLegend, San Diego, CA, USA) overnight at 4 °C. At the end of treatment, the platelets were again washed twice with T-TBS and were then probed with a secondary antibody, i.e., a goat anti-mouse IgG H&L antibody (conjugated with Alexa Flour 555; 1:50 dilution; Abcam, Cambridge, MA, USA), for 30 min at ambient temperature. Finally, after a subsequent PBS wash, the platelets were mounted with an antifade mounting medium (Vectashield; Vector laboratories, Burlingame, CA, USA), and CD41, CD62P, and CD63 expression levels were examined under a fluorescence microscope equipped with a cooled charge-coupled device (CCD) camera (Nikon, Tokyo, Japan).

Flow cytometric analysis
As described in the subsection above, the platelet fractions were prepared and treated with $CaCl_2$ in polypropylene sample tubes. At the end of incubation, the platelets were fixed with an equal volume of a commercial fixative, ThromboFix (Beckman-Coulter, Brea, CA, USA), for 30 min, washed twice with PBS, and probed simultaneously with phycoerythrin (PE)-conjugated mouse monoclonal anti-CD41 and FITC-conjugated anti-CD62P or FITC-conjugated CD63 antibodies (5 µL per 100 µL of a sample) (BioLegend) for 40 min at ambient temperature. After two washes with PBS, the platelets were analyzed on a flow cytometer (Cell Lab Quanta SC; Beckman-Coulter Inc., Brea, CA, USA) as described before [5]. For isotype controls, mouse IgG1 (BioLegend) was employed. The data were analyzed in the FlowJo software (FlowJo, LLC, Ashland, Oregon, USA).

Scanning electron microscopy (SEM)
As described above, to observe changes in platelet appearance, washed platelets were treated with 0.1% $CaCl_2$ in polypropylene sample tubes for up to 20 min and placed in polystyrene cell culture dishes where they were incubated for the last 5 min of treatment. Alternatively, to examine microparticles and platelet-derived fibrin fibers, washed platelets were treated with 0.1% $CaCl_2$ in polypropylene sample tubes, were immediately transferred onto specific filters (Sem Pore; JOEL, Akishima, Japan), and incubated for up to 15 min. At the end of treatment, the platelets were washed with PBS, fixed with 2.5%

neutralized glutaraldehyde, serially dehydrated in ethanol and *t*-butanol solutions, and freeze-dried.

Individual fibrin clots were compressed in a stainless steel compressor (JMR, Niigata, Japan) to eliminate abundant serum proteins with the exudate [11], washed three times with PBS, fixed with 2.5% neutralized glutaraldehyde, serially dehydrated in ethanol and *t*-butanol solutions, and freeze-dried.

After that, these samples were examined under a scanning electron microscope (TM-1000; Hitachi, Tokyo, Japan) at an accelerating voltage of 15 kV, as described previously [9].

Quantitative assessment of cell morphology by digital holographic microscopy (DHM)

As described in the section on SEM examination of platelets in cell culture dishes, washed platelets were treated with 0.1% Ca in sample tubes and plated in cell culture dishes (or in flasks) where they were incubated for the last 5 min of treatment. After fixation with 2.5%

neutralized glutaraldehyde, the platelets were washed with PBS and stored in PBS until DHM examination.

Imaging by DHM (HoloMonitor M4; Phase Holographic Imaging AB, Lund, Sweden) was performed as described elsewhere [12]. The data were analyzed using specialized software, HoloStudio M4 (Phase Holographic Imaging AB). For surface roughness and area analysis, after a series of images were captured, the grayscale images were converted to the black-and-white format by the Otsu method, and the cell identification and segmentation in the images were adjusted either automatically or manually.

Based on the accumulated data on the cell refractive index, the average refractive index for cultured monolayer cells was fixed at 1.38 (Phase Holographic Imaging AB, *personal communication*). This value was applied to platelets. The refractive index of the surrounding medium is 1.34 and should not excessively deviate (± 0.08) from the cell refractive index.

On the basis of our preliminary data, we focused on the parameters related to the cell area and roughness

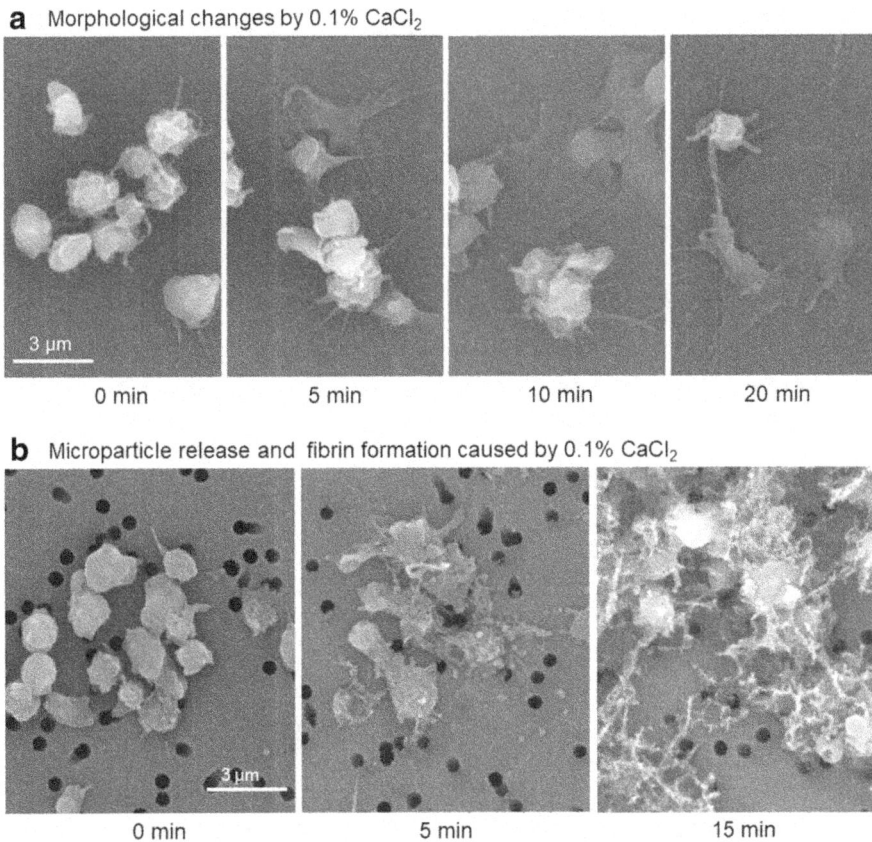

Fig. 1 Morphological changes of (and microparticle release and fibrin formation by) Ca^{2+}-stimulated platelets. **a** Washed platelets were treated with 0.1% CaCl$_2$ in sample tubes and then in culture dishes for 5, 10, and 20 min in total. **b** Washed platelets were treated with 0.1% CaCl$_2$ in sample tubes, immediately transferred onto filters, and incubated for 5 and 15 min in total. Control platelets were directly placed in culture dishes or filters and fixed. Similar results were obtained from samples of three other donors

and examined at least 4000–8000 platelets in each platelet population.

Determination of prothrombin time

This parameter was determined by means of a Coaguchek XS system (Roche Diagnostics International Ltd., Basel, Switzerland). For citrated samples, 500 µL of whole-blood samples was pre-warmed at 37 °C for 5 min, mixed well with 10 µL of 10% $CaCl_2$ by gentle inverting, and incubated for 5 min prior to the analysis.

A clot formation assay

Next, PRP fractions were centrifuged at $1060 \times g$ for 5 min to fractionate platelet-poor plasma (PPP). PRP or PPP (1.5 mL) was mixed with 10% $CaCl_2$ in the ratio mentioned for whole-blood samples on a watch glass or in a plastic dish. To activate platelets, small cut pieces of a collagen sponge composed of collagen microfibers (Integran®; Koken, Tokyo, Japan) were added to PRP in the plastic dish. Time for complete clot formation was determined.

Statistical analysis

The data were expressed as mean ± standard deviation (SD). For multigroup comparisons, statistical analyses were conducted to compare the mean values by one-way analysis of variance (ANOVA), followed by Dunn's multiple-comparison test (SigmaPlot 12.5; Systat Software, Inc., San Jose, CA, USA). Differences with P values of < 0.05 were considered statistically significant.

Results

Morphological changes of (and microparticle release and fibrin formation by) Ca^{2+}-stimulated platelets are shown in Fig. 1. When washed platelets were treated with 0.1% $CaCl_2$ in sample tubes and plated in culture dishes for the last 5 min of treatment (control, 2 min), platelets' ability to adhere to the dish bottom surface increased with the duration of Ca^{2+} treatment (Fig. 1a). On the

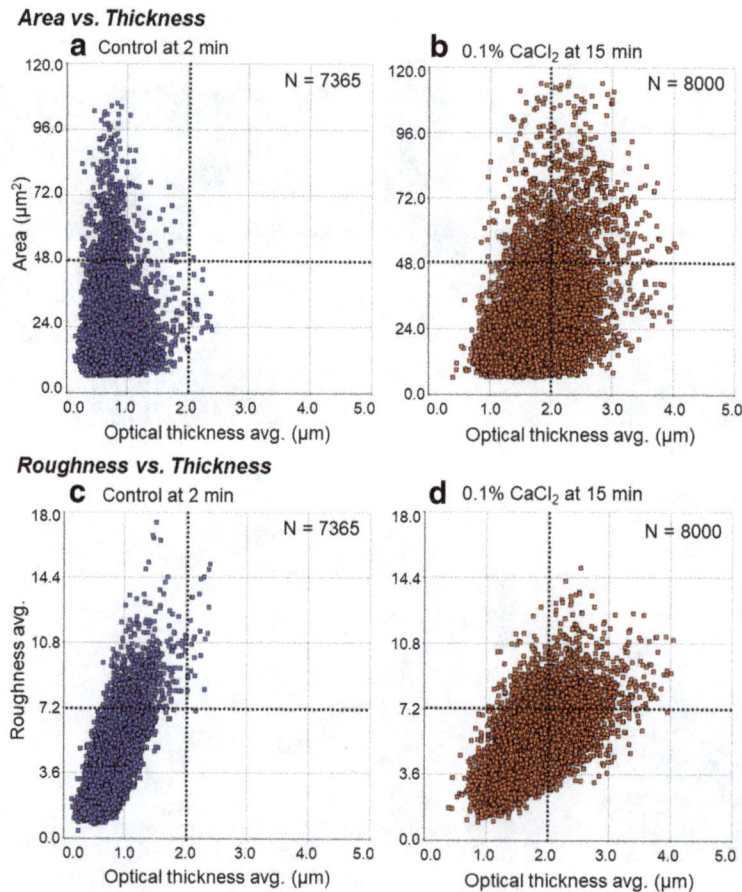

Fig. 2 DHM examination of changes in attachment area, optical thickness, and surface roughness of Ca^{2+}-simulated platelets. Washed platelets were treated with 0.1% $CaCl_2$ for 15 min (**b**, **d**) on culture flasks, fixed, and subjected to DHM examination. Control was no treatment at 2 min (**a**, **c**). Each platelet was plotted in the scatter plots of "Area vs. Thickness" (**a**, **b**) or "Roughness vs. Thickness". Similar results were obtained from samples of two other donors

other hand, when washed platelets were treated with 0.1% CaCl$_2$ in sample tubes, immediately transferred onto percolated filters, and incubated for up to 15 min, the platelets were found to release microparticles and fibrinogen, which was converted to fibrin even in the absence of plasma components (Fig. 1b).

Changes in attachment area, optical thickness on average, and surface roughness of Ca^{2+}-simulated platelets are shown in Fig. 2. In the control, i.e., resting platelets, the average thickness of almost all platelets was within 2 μm. Among the platelets stimulated by 0.1% Ca^{2+} for 15 min, approximately 50% of the cells increased their apparent thickness beyond 2 μm. Attachment area was also significantly enlarged by added Ca^{2+}, but roughness was not changed. In this case, enlarged platelets in terms of both thickness and area definitely represent aggregated platelets, but, probably, thicker platelets also represent aggregated platelets.

Immunofluorescent (IF) evaluation of changes in surface marker expression in Ca^{2+}-stimulated platelets is shown in Fig. 3. When washed platelets were treated with 0.1% CaCl$_2$ in sample tubes, immediately placed in culture dishes, and incubated for 15 min, CD62P and CD63, but not CD41, were substantially upregulated.

Flow cytometric analysis of changes in surface marker expression in Ca^{2+}-stimulated platelets is presented in Fig. 4. When washed platelets were treated with 0.1% CaCl$_2$ in sample tubes for up to 30 min, CD62P$^+$ platelet counts in CD41$^+$ platelet populations increased time-dependently. Similarly, platelet volume, as assessed by impedance, increased with the duration of Ca^{2+} treatment.

Because these findings taken together implied that exogenously added Ca^{2+} beyond physiological in vivo levels (approximately 9.0 vs. 2.5 mM) directly activates platelets in the absence of plasma components, platelets'

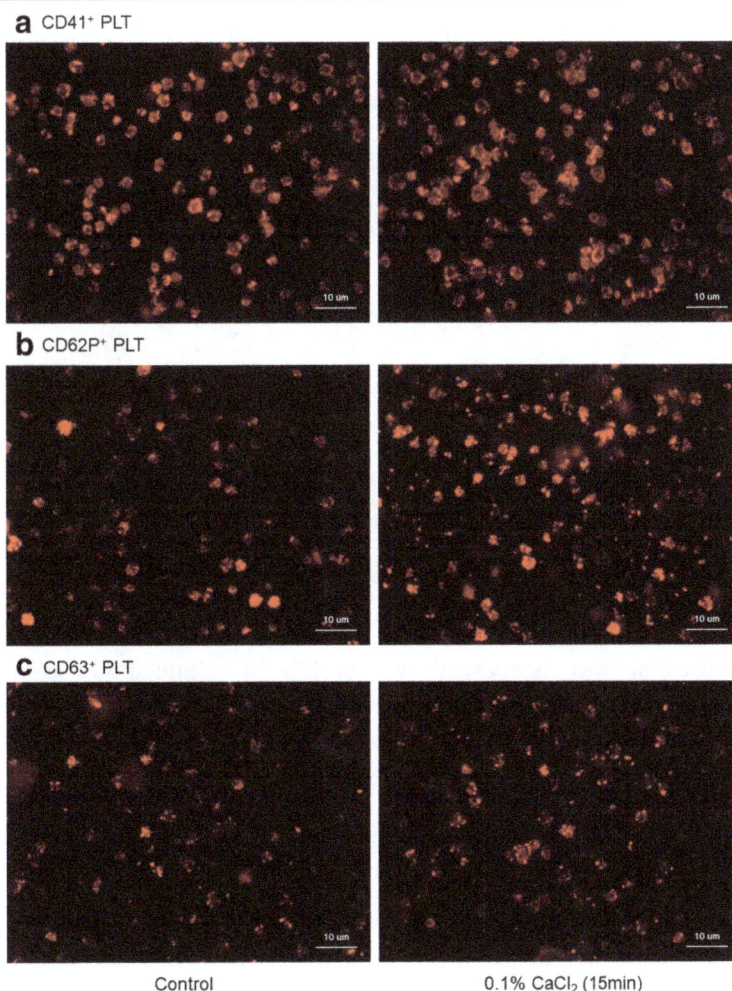

Fig. 3 Immunofluorescent (IF) evaluation of changes in surface marker expression—CD41 (**a**), CD62P (**b**), and CD63 (**c**)—in Ca^{2+}-stimulated platelets. PLT platelets. Washed platelets were treated with 0.1% CaCl$_2$ in culture dishes and subjected to IF staining. Similar results were obtained from samples of three other donors

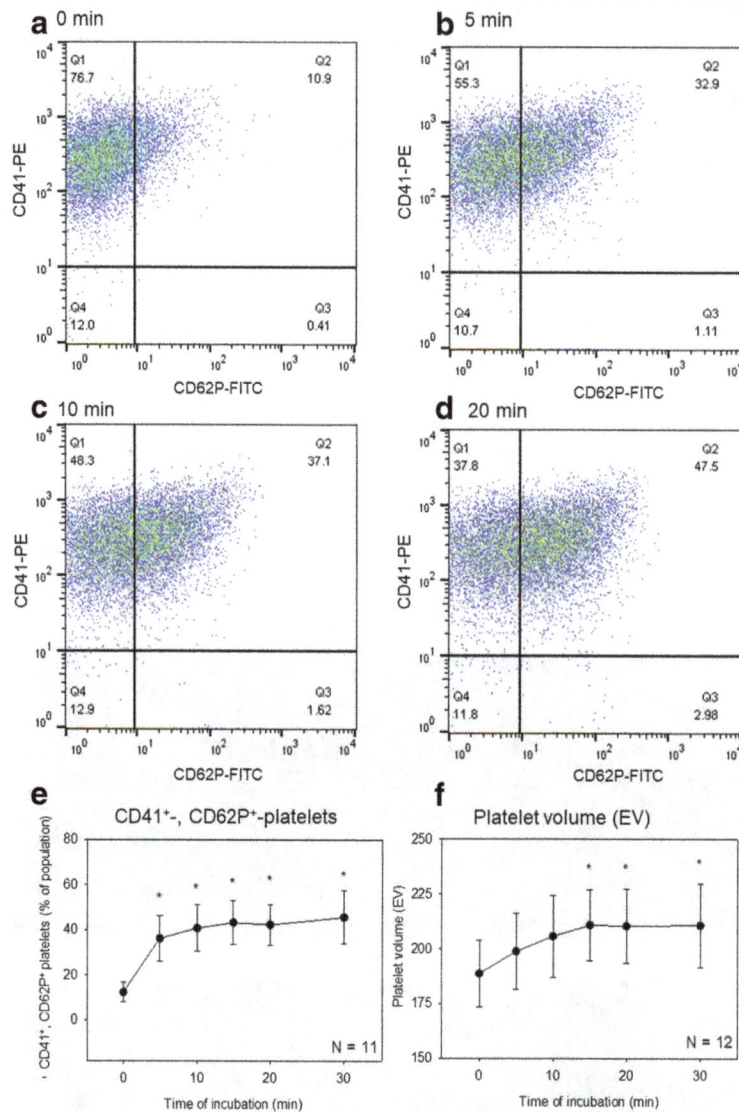

Fig. 4 Flow cytometric analysis of changes in surface marker expression in Ca^{2+}-stimulated platelets. Washed platelets were prepared and treated as described in the caption of Fig. 1a. **a–d** Representative scatter plots of CD41[+] and CD62P[+] platelets. **e** Effects of Ca^{2+} on percentages of double-positive platelets in whole platelet populations ($N = 11$). **f** Effects of Ca^{2+} on platelet volume ($N = 12$). Asterisks indicate statistically significant differences between the control data and treatment data

direct involvement in coagulation was then examined using platelet-rich and platelet-poor plasma. Effects of $CaCl_2$ on fibrin clot formation on watch glasses and in polystyrene culture dishes are shown in Fig. 5. On watch glasses (panel a, control), addition of 0.1% $CaCl_2$ most rapidly formed loop-like substances (in a dashed-line circle) and subsequently fibrin clots in PRP at 8 min of treatment (Fig. 5a). Polystyrene culture dishes, whose surface is optimized for adherent cells, significantly delayed Ca^{2+}-induced clot formation in PRP from 8 to 19 min (Fig. 5b). When the treatment was carried out in PPP, clot formation was also significantly delayed (Fig. 5c). Nonetheless, in the presence of the collagen sponge, Ca^{2+} addition caused formation of a fibrin clot

in PRP in culture dishes as rapidly as in the control (Fig. 5d vs. a).

The surface microstructures of the formed fibrin clots are depicted in Fig. 6. The loop-like substances that initially formed in PRP on watch glasses were composed of abundant aggregated platelets, and relatively smaller amounts of fibrin fibers were deposited around platelet aggregates (Fig. 6a). By contrast, in the final version of fibrin clots, platelet aggregates were hardly detectable and most parts consisted of fibrin fibers (Fig. 6b). Compared with the control clots, those formed in culture dishes were enriched in platelets although either thickness or cross-link density of fibrin fibers was apparently similar to that in the control clots (Fig. 6c). Fibrin clots

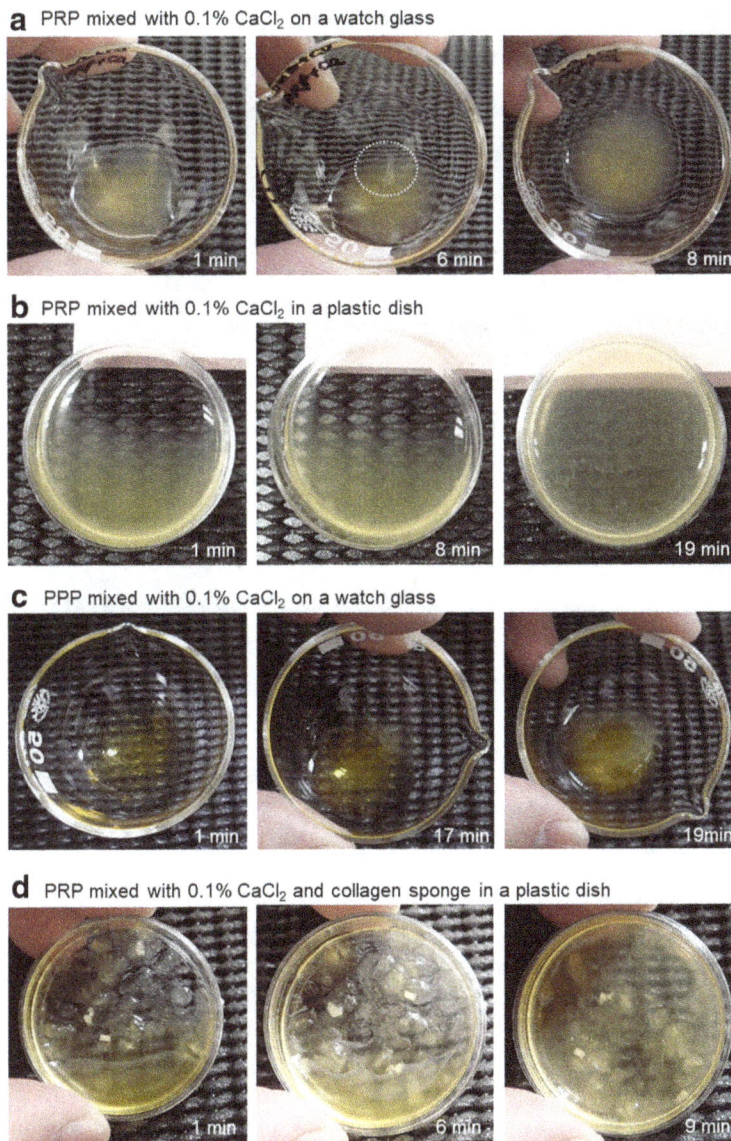

Fig. 5 Effects of CaCl$_2$ on fibrin clot formation on watch glasses and polystyrene culture dishes. **a** PRP mixed with 0.1% CaCl$_2$ on a watch glass. **b** PRP mixed with 0.1% CaCl$_2$ in a plastic dish. **c** PPP mixed with 0.1% CaCl$_2$ on a watch glass. **d** PRP mixed with 0.1% CaCl$_2$ and a collagen sponge in a plastic dish. Similar results were obtained from three other donors

formed from PPP on watch glasses and from PRP in culture dishes with collagen sponges were similar to the control clots.

Finally, effects of storage time on coagulation activity and platelet functions were examined. Effects of Ca^{2+} on prothrombin time and clot formation of stored whole-blood samples are shown in Fig. 7a, b. Because we preliminarily confirmed that reconstitution of citrated blood with CaCl$_2$ can recover the conditions applicable to the prothrombin time assay, we evaluated prothrombin time of citrated whole-blood samples stored for up to 6 days. Prothrombin time increased with the duration of storage. Effects of Ca^{2+} on CD62P and

CD63 expression in platelets isolated from citrated whole-blood samples stored for up to 6 days are presented in Fig. 7c, d. The responsiveness to Ca^{2+} in terms of both CD62P and CD63 at 15 min seemed to somewhat decrease with storage time; however, even after 6-day storage, platelets maintained their response to added Ca^{2+}: upregulation of CD62P and CD63 (vs. control levels).

Discussion

It is well known that platelets are activated by adenosine diphosphate (ADP), thrombin, epinephrine, thromboxane A$_2$, collagen, and many other compounds and

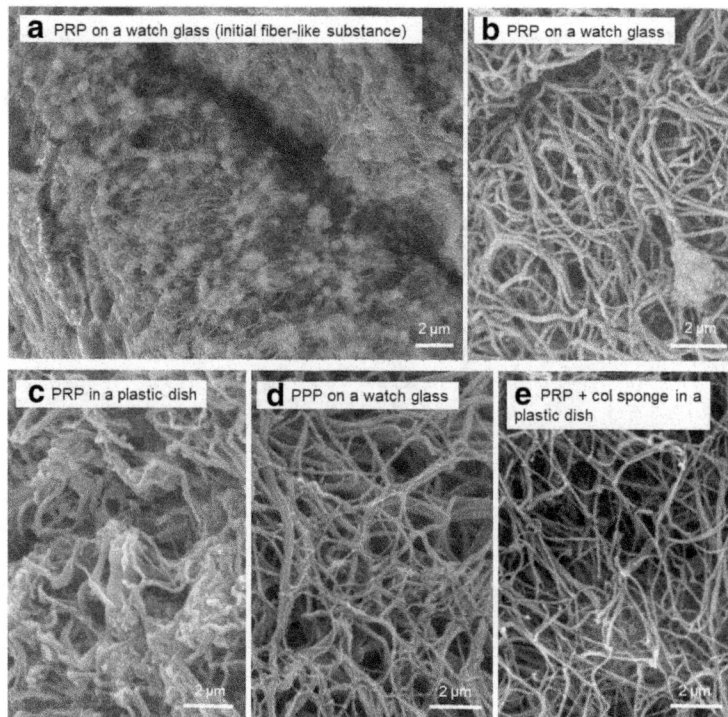

Fig. 6 SEM analysis of the surface microstructures of formed fibrin clots. **a** A fiber-like substance initially formed in Ca^{2+}-treated PRP on a watch glass. **b** The fibrin clot formed in Ca^{2+}-treated PRP on a watch glass. **c** The fibrin clot formed in Ca^{2+}-treated PRP in a plastic culture dish. **d** The fibrin clot formed in PPP on a watch glass. **e** The fibrin clot formed in PRP in the presence of a collagen sponge in a plastic dish. Similar results were obtained from three other donors

thus aggregate through binding of fibrinogen and glycoprotein IIb/IIIa receptors and upregulate surface antigens known as "platelet activation markers": CD62P and CD63 [13, 14]. During activation, platelet morphology generally changes from a disc-shaped appearance (resting) to a rolling ball-shaped appearance, hemisphere-shaped appearance, and finally spreading adhesion appearance [15]. To our knowledge, however, increased extracellular free Ca^{2+} levels have not been sufficiently studied as an activator of platelets probably because free Ca^{2+} levels are maintained within some range, but not depleted, under pathological conditions of plasma and tissues.

Compared with the in vivo settings, citrated whole blood provides totally different conditions to platelets: extracellular free Ca^{2+} is chelated by citrate. The primary purpose of addition of Ca^{2+}-chelating anticoagulants is to inhibit serial reactions of the coagulation pathway. Nevertheless, it is known that this chelation also suppresses various platelet functions related to aggregation [16]. Platelet activators mentioned above elevate intracellular Ca^{2+} concentrations, either by releasing Ca^{2+} from intracellular stores or by increasing Ca^{2+} influx across the plasma membrane [17]. Conversely, acute chelating of extracellular Ca^{2+} by EGTA inhibits the

platelet ability to adhere to glass and to aggregate in response to ADP or other platelet activators [16].

The mechanism of Ca^{2+}-induced platelet activation is discussed below. We preliminarily postulated expression of Ca^{2+}-sensing receptors (CaSR) but failed to detect this type of receptor by the methods of flow cytometry and IF staining with a mouse monoclonal anti-CaSR antibody (cat. # ab19347; Abcam). No appreciable specific binding was observed in IF staining, and fewer than 5% of platelets tested positive in the flow cytometric analysis. Therefore, because this CaSR antigen is known to be expressed in the brain, kidneys, lungs, liver, heart, skeletal muscle, and placenta [18], but not in platelets, it is reasonable to rule out the participation of CaSR in Ca^{2+}-induced platelet activation in our study.

An alternative possibility may be related to the status of platelets stored in a low-Ca^{2+} environment: platelets constantly increase thromboxane A_2 (TXA_2) production and tend to easily aggregate under the influence of the TXA_2 autocrine loop [19]. Therefore, it is thought that platelets prepared from citrated whole-blood samples continuously repeat Ca^{2+} discharge from intracellular Ca^{2+} stores and Ca^{2+} efflux across the plasma membrane [20] in response to endogenously produced TXA_2. In addition, even though the autocrine loop of TXA_2 does

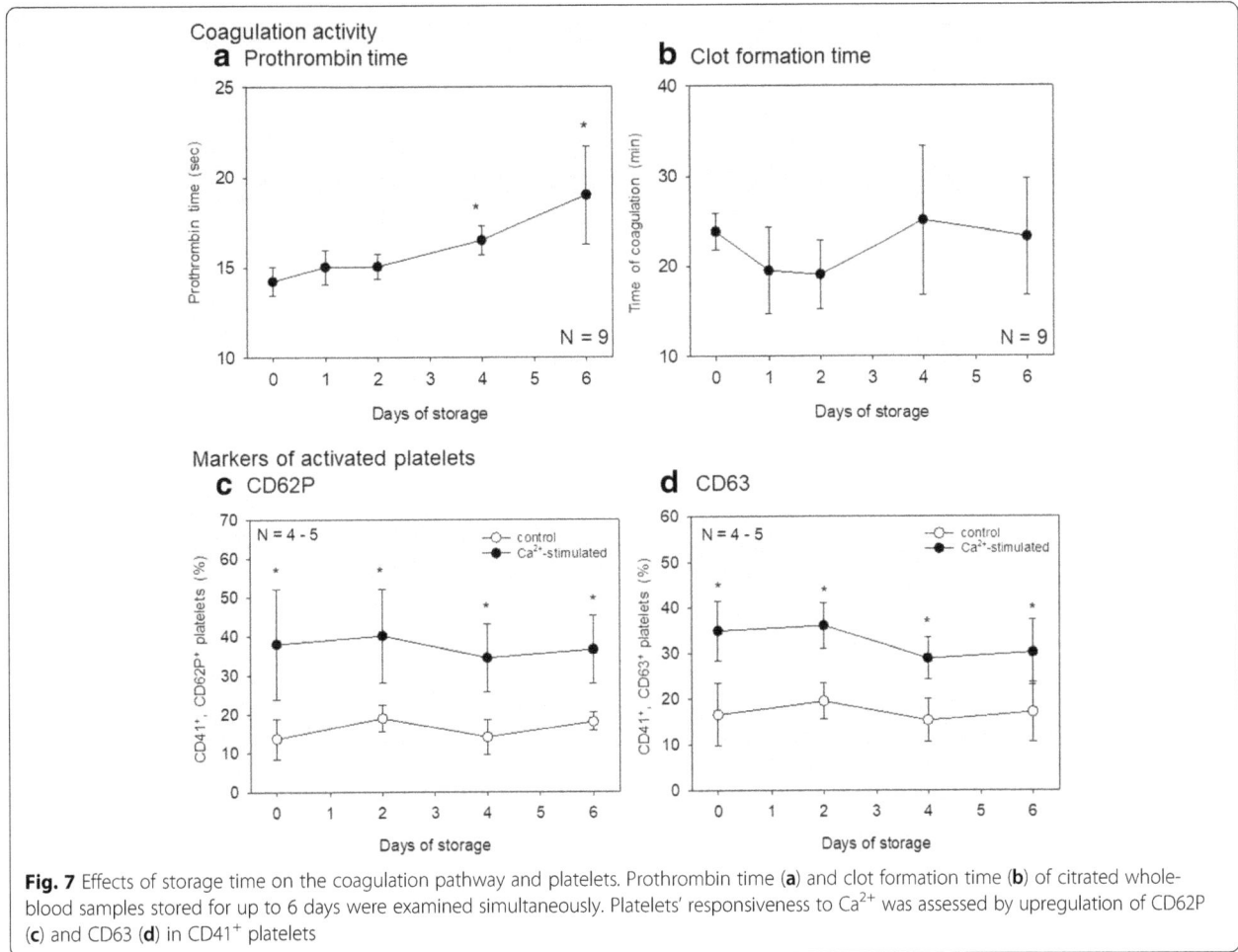

Fig. 7 Effects of storage time on the coagulation pathway and platelets. Prothrombin time (**a**) and clot formation time (**b**) of citrated whole-blood samples stored for up to 6 days were examined simultaneously. Platelets' responsiveness to Ca^{2+} was assessed by upregulation of CD62P (**c**) and CD63 (**d**) in $CD41^+$ platelets

not function actively, intracellular free Ca^{2+} levels of platelets (~ 100 nM at actual resting levels) are maintained also by a balance between the "passive" leak of Ca^{2+} into platelets and the concurrent efflux of Ca^{2+} across the plasma membrane and accumulation in intracellular stores [21]. Therefore, in a citrated medium, it is plausible that intracellular free Ca^{2+} in platelets is depleted gradually by repeated Ca^{2+} discharge from intracellular stores and passive and active Ca^{2+} flux across the plasma membrane. We can speculate that Ca^{2+} addition may promptly enable Ca^{2+} entry via the Ca^{2+} leak pathway and subsequently activate platelets by the autocrine pathway of TXA_2 or activators stored in α-granules, such as ADP and thrombin. In support of this possibility, Aoki et al. demonstrated that added Ca^{2+} increases thrombin production by washed platelets [22]. Further investigation is needed to clarify the mechanism of Ca^{2+}-induced platelet activation.

The mechanism of Ca^{2+}-induced clot formation is worthier of discussion. In the human body, two types of thrombosis are known: white and red thrombi [23]. According to this definition, a fibrin mesh is deposited on platelet aggregates in a white thrombus, whereas platelets (and red blood cells) are trapped and aggregated by the fibrin mesh in a red thrombus. In this study, we found that platelet aggregates function like nuclei of clot formation. Therefore, platelets are located mainly near the center or in a deep region of a clot, and this clot may be classified essentially as a "white thrombus." In this case, growth factors stored in platelets can be assumed to be retained for a relatively long time. It is possible that this type of clot functions as a long-lasting carrier with a better regenerative potential.

On the other hand, in PRF prepared from fresh whole-blood without anticoagulants, it is thought that the centrifugal force increases the contact of factor XII with a glass surface, thereby primarily forming fibrin clots. Although platelets can also be activated by a glass surface, the centrifugal force accumulates platelets at and just below the interface between the red blood cell fraction and plasma fraction as well as in the surface area of PRF preparations [11]. Even though only a few red blood cells are embedded in the clot, in terms of the formation mechanism, this clot could be classified as a

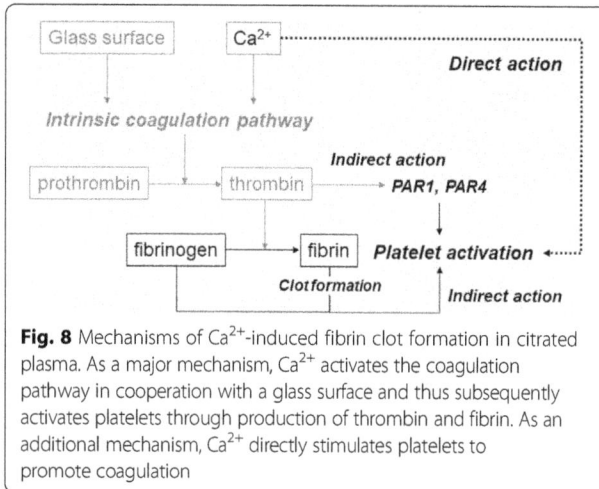

Fig. 8 Mechanisms of Ca^{2+}-induced fibrin clot formation in citrated plasma. As a major mechanism, Ca^{2+} activates the coagulation pathway in cooperation with a glass surface and thus subsequently activates platelets through production of thrombin and fibrin. As an additional mechanism, Ca^{2+} directly stimulates platelets to promote coagulation

"red thrombus." Therefore, it is plausible that growth factors that are stored in the platelets trapped in fibrin mesh may be released at early phases of degradation.

As described previously [24], glass tube production is no longer practiced by major manufacturers of medical equipment in Japan and in major Western countries. One of the possible solutions (when glassware is needed) is to coat the inner wall of plastic tubes with micronized silica particles, as in Greiner Bio-One Serum Clot Activator Tubes (Greiner Bio-One North America Inc., Monroe, NC, USA). Likewise, various types of plastic vacuum blood collection tubes containing a coagulation-activating film are produced by several manufacturers. Nevertheless, these products are intended for routine clinical examination, and their quality, especially safety, has never been ensured for preparation and implantation of platelet concentrates.

If platelet activity can be controlled in well-qualified plastic tubes, it is expected that safer PRF will be provided to patients without activation of the intrinsic coagulation pathway. In this study, we demonstrated that a collagen sponge can rapidly facilitate fibrin clot formation (without the aid of glassware) probably via activation of platelets. On the basis of this concept, we recently developed a PRF kit composed of plastic tubes containing a synthetic, RGD motif-enriched collagen-like peptide (RCP; FUJIFILM, Tokyo, Japan) and validated its utility in PRF preparation and its efficacy in bone regeneration [Tsukioka et al., manuscript submitted]. This fibrin clot formation is triggered by activated platelets.

Conclusions
In addition to the well-known intrinsic coagulation pathway, which activates platelets via thrombin conversion, added Ca^{2+} may directly activate washed platelets and promote clot formation alone and in cooperation with the coagulation pathway as illustrated in Fig. 8.

Therefore, it is possible to control platelet activation levels and the consequent growth factor release by modulating not only indirect but also direct activation pathways.

Abbreviations
ACD: Acid citrate dextrose solution; ADP: Adenosine diphosphate; CaSR: Calcium-sensing receptor; DHM: Digital holographic microscopy; PBS: Phosphate-buffered saline; PPP: Platelet-poor plasma; PRF: Platelet-rich fibrin; PRP: Platelet-rich plasma; SEM: Scanning electron microscope; TBS: Tris-buffered saline; TXA_2: Thromboxane A_2

Acknowledgements
The authors appreciate Shoshin EM (Okazaki, Japan) for giving an opportunity to use DHM.

Authors' contributions
TT, KI, TT, and TK conceived and designed the study, performed the experiments and data analysis, and wrote the manuscript. YK, FO, TW, MN, and YK designed and performed the experiments and data analysis. HO and KN conceived the study and participated in the discussion of the results and manuscript preparation. All authors read and approved the final version of the manuscript.

Competing interests
Toshihisa Toyoda, Kazushige Isobe, Tetsuhiro Tsujino, Yasuo Koyata, Fumitaka Ohyagi, Taisuke Watanabe, Masayuki Nakamura, Yutaka Kitamura, Hajime Okudera, Koh Nakata, and Tomoyuki Kawase declare that they have no competing interests.

Author details
[1]Tokyo Plastic Dental Society, Kita-ku, Tokyo, Japan. [2]Bioscience Medical Research Center, Niigata University Medical and Dental Hospital, Niigata, Japan. [3]Division of Oral Bioengineering, Institute of Medicine and Dentistry, Niigata University, Niigata, Japan.

References
1. Marx RE, Carlson ER, Eichstaedt RM, Schimmele SR, Strauss JE, Georgeff KR. Platelet-rich plasma: growth factor enhancement for bone grafts. Oral Surg Oral Med Oral Pathol Oral Radiol Endod. 1998;85:638–46.
2. Anitua E. Plasma rich in growth factors: preliminary results of use in the preparation of future sites for implants. Int J Oral Maxillofac Implants. 1999;14:529–35.
3. Masuki H, Okudera T, Watanabe T, Suzuki M, Nishiyama K, Okudera H, Nakata K, Uematsu K, Su CY, Kawase T. Growth factor and pro-inflammatory cytokine contents in PRP, plasma rich in growth factors (PRGF), advanced-platelet-rich fibrin (A-PRF) and concentrated growth factors (CGF). Int J Implant Dent. 2016;2:19.
4. Isobe K, Suzuki M, Watanabe T, Kitamura Y, Suzuki T, Kawabata H, Nakamura M, Okudera T, Okudera H, Uematsu K, Nakata K, Tanaka T, Kawase T. Platelet-rich fibrin prepared from stored whole-blood samples. Int J Implant Dent. 2017;3:6.
5. Kawabata H, Isobe K, Watanabe T, Okudera T, Nakamura M, Suzuki M, Ryu J, Kitamura Y, Okudera H, Okuda K, Nakata K, Kawase T. Quality assessment of platelet-rich fibrin-like matrix prepared from whole blood samples after extended storage. Biomedicine. 2017;5(57). http://www.mdpi.com/2227-9059/5/3/57.
6. Margolis J. Glass surface and blood coagulation. Nature. 1956;178:805–6.
7. Goldsack NR, Chambers RC, Dabbagh K, Laurent GJ. Molecules in focus thrombin. Int J Biochem Cell Biol. 1998;30:641–6.
8. Posma JJ, Posthuma JJ, Spronk HM. Coagulation and non-coagulation effects of thrombin. J Thromb Haemost. 2016;14:1908–16.
9. Isobe K, Watanabe T, Kawabata H, Kitamura Y, Okudera T, Okudera H, Uematsu K, Okuda K, Nakata K, Tanaka T, Kawase T. Mechanical and

degradation properties of advanced platelet-rich fibrin (A-PRF), concentrated growth factors (CGF), and platelet-poor plasma-derived fibrin (PPTF). Int J Implant Dent. 2017;3:17.

10. Watanabe T, Isobe K, Suzuki T, Kawabata H, Nakamura M, Tsukioka T, Okudera T, Okudera H, Uematsu K, Okuda K, Nakata K, Kawase T. An evaluation of the accuracy of the subtraction method used for determining platelet counts in advanced platelet-rich fibrin and concentrated growth factor preparations. Dentistry Journal. 2017;5:7.

11. Kobayashi M, Kawase T, Horimizu M, Okuda K, Wolff LF, Yoshie H. A proposed protocol for the standardized preparation of PRF membranes for clinical use. Biologicals. 2012;40:323–9.

12. Kawase T, Okuda K, Nagata M, Tsuchimochi M, Yoshie H, Nakata K. Non-invasive, quantitative assessment of the morphology of gamma-irradiated human mesenchymal stem cells and periosteal cells using digital holographic microscopy. Int J Radiat Biol. 2016;92:796–805.

13. Taylor ML, Misso NL, Stewart GA, Thompson PJ. Differential expression of platelet activation markers CD62P and CD63 following stimulation with PAF, arachidonic acid and collagen. Platelets. 1995;6:394–401.

14. Choudhury A, Chung I, Blann AD, Lip GY. Platelet surface CD62P and CD63, mean platelet volume, and soluble/platelet P-selectin as indexes of platelet function in atrial fibrillation: a comparison of "healthy control subjects" and "disease control subjects" in sinus rhythm. J Am Coll Cardiol. 2007;49:1957–64.

15. Kuwahara M, Sugimoto M, Tsuji S, Matsui H, Mizuno T, Miyata S, Yoshioka A. Platelet shape changes and adhesion under high shear flow. Arterioscler Thromb Vasc Biol. 2002;22:329–34.

16. Zucker MB, Grant RA. Nonreversible loss of platelet aggregability induced by calcium deprivation. Blood. 1978;52:505–13.

17. Jy W, Haynes DH. Intracellular calcium storage and release in the human platelet. Chlorotetracycline as a continuous monitor. Circ Res. 1984;55:595–608.

18. Riccardi D, Kemp PJ. The calcium-sensing receptor beyond extracellular calcium homeostasis: conception, development, adult physiology, and disease. Annu Rev Physiol. 2012;74:271–97.

19. Hu H, Forslund M, Li N. Influence of extracellular calcium on single platelet activation as measured by whole blood flow cytometry. Thromb Res. 2005;116:241–7.

20. Varga-Szabo D, Braun A, Nieswandt B. Calcium signaling in platelets. J Thromb Haemost. 2009;7:1057–66.

21. Roberts DE, McNicol A, Bose R. Mechanism of collagen activation in human platelets. J Biol Chem. 2004;279:19421–30.

22. Aoki I, Aoki N, Kawano K, Shimoyama K, Maki A, Homori M, Yanagisawa A, Yamamoto M, Kawai Y, Ishikawa K. Platelet-dependent thrombin generation in patients with hyperlipidemia. J Am Coll Cardiol. 1997;30:91–6.

23. Blitz A. Pump thrombosis—a riddle wrapped in a mystery inside an enigma. Ann Cardiothor Surg. 2014;3:450–71.

24. Kawase T, Watanabe T, Okuda K. Platelet-rich plasma and its derived platelet concentrates: what dentists involved in cell-based regenerative therapy should know. Nihon Shishubyou Gakkai Kaishi. 2017;59:68–76. (in Japanese)

9

Biomechanical properties of polymer-infiltrated ceramic crowns on one-piece zirconia implants after long-term chewing simulation

Pia Baumgart[1], Holger Kirsten[2,3], Rainer Haak[4] and Constanze Olms[5]*

Abstract

Background: Implant and superstructure provide a complex system, which has to withstand oral conditions. Concerning the brittleness of many ceramics, fractures are a greatly feared issue. Therefore, polymer-infiltrated ceramic networks (PICNs) were developed. Because of its high elastic modulus, the PICN crown on a one-piece zirconia implant might absorb forces to prevent the system from fracturing in order to sustain oral forces. Recommendations for the material of superstructure on zirconia implants are lacking, and only one study investigates PICN crowns on these types of implants.

Accordingly, this study aimed to examine PICN crowns on one-piece zirconia implants regarding bond strength and surface wear after long-term chewing simulation (CS).

Methods: Twenty-five hybrid ceramic crowns (Vita Enamic, Vita Zahnfabrik) were produced using computer-aided design/computer-aided manufacturing (CAD/CAM) technology and adhesively bonded (RelyX™ Ultimate, 3M ESPE) to zirconia implants. Twenty of the specimens underwent simultaneous mechanical loading and thermocycling simulating a 5-year clinical situation (SD Mechatronik GmbH). Wear depth and wear volume, based on X-ray micro-computed tomography volume scans (Skyscan 1172-100-50, Bruker) before and after CS, were evaluated.

All crowns were removed from the implants using a universal testing machine (Z010, Zwick GmbH&Co.KG). Subsequently, luting agent was light microscopically localized (Stemi 2000-C, Zeiss).

With a scanning electron microscope (SEM, Phenom™ G2 pro, Phenom World), the area of abrasion was assessed.

Results:

1. After CS, none of the tested crowns were fractured or loosened.
2. The maximum vertical wear after CS was $M = 0.31 \pm 0.04$ mm (mean $\pm$ standard deviation), and the surface wear was $M = 0.74 \pm 0.23$ mm^3.
3. The pull-off tests revealed a 1.8 times higher bond strength of the control group compared to the experimental group ($t(23) = 8.69$, $p < 0.001$).
4. Luting agent was mostly located in the crowns, not on the implants.
5. The area of abrasion showed avulsion and a rough surface.

Conclusions: PICN on one-piece zirconia implants showed high bond strength and high wear after CS.

Keywords: Hybrid ceramic, Polymer-infiltrated ceramic network, PICN, Implant, One-piece, Zirconia

* Correspondence: constanze.olms@medizin.uni-leipzig.de
[5]Department of Dental Prosthodontics and Materials Science, University of Leipzig, Liebigstraße 12, Haus 1, 04103 Leipzig, Germany
Full list of author information is available at the end of the article

Background

The demand for tooth-colored dental restorations has increased rapidly within the last few years. Ceramic restorations can often meet these requirements. In dental implantology, zirconia especially—due to its esthetical advantage as well as high flexural strength and outstanding biocompatibility—has gained importance [1]. On the other hand, one-piece zirconia implants are not yet commonly used because the surgical possibilities do not always meet the prosthodontics requirements. Besides, angled one-piece zirconia implants are not yet available. The superstructure can only be cemented to the zirconia implant which may result in remaining excess cement and peri-implant inflammation [2].

Implant and superstructure provide a complex system, which has to withstand oral conditions. Concerning the brittleness of many ceramics, fractures are a greatly feared issue. Therefore, PICNs were developed. They are composed of a ceramic and a composite network and are supposed to combine the advantages of both materials [3]. One of these PICN materials is known under the trade name Vita Enamic (VE) (Vita Zahnfabrik, Bad Säckingen, Germany). It consists of 86 wt% feldspathic ceramic and 14 wt% polymer network. The two networks entirely interpenetrate one another which is supposed to result in a high fracture resistance [4].

Low hardness and high fracture stability differentiate PICNs from conventional feldspathic ceramics [5]. Because of a high elastic modulus [6], PICN crowns on one-piece zirconia implants could absorb forces to prevent the system from fracturing when sustaining oral forces. Recommendations for the material of superstructures on zirconia implants are still lacking, and only one study investigates PICN crowns on these types of implants [5].

Accordingly, this study aimed to examine PICN crowns on one-piece zirconia implants regarding bond strength and surface wear after long-term chewing simulation. The number of cycles during chewing simulation (CS) corresponds roughly to an in vivo load of 5 years [7].

Methods

Specimen preparation

Twenty-five PICN crowns (Vita Enamic, Vita Zahnfabrik, Bad Säckingen, Germany) for premolars were produced using CAD/CAM technology and polished with the Vita Enamic Polishing Set Technical (Vita Zahnfabrik) as recommended by the manufacturer. All crowns were bonded to identical one-piece zirconia testing implants. The implants were turned from pre-sintered zirconia blocks (VITA In-Ceram® 2000 YZ–55, VITA Zahnfabrik) by the faculty of physics and geosciences at the University of Leipzig. Subsequently, the implants were sintered in a dental laboratory. The abutment had a cone angle of 3 °, while the length of the implant totaled up to 21.5 mm.

The abutment length was 6 mm. The thread was conceived schematically.

Twenty of the specimens belonged to the experimental group ($n = 20$) and underwent mechanical loading and wear behavior tests, whereas five of the specimens ($n = 5$) only underwent the pull-off tests.

Five specimens fit into the chewing simulator which is why five specimens were prepared at a time. Therefore, four rounds of CS were performed.

All steps of the bonding procedure followed the manufacturer's instructions: the bonding surface of the crown was degreased with alcohol and conditioned with 5 % hydrofluoric acid gel for 60 s (Vita Ceramics Etch, Vita Zahnfabrik). The hydrofluoric acid gel was removed with water spray and the bonding surface was dried for 20 s. Conditioning of the bonding surface of the implant was ensured by sandblasting with aluminum oxide (Al_2O_3) 110 μm at 1 bar and cleaning with alcohol. After that, a bonding agent (Scotchbond Universal, 3M ESPE, St. Paul, MN, USA) was applied to the surfaces to bond the crown and the implant and both dried with air. The crowns were adhesively bonded (RelyX™ Ultimate, 3M ESPE) to the one-piece zirconia implants. Photopolymerization of the luting agent was carried out by a dental curing light for 40 s on each surface.

All specimens were embedded in acrylic resin (Technovit 4000, Heraeus Kulzer GmbH, Wehrheim, Germany) with a parallelometer for the exact vertical orientation. Epoxy was prepared according to manufacturer's data, and the specimens were embedded directly into the sample holder of the chewing simulator. Figure 1 shows a luted crown on an embedded implant ready for CS.

The specimens attached to the parallelometer were perpendicularly recessed until only the upper coils of the implants were on view.

To produce replicas of the specimens from the experimental group, the crowns' occlusal was cast using VPS Hydro Putty und VPS Hydro Light Body (Henry Schein Inc., New York, USA) before and after CS. The impression was grouted with Stycast 1266 (Loctite Henkel Electronic Materials, Westerlo, Belgium). The replicas could be scanned by X-ray micro-computed tomography (Micro-CT, Skyscan 1172-100-50, Bruker microCT, Kontich, Belgium). Table 1 shows the scanning parameters of the replicas before and after CS.

Chewing simulation

The specimens of the experimental group underwent long-term chewing simulation (SD Mechatronik GmbH, Feldkirchen-Westerham, Germany): 1,200,000 cycles, 50 N, and simultaneous thermocycling of 5500 cycles with changing temperatures of 4 and 56 °C for 60 s each. Hydroxyapatite steatite indenters (6.35 mm diameter) were used as antagonists and were replaced for each

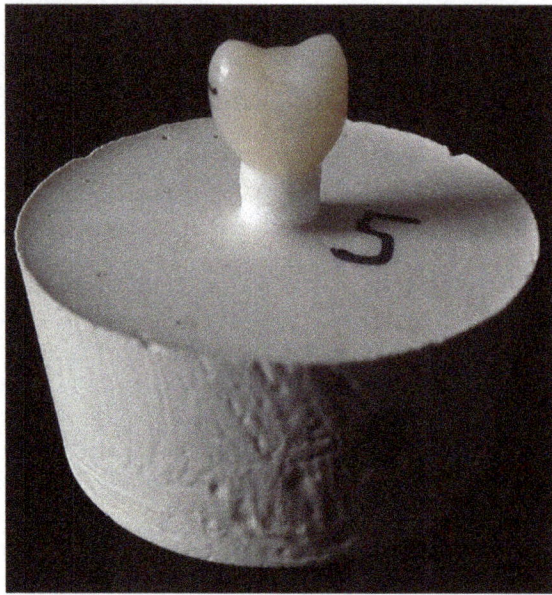

Fig. 1 Luted crown on embedded implant before chewing simulation

specimen. The indenter slid 1.5 mm down the inner cliff of the vestibular cusp and 0.5 mm horizontally toward the central fossa at a speed of 60 mm/s each. Five specimens underwent CS at the same time.

The specimens from the control group did not undergo CS. Failure was defined as fracture within the system (crown or implant) or loosening of the crowns during or after CS.

Wear behavior after long-term mechanical loading

After CS, replicas were produced in the same way as before CS. A commercially available dough, aluminum holder (SEM Specimen Stubs, Agar Scientific, Essex, UK), and foam pellets allowed four replicas to be attached at the same time to the tubes of the Micro-CT (Fig. 2). One single specimen could not be scanned due to a mistake during grouting.

For the generation of 3D data sets from the scans of the Micro-CT, the program NRecon v.1.6.10.4 (Bruker

Table 1 Micro-CT scanning parameters of the replicas before and after CS

Voltage	60 kV
Amperage	167 µA
Filter	No filter
Angle step	0.7°
Scanning resolution	Large pixel scan, 960 × 666 pixels
Rotation angle	180 °
Voxel size	14.985 µm
Frame averaging	20
Random shift	10

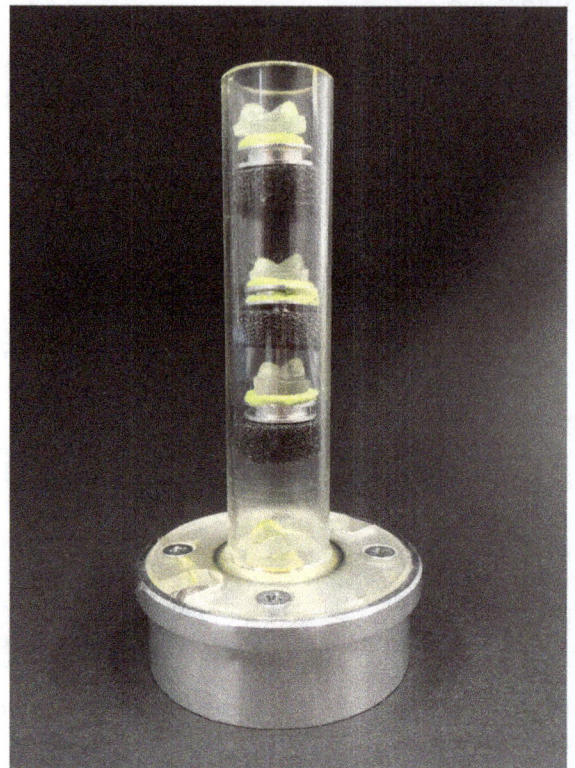

Fig. 2 Four replicas on specimen stubs and foam pellets in the sample holder of the Micro-CT

microCT) was employed. The software could reduce ring artifacts by 20 (Ring Artifact Correction). Beam hardening correction was set to 60 %.

For volume assessment of abrasion, each 3D data set was segmented before and after CS in CTAn (CTAnalyzer V.1.15.4.0, Bruker microCT). Both data sets were overlapped, and the remaining volume of abrasion quantified in pixels and converted into cubic millimeters.

The maximum wear depth was determined by "blowing up" virtual bullets within the surface of abrasion. The diameter of the most massive bullet (at the spot of maximum wear depth) was measured in pixels and converted into millimeters.

The arrow in Fig. 3 shows the maximum wear depth after CS. Volume wear is demonstrated as a yellow surface. Descriptive statistical analysis was applied.

In addition to quantifying wear behavior, one specimen from the test group was randomly selected for analyzing qualitative wear behavior with a scanning electron microscope (SEM, REM, Phenom™ G2 pro, Phenom-World). Before SEM imaging, the crown was gold-coated (2 nm, Sputter Coater MSC1, Ingenieurbüro Peter Liebscher, Wetzlar, Germany) to prevent accumulation of electrostatic charge.

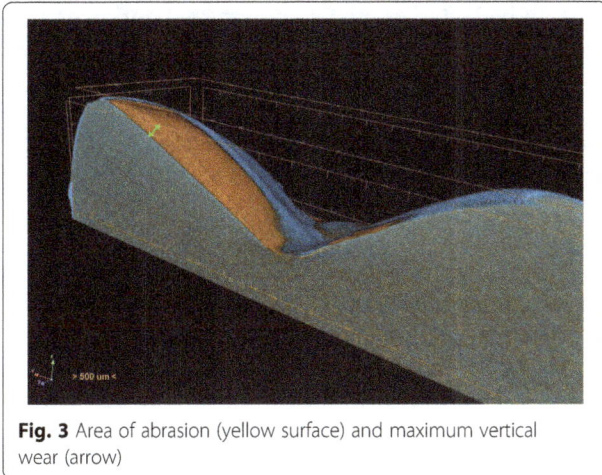

Fig. 3 Area of abrasion (yellow surface) and maximum vertical wear (arrow)

Pull-out forces and localization of luting agent

The crowns were removed from the implants using a universal testing machine (Z010, Zwick GmbH&Co.KG, Ulm, Germany). To do so, the embedded specimens (crown + implant) were placed in a specially built device and covered with a base metal alloy which was specially created as well. A preload of 1 N was applied vertically to the crown followed by traction of 0.75 mm/min. Load at breakage/removal was recorded. The bond strength from the specimens from both the control group without CS ($n = 5$) and the experimental group after CS ($n = 20$) was measured.

Luting agents on both the crown and the implant after CS were localized under a stereomicroscope (Stemi 2000-C, Zeiss, Karlsruhe, Germany). Representative pictures of each crown and implant were taken, and a percentage of luting agent on crown and implant was recorded descriptively.

Statistical analysis

The statistical analyses were performed using GNU Project (2015) (GNU PSPP (Version 0.8.5) [Computer Software]. Free Software Foundation. Boston, MA). The Kolmogorov-Smirnov test, visual inspection of the distribution of the data in histograms as well as in quantile-quantile plots, was applied to verify if the data were normally distributed. The ANOVA test was used to analyze the differences in the mean level of the four rounds of CS concerning bond strength, maximum vertical wear, and volume wear of the experimental groups. A t-test for independent samples was performed to find differences in bond strength between the experimental and the control group. Student's t-test was applied assuming no different variants between control and experimental group as no empirical difference of the variances was observed ($p = 0.755$, Levene's test). The exact confidence interval was calculated according to Clopper-Pearson.

Results

1. No failure occurred as none of the tested crowns or implants was fractured or loosened during or after CS.
2. The tested crowns showed a maximum wear depth of $M = 0.31 \pm 0.04$ mm (mean ± SD) and volume wear of $M = 0.74 \pm 0.23$ mm^3 (mean ± SD). Table 2 shows the mean and standard deviation of assessed parameters (pull-out forces, maximum wear, volume wear) of each round of CS. Abrasion was macroscopically observed.
   The Kolmogorov-Smirnov test and a visual inspection of the histograms and the quantile-quantile plot showed no significant divergence from the normal distribution in any of the groups (maximum wear depth after CS, volume wear after CS, pull-off forces without and after CS).
3. One-way ANOVA showed differences neither in pull-out forces $F(3,16) = 0.02$, $p = 0.997$, nor in maximum wear $F(3,15) = 0.39$, $p = 0.764$, or volume wear $F(3,15) = 0.77$, $p = 0.530$, among the four rounds of CS (Table 3), thereby demonstrating stable and comparable conditions within all rounds of CS.
4. In the pull-out tests, the crowns from the control group were removed from the implants at a 1.8 times higher load ($M = 588.4 \pm 57.7$ N) than the crowns of the experimental group ($M = 322.8 \pm 61.9$ N). Therefore, the bond strength of the control group was significantly higher than the bond strength of the experimental group ($t(23) = 8.69$, $p < 0.001$). Table 4 shows the resulting characteristics of PICN crowns on one-piece zirconia implants.
5. Under the stereomicroscope, approximately 90% of the luting agent could be stereomicroscopically located in the crowns, not on the implants. Figure 4 shows the luting agent situated mostly in the crown (a) and only sparsely on the implant (b).
6. The crowns' surface of abrasion revealed avulsion and a rough surface under SEM. The polished surface and the surface of abrasion do not appear similar. Figure 5 shows SEM images of the mesial margin of abrasion under topography (a) and material contrast (b).

Table 2 Mean (standard deviation) of assessed parameters

CS round (n)	Pull-out forces	Maximum wear	Volume wear
#1 (5)	319.6 (75.4)	0.33 (0.05)	0.88 (0.31)
#2 (5)	326.2 (75.0)	0.30 (0.04)	0.71 (0.20)
#3 (5)	319.4 (43.9)	0.32 (0.03)	0.68 (0.18)
#4 (5)	325.9 (69.8)	0.31 (0.07)*	0.69 (0.27)*

*Only four specimens could be analyzed due to a mistake during grouting
n number of samples per round

Table 3 Stability of conditions across four CS rounds

ANOVA results	Pull-out forces	Maximum wear	Volume wear
F (df)	0.02 (3, 16)	0.39 (3, 15)	0.77 (3, 15)
p value	0.997	0.764	0.530

No statistically significant differences were observed between rounds (testing the null hypothesis that means are similar across all four rounds of CS). This supports stability and comparability of the experiments

Discussion

To the best of our knowledge, it was the first time that the biomechanical properties of polymer-infiltrated ceramic crowns on one-piece zirconia implants after long-term chewing simulation were examined. The present in vitro study investigated the biomechanical properties concerning surface wear and bond strength. No fractures occurred during long-term chewing simulation, and the abrasion of the crowns was macroscopically visible. There are several reasons for the fracture resistance:

Firstly, the layer thickness prescribed by the manufacturer could be strictly adhered to.

Due to the sizes of the probational implants, enough friction surfaces on the implants could be ensured and fracture and debonding was less likely.

Lastly, the occlusal force of 50 N appointed in the chewing simulator is distinctly lower than the maximum in vivo bite force of approximately 700 N [8]. 50 N roughly imitates light biting [9].

El Zhawi et al. also investigated wear and fatigue fracture of PICN crowns (Vita Enamic) but attached to composite abutments instead of zirconia implants [10]. They tested VE crowns after long- and short-term biomechanical loading. The specimens from the long-term mechanical loading group, which are most likely to be compared to our study, did not undergo any pull-off

Table 4 Characteristics of polymer-infiltrated ceramic crowns on one-piece zirconia implants

Characteristics	Total n	Observations
With CS		
System fractured	20	0% (95% CI 0–16.8%)
Crowns loosened	20	0% (95% CI 0–16.8%)
Maximum wear depth	19	0.31 mm (0.04 mm)
Volume wear	19	0.74 mm^3 (0.23 mm^3)
Bond strength (pull-out test)	20	322.8 N (61.9 N)*
Without CS		
Bond strength (pull-out test)	5	588.4 N (57.7 N)*

If not stated otherwise, means (standard deviations) of assessed parameters are shown

*$p < 0.001$ for comparing the effect of performing a CS (experimental group) vs. performing no CS (control group) on bond strength according to the null hypothesis of no difference between both groups

tests. In both studies, no failure occurred during or after mechanical loading. A remarkable difference between the results of both studies was seen in surface wear of the crowns which was much higher in our study despite the lower load of 50 N instead of 200 N. The materials' characteristics may explain the relatively high wear of the crowns. Compared to composites and dentin-like materials, zirconia is a very rigid material. During chewing simulation, the implant does not move so there is only one component of the system to absorb the occlusal force which may result in high wear. Even though surface wear was macroscopically visible, abrasion may also prevent the system from catastrophic failure, namely, fractures in the implant.

In the study of Naumova et al., volume and vertical wear of PICN crowns, compared to other materials such as a nanoceramic resin and a lithium silicate reinforced ceramic after CS, were tested [11]. They used the same settings of CS as in the present study, but the crowns were luted to extracted molars instead of implants and extracted molars as antagonists were used as well. Concerning volume and vertical wear after CS, PICN crowns showed the lowest cusp abrasion, much lower than in our study. Due to the use of abutment teeth instead of dental implants, the results cannot be compared to ours.

Mörmann et al. compared the surface wear of different dental ceramics including Vita Enamic [12] after the same type of mechanical loading as in the present study. The results showed similar wear to other CAD/CAM materials as well as to human enamel. Since enamel of extracted molars was used as indenters in this study, it cannot be compared directly to our procedure. Nevertheless, a remarkable difference could be found in the results of the SEM images. Mörmann et al. described the surface of abrasion as similar to the polished surface [12], which cannot be found in our specimen.

According to Lauvahutanon et al., PICN crowns show minor wear compared to direct restorations made of composite [13].

Until now, there have been numerous publications on VE [3–6, 10–24] but only one study has investigated the combination with zirconia implants [5] where fracture strength of VE and feldspathic ceramic on zirconia implants was compared using different luting agents. Fracture strength was tested by applying an axial force to the specimen until fracture. The results showed higher fracture strength of VE. The samples were placed in distilled water for 24 h after cementing, so no dynamic loading occurred. Due to the different study designs—no pull-off forces, no dynamic loading, and no wear tests—it cannot be compared to ours.

The missing comparison to other PICN materials can be considered a limitation of the study. Since VE is a

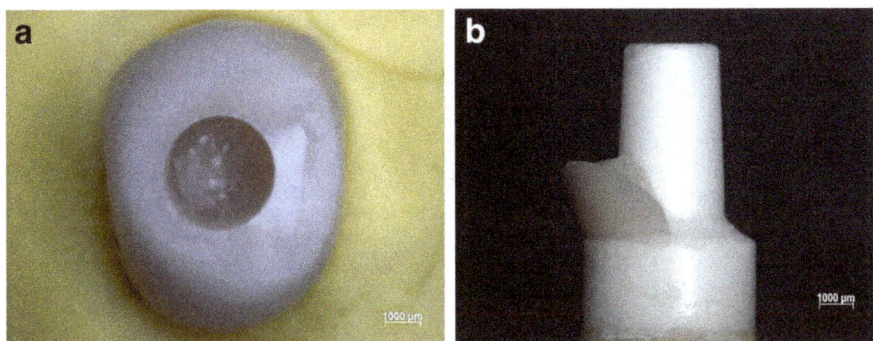

Fig. 4 Luting agent located mostly in the crown (**a**) and only sparsely on the implant (**b**). A crown fragment is remaining on the implant

unicum in the family of PICN materials, it is difficult to find an appropriate material of comparison, especially since Lava Ultimate (3M Espe), a resin nanoceramic, is no longer indicated as a crown material due to a high rate of loosening. The review of Mainjot et al. reported that the loosening has mostly occurred when bonded to zirconia and that there is a lack of studies concerning bonding of VE to other ceramics [25].

Although the sample size of this pilot study is limited (due to the practicability reasons associated with the applied procedures), the standard deviations are low, which improved the statistical power of our analysis.

Surface wear of replicas of the superstructure's occlusal was assessed by Micro-CT instead of the crowns themselves. This was done to entrench the Micro-CT as a clinical method to quantify abrasion. Using a Micro-CT for quantifying abrasion could be a non-invasive option without radiation exposure for the patient. Additionally, the grouting material (Stycast Epoxidharz) exhibits a very low viscosity of 0.65 Pa s [26] and therefore a high flowability even in small volumes which can result in exact replicas.

The use of spherical steatite indenter during CS instead of natural teeth with their anatomy and composition may be a limitation of the study.

Abrasion may depend on the type of construction as well. Wear of VE crowns on one-piece zirconia implants seems different from wear of VE crowns on dentin-like materials [10]. This aspect should be investigated in further studies.

Conclusions

The present study demonstrates that elastic PICN crowns on rigid one-piece zirconia implants seem to be a promising material combination for clinical practice. Though the crowns suffered major wear after CS, the stability was not affected, and no catastrophic failure occurred. However, clinical trials are essential to examine the behavior of the material combination, especially in comparison to other restorative materials.

Micro-CT for replicas proved to be able to measure surface wear of dental restorations.

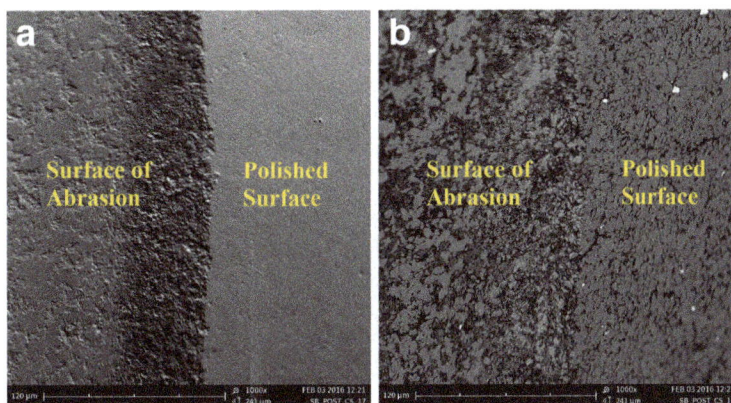

Fig. 5 SEM images of the mesial margin of abrasion under topography contrast (**a**) and material contrast (**b**)

Abbreviations

3D: Three-dimensional space; ANOVA: Analysis of variance; CAD/CAM: Computer-aided design/computer-aided manufacturing; CI: confidence interval (exact) according to Clopper-Pearson; CS: Chewing simulation; df: degrees of freedom; et al.: Et alii/et aliae/et alia; F: F test; M: Mean; Micro-CT: X-ray micro-computed tomography; n: Number; p: p value; PICN: Polymer-infiltrated ceramic network; SD: Standard deviation; SEM: Scanning electron microscope; VE: Vita Enamic

Acknowledgements

The authors would like to thank T. Meißner for the lab support.

Funding

Not applicable

Authors' contributions

PB carried out the material studies, participated in the statistical analyses, collaborated the manuscript, and made revision. HK performed the statistical analysis. RH was revising it critically for important intellectual content. CO conceived of the study, participated in its design and coordination, drafted the manuscript, and made revision. All authors read and approved the final manuscript.

Competing interests

Pia Baumgart, Holger Kirsten, Rainer Haak, and Constanze Olms declare that they have no competing interests.

Author details

[1]Department of Dental Prosthodontics and Materials Science, University of Leipzig, Liebigstraße 12, Haus 1, 04103 Leipzig, Germany. [2]Institute for Medical Informatics, Statistics, and Epidemiology (IMISE), Haertelstraße 16-18, 04107 Leipzig, Germany. [3]LIFE Research Center for Civilization Diseases, University of Leipzig, Philipp-Rosenthal-Straße 27, 04103 Leipzig, Germany. [4]Department of Cariology, Endodontology and Periodontology, University of Leipzig, Liebigstraße 12, Haus 1, 04103 Leipzig, Germany. [5]Department of Dental Prosthodontics and Materials Science, University of Leipzig, Liebigstraße 12, Haus 1, 04103 Leipzig, Germany.

References

1. Guess PR, Att W, Strub JR. Zirconia in Fixed Implant Prosthodontics. Clin Implant Dent Relat Res. 2012;14:633-45
2. Wilson TG Jr. The Positive Relationship Between Excess Cement and Peri-Implant Disease: A prospective Clinical Endoscopic Study. J Periodontol. 2009;80:1388-92.
3. Schwenter J, Schmidli F, Weiger R, Fischer J. Adhesive bonding to polymer infiltrated ceramic. Dent Mater J. 2016;35:796-802.
4. Coldea A, Swain MV, Thiel N. Hertzian contact response and damage tolerance of dental ceramics. J Mech Behav Biomed Mater. 2014;34:124-33.
5. Rohr N, Coldea A, Zitzmann NU, Fischer J. Loading capacity of zirconia implant-supported hybrid ceramic crowns. Dent Mater. 2015;31:279-88.
6. He L-H, Swain M. A Novel polymer infiltrated ceramic dental material. Dent Mater. 2011;27:527-34.
7. Ali SAM, Manoharan PS, Shekhawat KS, Deb S, Chidambaram S, Konchada J, et al. Influence of full veneer restoration on fracture resistance of three different core materials: an in vitro study. J Clin Diagn Res. 2015;9:12-5.
8. Xu L, Fan S, Cai B, Fang Z, Jiang X. Influence of sustained submaximal clenching fatigue test on electromyographic activity and maximum voluntary bite forces in healthy subjects and patients with temporomandibular disorders. J Oral Rehabil. 2017;44:340-6.
9. Kayumi S, Takayama Y, Yokoyama A, Ueda N. Effect of bite force in occlusal adjustment of dental implants on the distribution of occlusal pressure: comparison among three bite forces in occlusal adjustment. Int J Implant Dent. 2015;1:14.
10. El Zhawi H, Kaizer MR, Chughtai A, Moraes RR, Zhang Y. Polymer infiltrated ceramic network structures for resistance to fatigue fracture and wear. Dent Mater. 2016;32:1352-61.
11. Naumova EA, Schneider S, Arnold WH, Piwowarczyk A. Wear behavior of ceramic CAD/CAM crowns and natural antagonists. Materials (Basel). 2017;10:244.
12. Mörmann WH, Stawarczyk B, Ender A, Sener B, Attin T, Mehl A. Wear characteristics of current aesthetic dental restorative CAD/CAM materials: two-body wear, gloss retention, roughness and Martens hardness. J Mech Behav Biomed Mater. 2013;20:113-25.
13. Lauvahutanon S, Takahashi H, Oki M, Arksornnukit M, Kanehira M, Finger W. In vitro evaluation of the wear resistance of composite resin blocks for CAD/CAM. Dent Mater J. 2015;34:495-502.
14. Coldea A, Swain MV, Thiel N. Mechanical properties of polymer-infiltrated-ceramic-network materials. Dent Mater. 2013;29:419-26.
15. Dirxen C, Blunck U, Preissner S. Clinical performance of a new biomimetic double network material. Open Dent J. 2013;7:118-22.
16. Della Bona A, Corazza PH, Zhang Y. Characterization of a polymer-infiltrated ceramic-network material. Dent Mater. 2014;30:564-9.
17. Keul C, Muller-Hahl M, Eichberger M, Liebermann A, Roos M, Edelhoff D, et al. Impact of different adhesives on work of adhesion between CAD/CAM polymers and resin composite cements. J Dent. 2014;42:1105-14.
18. Albero A, Pascual A, Camps I, Grau-Benitez M. Comparative characterization of a novel cad-cam polymer-infiltrated-ceramic-network. J Clin Exp Dent. 2015;7:495-500.
19. Elsaka SE. Repair bond strength of resin composite to a novel CAD/CAM hybrid ceramic using different repair systems. Dent Mater J. 2015;34:161-7.
20. Frankenberger R, Hartmann VE, Krech M, Krämer N, Reich S, Braun A, Roggendorf M. Adhesive luting of new CAD/CAM materials. Int J Comput Dent. 2015;18:9-20.
21. Aboushelib MN, Elsafi MH. Survival of resin infiltrated ceramics under influence of fatigue. Dent Mater. 2016;32:529-34.
22. Güngör MB, Nemli SK, Bal BT, Ünver S, Doğan A. Effect of surface treatments on shear bond strength of resin composite bonded to CAD/CAM resin-ceramic hybrid materials. J Adv Prosthodont. 2016;8:259-66.
23. Özarslan MM, Büyükkaplan UŞ, Barutcigil Ç, Arslan M, Türker N, Barutcigil K. Effects of different surface finishing procedures on the change in surface roughness and color of a polymer infiltrated ceramic network material. J Adv Prosthodont. 2016;8:16-20.
24. Tassin M, Bonte E, Loison-Robert LS, Nassif A, Berbar T, Le Goff S, et al. Effects of high-temperature-pressure polymerized resin-infiltrated ceramic networks on oral stem cells. PLoS One. 2016;11
25. Mainjot AK, Dupont NM, Oudkerk JC, Dewael TY, Sadoun MJ. From artisanal to CAD-CAM blocks: state of the art of indirect composites. J Dent Res. 2016;95:487-95.
26. Emerson & Cuming: STYCAST® 1266. Two component, low viscosity, epoxy encapsulant 2003.

10

Effectiveness and compliance of an oscillating-rotating toothbrush in patients with dental implants

Giuseppe Allocca[1], Diana Pudylyk[1], Fabrizio Signorino[1*] ⓘ, Giovanni Battista Grossi[2] and Carlo Maiorana[1]

Abstract

Background: The aim of this randomized clinical trial was to assess the efficacy of an oscillating-rotating toothbrush in reducing plaque and inflammation around dental implants.

Methods: Eighty patients presenting dental implants were enrolled in this study and assigned randomly to two different groups: 40 patients in the test group and 40 in the control one. Each patient in the test group received an oscillating-rotating toothbrush while in the control group patients kept using the manual toothbrush. Furthermore, the test group received a special toothbrush head designed for dental implants and another one for natural teeth. Domiciliary oral hygiene instructions were given to both groups. Periodontal parameters like plaque index (PI), bleeding on probing (BoP), and probing pocket depth (PPD) were recorded at the baseline and after 1 and 3 months.

Results: At the end of the study, the difference of plaque and bleeding indices with the baseline was statistically significant for both test and control groups ($P < 0.0001$). Implant sites showed higher values of both BoP and PI when compared to the natural teeth. In the second part of the study, comparing the 1–3-month period, the oscillating-rotating toothbrush was effective in reducing new plaque formation ($P < 0.0001$) and bleeding ($P < 0.0001$) both at the implant sites and the dental sites comparing to manual ones ($P > 0.05$). No significant differences were appreciated concerning the PPD.

Conclusions: The oscillating-rotating toothbrush can be successfully used for the plaque and bleeding control of the peri-implant tissues.

Keywords: Dental implant, Domiciliary hygiene, Electric toothbrush, Implant maintenance, Oral hygiene

Background

Dental implants became one of the most accepted treatments for the rehabilitation of partial or complete edentulism [1]. However, inflammatory processes may still occur due to the presence of the implant itself [2]. It is well known that peri-mucositis and peri-implantitis are strictly related to the presence of plaque on the surface of the implant-prosthetic complex, which lead respectively to the inflammation of peri-implant soft tissues and the bone loss around the implant neck area [3, 4]. The problem of implant maintenance must be taken in serious consideration even before the dental implant placement. Many risk factors have been associated to peri-implantitis such as smoke, diabetes, and a history of periodontal disease [5–8]. Furthermore, the prevalence of this pathology is rising. It has been estimated, in fact, that a range from 10 to 43% of all implants placed today will have some form of peri-implantitis in about 10 years [9, 10]. Many authors associated the microbiological flora responsible of peri-implantitis to the one associated to periodontal disease, while others confuted this hypothesis [11].

---

* Correspondence: fabroski@hotmail.it
[1]Center for Edentulism and Jaw Atrophies, Maxillofacial Surgery and Dentistry Unit, Fondazione IRCCS Cà Granda – Ospedale Maggiore Policlinico, University of Milan, Via Commenda 10, 20122 Milan, Italy

Many techniques and protocols have been introduced for the treatment of peri-implantitis; however, the topic is still debated and the different rates of success of various treatments still suggest that a good prevention must still be preferred [12]. The presence of bacterial microfilm on the implant surface has been individuated as the primary cause of the pathologic mechanism. As well as in the teeth, mechanical removal represents the only treatment able to remove the microfilm and toothbrush and dental floss are the only effective domiciliary devices able to remove plaque from the teeth and dental implant. Mouth rinses or other methods may enhance periodontal indices but only when associated to an effective primary mechanic removal device. It has also been proved how both manual and electric toothbrushes are effective in the plaque removal [13]. Several authors comparing the two devices were not able to find any differences in term of clinical results, while others found advantages for one technique with respect to the other [14–17]. Patients with motor problems and elderly may found benefit in using the electric toothbrush, which does not require the same level of manual skills as the manual one [18, 19]. Recently, there has been introduced a new type of electric toothbrush, with a visual-sound system, showing the correct pressure to apply when brushing and the exact amount of time necessary to complete one or half dental arch. Special designed toothbrush heads for different areas of the mouth and different surfaces, like dental implants, have recently been introduced for electric toothbrushes without a clear scientific support. The present study aims to investigate the efficacy of an oscillating-rotating toothbrush using a dedicated designed head, in patients with dental implants.

Methods

The study was conducted between September 2015 and June 2017 at Implantology Department of Policlinic Hospital, University of Milan, Milan. It was designed as a monocentric randomized clinical study according to the STROBE criteria. Eighty patients who underwent dental implant rehabilitation were selected for this study. At the screening visit, subjects were asked to read and sign a written informed consent and personal medical history and demographic information was obtained. Dental implants must have been placed at least 1 year before the recruitment; other inclusion criteria were age between 18 and 90 and a good general health. Patients with orthodontic therapy or removable prosthesis, including overdenture type, were not included in the study as well as non-controlled diabetic or heavy smoker (> 10 cigarettes) patients. The patients were already following a maintenance program after the implant placement; however, all of them

were using the manual toothbrush for domiciliary oral hygiene. After being included in the study, each patient underwent periodontal (North Carolina) and peri-implant (perio probe) charting and recording of bleeding and plaque indexes (gingival bleeding index and plaque control record). Gingival bleeding index and plaque control record were recoded as the presence/absence of bleeding or plaque on four sites per tooth/implant. In order to detect the plaque, a disclosing agent was used. Sequentially, dental hygienist performed professional prophylaxis to establish a plaque free dentition. A software program randomly assigned 40 patients for both test and control groups. The electric toothbrush (Oral-B® ProfessionalCare 6000 with Bluetooth; Oral-B®, Procter & Gamble, Cincinnati, OH, United States) was introduced to patients of the test group, and instructions were given. According to the producer instruction, the procedure must have lasted not less than 2 min, using a timer set on 30 s for quadrant, twice/day. Furthermore, all the patients received a special toothbrush head designed for dental implants (Interspace; Oral-B®) together with another one for the natural teeth (Precision clean; Oral-B®) (Fig. 1). The patients of the control group did not change the manual toothbrush as a domiciliary oral hygiene device and received instructions of the modified Bass technique. The recommended time for toothbrushing was at least 90 s, twice a day. Patients of both groups received all the information in a paper copy. Once verified that the patients understood the instructions, new appointments were scheduled after 1 and 3 months. Bleeding on probing, plaque index, and probing depth were recorded at each visit on both dental implants and natural teeth. The entire

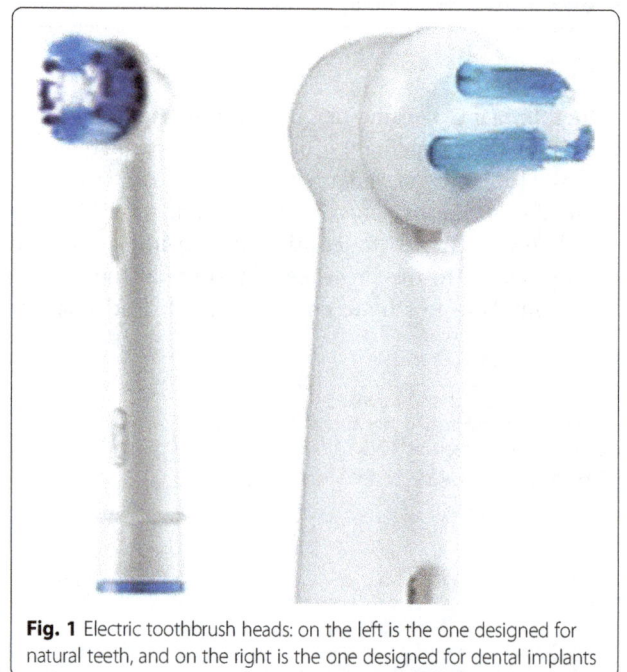

Fig. 1 Electric toothbrush heads: on the left is the one designed for natural teeth, and on the right is the one designed for dental implants

sample had to use the same toothpaste to reduce the variability of the results.

Statistical analysis

Mean scores of all clinical indices for each subject were calculated separately for dental implants and natural teeth. The final data analysis was performed for those subjects who completed the study. The Student's t test and the Mann-Whitney U test were used to evaluate whether any statistically significant differences were present between the two groups at each time point, and the Wilcoxon signed-rank test was performed to verify if any statistically significant changes occurred from baseline within each group. A total sample size of 74 patients (37 per group) achieves 81% power to detect a difference of 0.2 between the differences of group means with group standard deviations of 0.3. P values < 0.05 were considered statistically significant.

Results

Seventy-eight patients successfully completed the study (45 women and 33 men aged from 31 to 76 years old) (Fig. 2). Two patients of test group did not show up both at the first and second controls. No patients were excluded or showed complications or adverse reaction. Results are shown in Table 1. The average number of implants per patients was 4.8 ± 3.4 in the control group and 4.4 ± 2.9 in the test one. Single crowns, implant-supported bridges, and Toronto bridge were included in both of the study groups. The values taken in consideration were recorded for both the dental implants and the rest of the dentition and compared at each time. All dental implant index values were higher when compared to the natural teeth ones while no differences were appreciable concerning the PPD. The study provided data for the test and control

groups at three different time points. Analyzing the results, it can be observed for both groups a high decrease of BoP and PI values after 1 month after the baseline, related to the prophylaxis performed by dental hygienist.

The second part of the study described the re-colonization of dental implants and teeth surfaces: this was related to the proper use of oral hygiene devices, showing the effective difference of the manual and electric toothbrushes in preventing the new plaque formation and the consequent inflammation status.

Plaque index

The difference of PI recorded around implants at the beginning and the end of the study was statistically significant for both control and test groups ($P < 0.0001$). Observing in detail the second part of the study in Fig. 3, it was possible to observe how the test group kept reducing ($P < 0.0001$) while the control showed a mild increase ($P = 0.68$). Comparison at 3 months showed statistical significance ($P < 0.05$).

In Fig. 4 is shown the PI recorded around natural teeth: in this case, comparing the baseline with the data collected after 3 months was possible to observe high statistical significance only for the test ($P < 0.0001$) and significance for the control ($P < 0.05$; $P = 0.031$). Highlighting the second part, the different trend of test and control lines confirmed the higher performances of test devices ($P < 0.0001$) compared to the control that showed a mild increase ($P = 0.16$). Comparison between the two groups at 3 months was highly statistically significant ($P < 0.0001$).

Bleeding on probing

The difference between the BoP recorded on dental implant sites at baseline and the end of the study showed statistical significance for both the test and

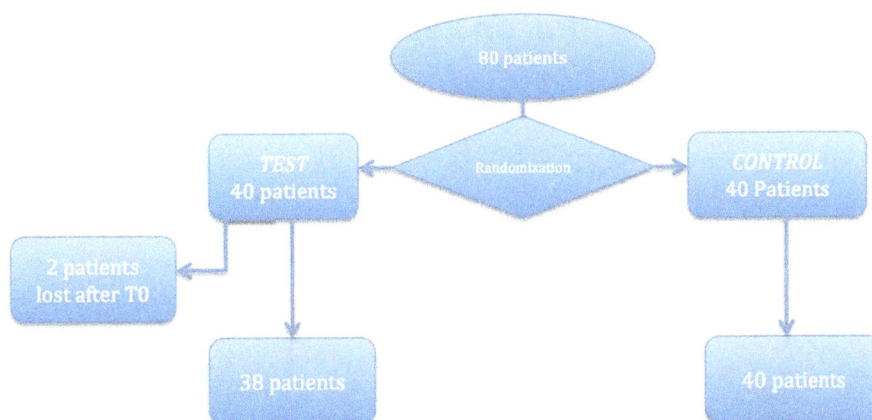

Fig. 2 Patients' population flow chart

Table 1 BoP, PI, and PPD mean values at baseline, 1 month, and 3 months

	Baseline	1 month	3 months
	T0	T1	T2
BoP implants, test	46.55% ± 18.41%	32.31% ± 13.27%	22.18% ± 11.06%
BoP implants, control	32% ± 24.88%	19.84% ± 15.52%	19.11% ± 17.30%
BoP teeth, test	18.81% ± 15.93%	8.76% ± 8.11%	6.5% ± 5.18%
BoP teeth, control	21.61% ± 15.38%	15.50% ± 12.21%	16.38% ± 11.79%
PI implants, test	53.71% ± 14.72%	33.65% ± 12.57%	15.52% ± 12.29%
PI implants, control	50.13% ± 27.39%	28.66% ± 16.26%	32.68% ± 16.02%
PI teeth, test	33.15% ± 13.49%	20.76% ± 10.16%	14.5% ± 6.74%
PI teeth, control	41.34% ± 17.20%	32.26% ± 15.02%	35.77% ± 15.80%
PPD implants, test	2.73 mm ± 0.59 mm	2.67 mm ± 0.5 mm	2.61 mm ± 0.54 mm
PPD implants, control	2.4 mm ± 0.97 mm	2.22 mm ± 0.57 mm	2.21 mm ± 0.66 mm
PPD teeth, test	1.7 mm ± 0.47 mm	1.69 mm ± 0.38 mm	1.69 mm ± 0.4 mm
PPD teeth, control	2.01 mm ± 0.67 mm	1.93 mm ± 0.58 mm	2.04 mm ± 0.52 mm

Data are shown as mean ± standard deviation
test electric toothbrush with the two different heads designed for dental implants and natural teeth, *control* manual toothbrush

control groups ($P < 0.0001$) (Fig. 5). Analyzing in detail the 1–3-month period, it was observed how only the test group showed a statistical significance ($P < 0.0001$) while the control lost it ($P = 0.709$). At 3 months, no significative differences between the two groups were observed ($P = 0.564$).

Analog situation could be observed in Fig. 6, representing BoP around the natural teeth. In this case, the difference with the baseline were significant for both groups ($P < 0.0001$ and $P = 0.007$ respectively for test and control). In the second part of the observation period (1–3-month period), it was possible to detect an increase for the control ($P = 0.342$) while the test kept decreasing, even if slightly ($P < 0.05$; $P = 0.0021$). The comparison between the test and

control groups after 3 months showed a statistical significance ($P < 0.05$).

Pocket probing depth

No differences during the time points were observed in both test and control groups as clearly shown in Figs. 7 and 8. It was possible to observe a reduction of PPD of 0.15 mm between the beginning and end of the study around dental implants on both test and control groups.

Discussion

This 3-month study aimed to demonstrate the efficacy of an electric toothbrush in reducing plaque and gingival inflammation around dental implants

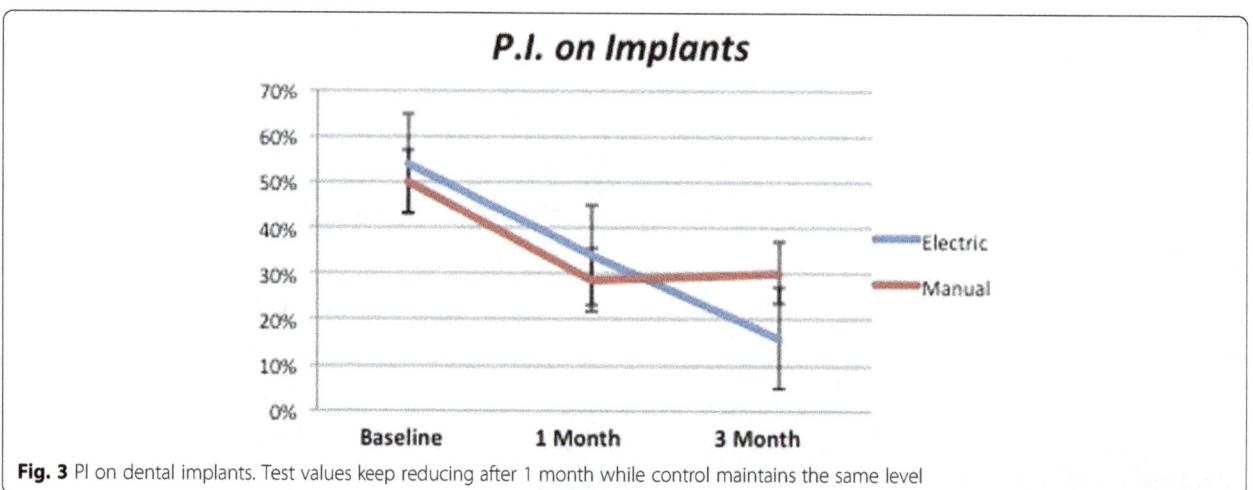

Fig. 3 PI on dental implants. Test values keep reducing after 1 month while control maintains the same level

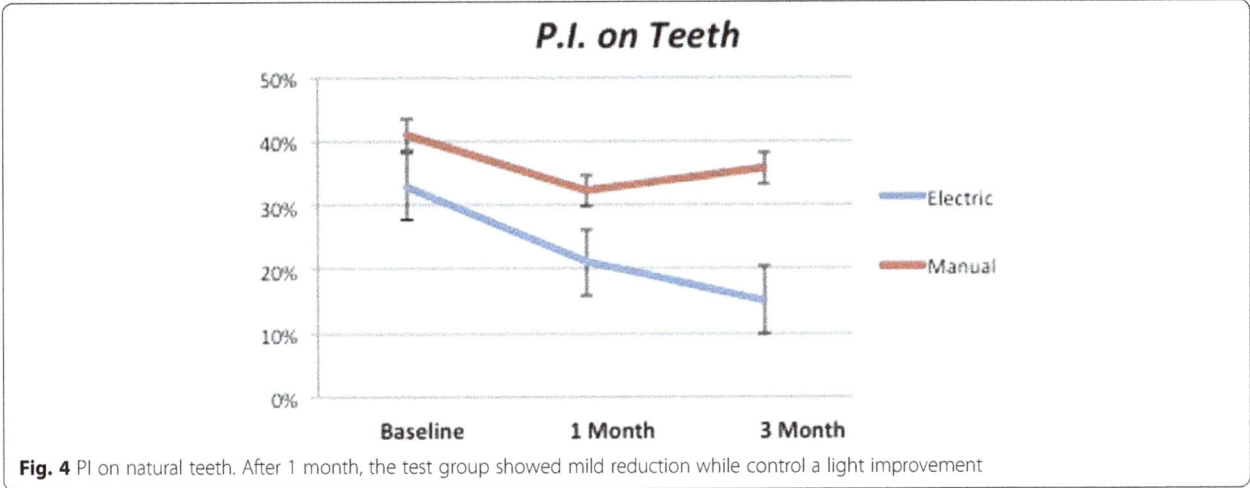

Fig. 4 PI on natural teeth. After 1 month, the test group showed mild reduction while control a light improvement

and natural teeth. To better understand the different data collected around two different anatomical structures, we decided to collect data separately. Analyzing our results, it is possible to observe how the mean values for probing, bleeding, and plaque index were bigger for dental implants. According to literature, it was expected to find deeper probing for dental implants [20]. Many authors associated this to the different kind of attachment and the different orientation of periodontal fiber around dental implants [21–23]. The electric toothbrush has widely been described as a preventive option in the maintenance of peri-implant tissues [24–28]. However, many authors did not observe any differences between the manual and electric toothbrush, and for this reason, the topic is still controversial [17, 19]. In the present study, the manual toothbrush seemed to maintain the

values achieved with the professional prophylaxes; however, a mild increase of both PI and BoP was detected after 3 months. The choice to perform prophylaxis on all patients after baseline index recording was done in order to bring the patients at the same level and reduce the variability of the study according to several authors [29, 30]. As a direct consequence, all the values recorded in both groups resulted to be extremely decreased at the second time point, after 1 month. However, the data collection at the third time point 3 months after the baseline made possible to analyze the new plaque formation trend in both groups and verify the different devices' efficacy on both teeth and implant. The evolution observed over time can be related also to the presence of peri-implant and periodontal pockets. Despite that the average values of PPD were lower

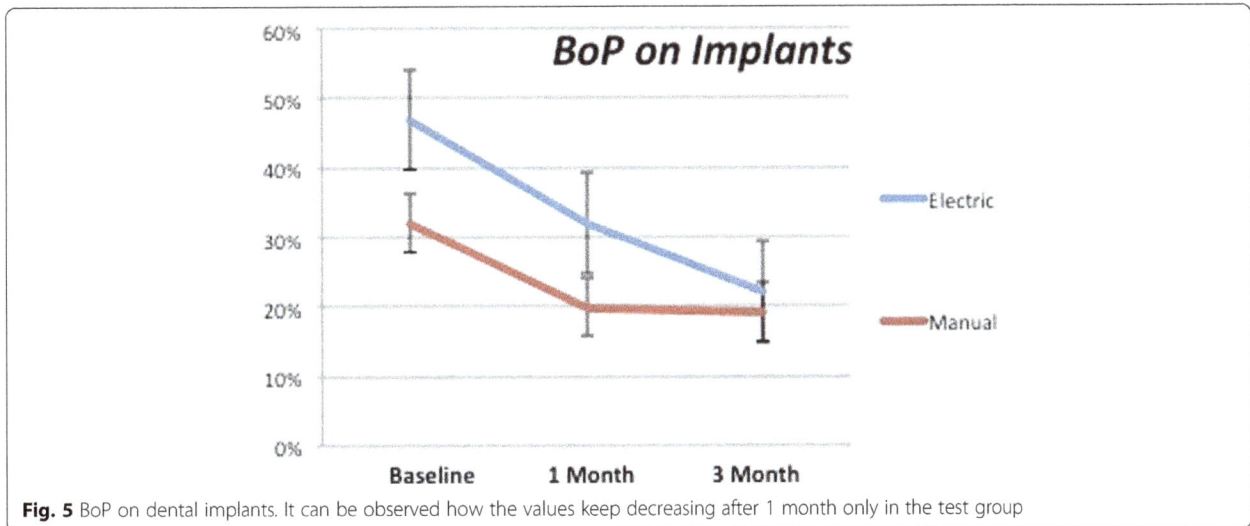

Fig. 5 BoP on dental implants. It can be observed how the values keep decreasing after 1 month only in the test group

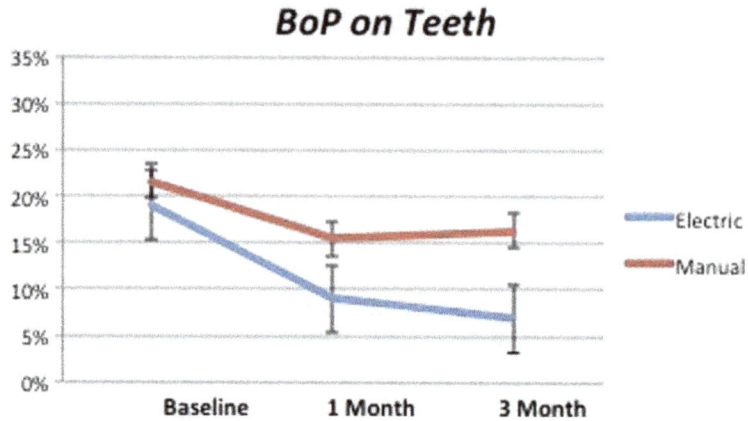

Fig. 6 BoP on natural teeth. While the control group shows a mild increase between 1 month and 3 months, the test group values decrease during all the duration of the study

than 3 mm, patients presenting deeper pockets were included, which might represent a limit of the study. The prophylaxis performed at the beginning of the study, in fact, could not remove adequately the plaque present in the deepest area of these pockets. This prevented the achievement of a "level 0" of PI and BoP and, at the same time, promoted a faster re-colonization. During this time, patients also improved their skills with the electric toothbrush, which have also might influence their motivation. These factors could explain the reduction of PI observed in the second part of the study on the electric toothbrush groups and, sequentially, of the BoP as inflammatory index caused by the presence of plaque itself. The efficacy of the electric toothbrush can be related to the easiness of use and the complexity of artificial movement (rotating-oscillatory), which has been demonstrated to be more effective in plaque removal with respect to the manual toothbrush as reported

by many authors [14, 25, 27]. Many authors observed a 0.3-mm reduction of probing depth after at least 12-month observation period in the patients using the electric toothbrush [26, 28]. Despite in the present study it was observed only 0.15 mm of mean probing reduction for dental implants, our observation was limited only to a 3-month period. This trend could be comparable to a 0.3-mm reduction in 12 months, as observed in the previous studies. However, a similar trend was also detected in the control group so the electric toothbrush cannot be directly related to the PPD reduction.

At the end of the present study, electric toothbrush groups showed plaque and bleeding values lower (PI and BoP on teeth) or at least without significative differences (BoP on implants) than the control group. These data may suggest how the use of electric toothbrush, associated to the dedicate heads, can be an effective method for plaque and bleeding reduction.

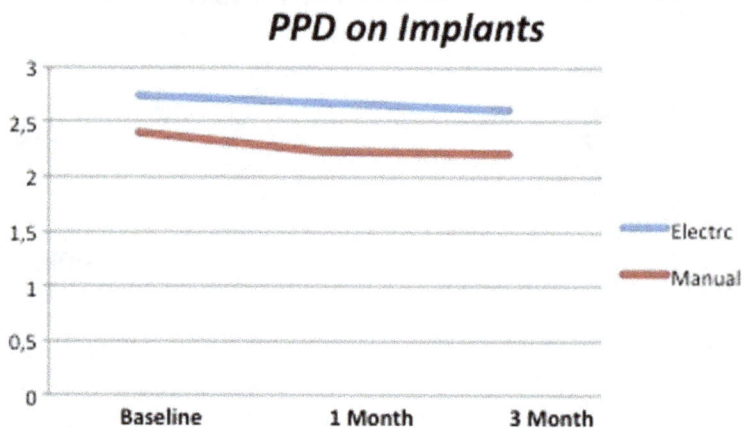

Fig. 7 PPD on dental implants. No significant differences appreciable

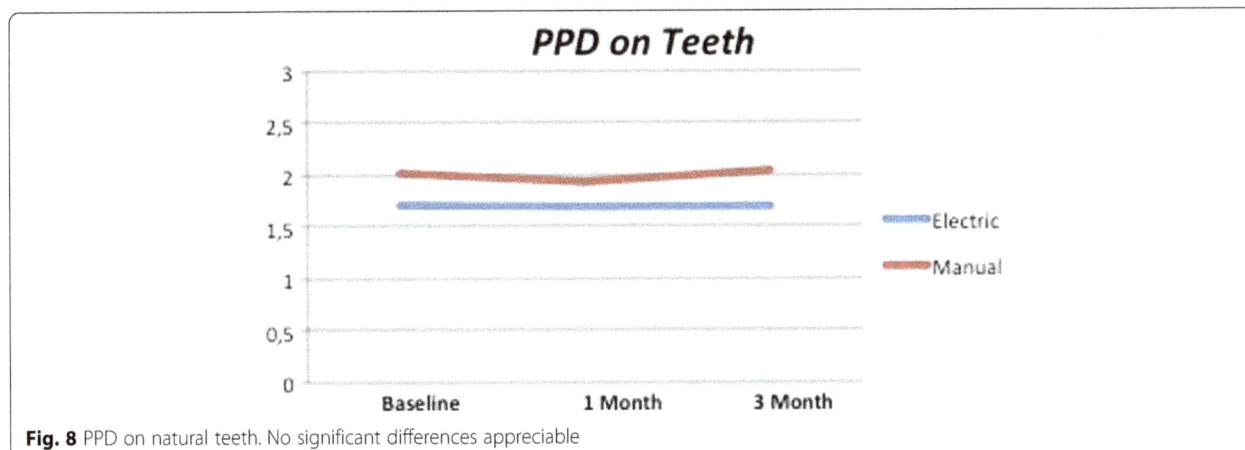

Fig. 8 PPD on natural teeth. No significant differences appreciable

Conclusion

The oscillating-rotating toothbrush can be used for the plaque and bleeding control around both natural teeth and dental implants. It has also been shown how the toothbrush head designed for dental implant can be effective in plaque removing of the peri-implant tissues.

Abbreviations
BoP: Bleeding on probing; PI: Plaque index; PPD: Pocket probing depth

Acknowledgements
Not applicable

Funding
The authors declare no funds for the research.

Authors' contributions
CM and FS designed the study; GA and DP performed the patient treatment and data collection. FS edited the manuscript. GBG performed the data analysis. All authors read and approved the final version of the manuscript.

Authors' information
Not applicable

Competing interests
Giuseppe Allocca, Diana Pudylyk, Fabrizio Signorino, Giovanni Battista Grossi, and Carlo Maiorana declare that they have no competing interests.

Author details
[1]Center for Edentulism and Jaw Atrophies, Maxillofacial Surgery and Dentistry Unit, Fondazione IRCCS Cà Granda – Ospedale Maggiore Policlinico, University of Milan, Via Commenda 10, 20122 Milan, Italy. [2]Oral Surgery, Maxillofacial Surgery and Dentistry Unit, Fondazione IRCCS Cà Granda – Ospedale Maggiore Policlinico, University of Milan, Via Commenda 10, 20122 Milan, Italy.

References
1. Pjetursson BE, Lang NP. Prosthetic treatment planning on the basis of scientific evidence. J Oral Rehabil. 2008;35(Suppl 1):72–9. https://doi.org/10.1111/j.1365-2842.2007.01824.x PubMed PMID: 18181936.
2. Jung RE, Pjetursson BE, Glauser R, Zembic A, Zwahlen M, Lang NP. A systematic review of the 5-year survival and complication rates of implant-supported single crowns. Clin Oral Implants Res. 2008;19(2):119–30. https://doi.org/10.1111/j.1600-0501.2007.01453.x Epub 2007/12/07. PubMed PMID: 18067597.
3. Zhuang LF, Watt RM, Mattheos N, Si MS, Lai HC, Lang NP. Periodontal and peri-implant microbiota in patients with healthy and inflamed periodontal and peri-implant tissues. Clin Oral Implants Res. 2016;27(1):13–21. https://doi.org/10.1111/clr.12508 Epub 2014/11/14. PubMed PMID: 25399962.
4. Lindquist LW, Rockler B, Carlsson GE. Bone resorption around fixtures in edentulous patients treated with mandibular fixed tissue-integrated prostheses. J Prosthet Dent. 1988;59(1):59–63 PubMed PMID: 3422305.
5. Karoussis IK, Kotsovilis S, Fourmousis I. A comprehensive and critical review of dental implant prognosis in periodontally compromised partially edentulous patients. Clin Oral Implants Res. 2007;18(6):669–79. https://doi.org/10.1111/j.1600-0501.2007.01406.x Epub 2007/09/13. PubMed PMID: 17868376.
6. van der Weijden GA, Hioe KP. A systematic review of the effectiveness of self-performed mechanical plaque removal in adults with gingivitis using a manual toothbrush. J Clin Periodontol. 2005;32(Suppl 6):214–28. https://doi.org/10.1111/j.1600-051X.2005.00795.x PubMed PMID: 16128840.
7. Dalago HR, Schuldt Filho G, Rodrigues MA, Renvert S, Bianchini MA. Risk indicators for peri-implantitis. A cross-sectional study with 916 implants. Clin Oral Implants Res. 2017;28(2):144–50. https://doi.org/10.1111/clr.12772 Epub 2016/01/11. PubMed PMID: 26754342.
8. Lindquist LW, Carlsson GE, Jemt T. A prospective 15-year follow-up study of mandibular fixed prostheses supported by osseointegrated implants. Clinical results and marginal bone loss. Clin Oral Implants Res. 1996;7(4):329–36 PubMed PMID: 9151599.
9. Fransson C, Lekholm U, Jemt T, Berglundh T. Prevalence of subjects with progressive bone loss at implants. Clin Oral Implants Res. 2005;16(4):440–6. https://doi.org/10.1111/j.1600-0501.2005.01137.x PubMed PMID: 16117768.
10. Costa FO, Takenaka-Martinez S, Cota LO, Ferreira SD, Silva GL, Costa JE. Peri-implant disease in subjects with and without preventive maintenance: a 5-year follow-up. J Clin Periodontol. 2012;39(2):173–81. https://doi.org/10.1111/j.1600-051X.2011.01819.x Epub 2011/11/23. PubMed PMID: 22111654.
11. Quirynen M, De Soete M, van Steenberghe D. Infectious risks for oral implants: a review of the literature. Clin Oral Implants Res. 2002;13(1):1–19 PubMed PMID: 12005139.
12. Roos-Jansåker AM, Renvert S, Egelberg J. Treatment of peri-implant infections: a literature review. J Clin Periodontol. 2003;30(6):467–85 PubMed PMID: 12795785.
13. Ho HP, Niederman R. Effectiveness of the Sonicare sonic toothbrush on reduction of plaque, gingivitis, probing pocket depth and subgingival bacteria in adolescent orthodontic patients. J Clin Dent 1997;8(1 Spec No):15–19. PubMed PMID: 9487840.
14. Wolff L, Kim A, Nunn M, Bakdash B, Hinrichs J. Effectiveness of a sonic toothbrush in maintenance of dental implants. A prospective study. J Clin Periodontol. 1998;25(10):821–8 PubMed PMID: 9797055.
15. Cronin M, Dembling W, Warren PR, King DW. A 3-month clinical investigation comparing the safety and efficacy of a novel electric toothbrush (Braun Oral-B 3D Plaque Remover) with a manual toothbrush. Am J Dent 1998;11(Spec No):S17–S21. PubMed PMID: 10530095.

16. Quirynen M, Vervliet E, Teerlinck J, Darius P, van Steenberghe D. Medium- and long-term effectiveness of a counterrotational electric toothbrush on plaque removal, gingival bleeding, and probing pocket depth. Int J Periodontics Restorative Dent. 1994;14(4):364–77 PubMed PMID: 7814228.

17. Swierkot K, Brusius M, Leismann D, Nonnenmacher C, Nüsing R, Lubbe D, et al. Manual versus sonic-powered toothbrushing for plaque reduction in patients with dental implants: an explanatory randomised controlled trial. Eur J Oral Implantol. 2013;6(2):133–44 PubMed PMID: 23926585.

18. Hellstadius K, Asman B, Gustafsson A. Improved maintenance of plaque control by electrical toothbrushing in periodontitis patients with low compliance. J Clin Periodontol. 1993;20(4):235–7 PubMed PMID: 8473531.

19. Tawse-Smith A, Duncan WJ, Payne AG, Thomson WM, Wennström JL. Relative effectiveness of powered and manual toothbrushes in elderly patients with implant-supported mandibular overdentures. J Clin Periodontol. 2002;29(4):275–80 PubMed PMID: 11966923.

20. Chang M, Wennström JL, Odman P, Andersson B. Implant supported single-tooth replacements compared to contralateral natural teeth. Crown and soft tissue dimensions. Clin Oral Implants Res. 1999;10(3):185–94 PubMed PMID: 10522178.

21. Berglundh T, Lindhe J. Dimension of the periimplant mucosa. Biological width revisited. J Clin Periodontol. 1996;23(10):971–3 PubMed PMID: 8915028.

22. Berglundh T, Lindhe J, Ericsson I, Marinello CP, Liljenberg B, Thomsen P. The soft tissue barrier at implants and teeth. Clin Oral Implants Res. 1991;2(2): 81–90 PubMed PMID: 1809403.

23. Berglundh T, Abrahamsson I, Welander M, Lang NP, Lindhe J. Morphogenesis of the peri-implant mucosa: an experimental study in dogs. Clin Oral Implants Res. 2007;18(1):1–8. https://doi.org/10.1111/j.1600-0501. 2006.01380.x PubMed PMID: 17224016.

24. Cagna DR, Massad JJ, Daher T. Use of a powered toothbrush for hygiene of edentulous implant-supported prostheses. Compend Contin Educ Dent. 2011;32(4):84–8 PubMed PMID: 21661663.

25. Truhlar RS, Morris HF, Ochi S. The efficacy of a counter-rotational powered toothbrush in the maintenance of endosseous dental implants. J Am Dent Assoc. 2000;131(1):101–7 PubMed PMID: 10649881.

26. Vandekerckhove B, Quirynen M, Warren PR, Strate J, van Steenberghe D. The safety and efficacy of a powered toothbrush on soft tissues in patients with implant-supported fixed prostheses. Clin Oral Investig. 2004;8(4):206–10. https://doi.org/10.1007/s00784-004-0278-z Epub 2004/07/28. . PubMed PMID: 15583919.

27. Kurtz B, Reise M, Klukowska M, Grender JM, Timm H, Sigusch BW. A randomized clinical trial comparing plaque removal efficacy of an oscillating-rotating power toothbrush to a manual toothbrush by multiple examiners. Int J Dent Hyg. 2016;14(4):278–83. https://doi.org/10.1111/idh. 12225 Epub 2016/05/06. PubMed PMID: 27151435.

28. Rasperini G, Pellegrini G, Cortella A, Rocchietta I, Consonni D, Simion M. The safety and acceptability of an electric toothbrush on peri-implant mucosa in patients with oral implants in aesthetic areas: a prospective cohort study. Eur J Oral Implantol. 2008;1(3):221–8 PubMed PMID: 20467624.

29. Parizi MT, Mohammadi TM, Afshar SK, Hajizamani A, Tayebi M. Efficacy of an electric toothbrush on plaque control compared to two manual toothbrushes. Int Dent J. 2011;61(3):131–5. https://doi.org/10.1111/j.1875-595X.2011.00029.x PubMed PMID: 21692783.

30. Heasman PA, Stacey F, Heasman L, Sellers P, Macgregor ID, Kelly PJ. A comparative study of the Philips HP 735, Braun/Oral B D7 and the Oral B 35 advantage toothbrushes. J Clin Periodontol. 1999;26(2):85–90 PubMed PMID: 10048641.

11

Segmental sandwich osteotomy and tunnel technique for three-dimensional reconstruction of the jaw atrophy

Mario Santagata[1,2*], Nicola Sgaramella[1], Ivo Ferrieri[1], Giovanni Corvo[1], Gianpaolo Tartaro[1] and Salvatore D'Amato[1]

Abstract

Background: A three-dimensionally favourable mandibular bone crest is desirable to be able to successfully implant placement to meet the aesthetic and functional criteria in the implant-prosthetic rehabilitation. Several surgical procedures have been advocated for bone augmentation of the atrophic mandible, and the sandwich osteotomy is one of these techniques. The aim of the present case report was to assess the suitability of segmental mandibular sandwich osteotomy combined with a tunnel technique of soft tissue. Based on our knowledge, nobody described before the sandwich osteotomy with tunnel technique to improve the healing of the wound and meet the dimensional requirements of preimplant bone augmentation in cases of a severely atrophic mandible.

Case presentation: A 59-year-old woman with a severely atrophied right mandible was treated with the sandwich osteotomy technique filled with autologous bone graft harvested by a cortical bone collector from the ramus. Clinical examination revealed that the mandible was edentulous bilaterally from the first molar to the second molar region. Radiographically, atrophy of the mandibular alveolar ridge in the same teeth site was observed. We began to treat the right side. A horizontal osteotomy of the edentulous mandibular bone was then made with a piezoelectric device after tunnel technique of the soft tissue. The segmental mandibular sandwich osteotomy (SMSO) was finished by two (mesial and distal) slightly divergent vertical osteotomies. The entire bone fragment was displaced cranially, and the desirable position was obtained. The gap was filled completely with autologous bone chips harvested from the mandibular ramus through a cortical bone collector. No barrier membranes were used to protect the grafts. The vertical incisions were closing with interruptive suturing of the flaps with a resorbable material. In this way, the suture will not fall on the osteotomy line of the jaw; the result will be a better predictability of soft and hard tissue healing.

Conclusions: Segmental mandibular sandwich osteotomy is an easy and safety technique that could be performed in an atrophic posterior mandible. Future studies involving long-term follow-up are needed to evaluate the permanence of these results.

Keywords: Sandwich osteotomy, Ridge augmentation, Tunnel technique

* Correspondence: mario.santagata@tin.it; mario.santagata@unicampania.it
[1]Multidisciplinary Department of Medical and Dental Specialties, Oral and Maxillofacial Surgery Unit, AOU - University of Campania "Luigi Vanvitelli", Naples, Italy
[2]Piazza Fuori Sant'Anna 17, 81031 Aversa, Italy

Background

In cases of atrophic mandible, the distance to the mandibular canal and the transverse decrease in bone is an anatomic limitation for prosthetic rehabilitation with dental implants. The gold standard for treatment of this mandibular atrophy continues to be autologous bone grafting [1, 2].

A relatively modern technique for vertical bone augmentation is sandwich osteotomy. Schettler and Holtermann first described this technique, with promising results [3]. The sandwich technique has been proved to be relatively safe, with successful long-term results, in both the mandible and the maxilla [4–10]. The technique is executed by segmentalising the alveolar bone through a minimal vestibular incision (similar to osteotomies such as alveolar distraction osteogenesis), transporting the segment attached to the periosteum to the desired three-dimensional planned area and fixing it with plate and screws. Most studies have used autogenous bone graft as the filler for the created gap.

To the best of our knowledge, the present study is the first to use sandwich osteotomy to obtain both vertical and transversal bone gain flapless; in more detail, the authors used the tunnel technique of the soft tissue without a full-thickness flap to perform the described mandibular osteotomy to improve hard and soft tissue healing.

Case report

A 59-year-old woman with a severely atrophied right mandible was treated with the sandwich osteotomy technique filled with autologous bone graft harvested by a cortical bone collector from the ramus.

The requirements of the Helsinki Declaration were observed, and the patient gave informed consent for all surgical procedures. After local infiltration of anaesthesia (mepivacaina plus adrenaline 1:200,000), buccally and lingually to the defect area, a single vertical incision was initiated at the distal margin of the mesial tooth (43) to the defect. The second incision was carried out distally about 3 cm far from the first (Fig. 1). The soft tissues were elevated from the bone through the tunnelling mechanism cranially, mesially and distally in a subperiosteal plane. The elevator of Zucchelli (Stoma®—Storz am Mark GmbH, Emmingen-Liptingen, Germany) was used for the subperiosteal dissection.

However, the entire periosteum could be preserved to ensure adequate vascularisation of the future bone cranial segment.

A horizontal osteotomy of the edentulous mandibular bone was then made with a piezoelectric device (Mectron Medical, GE, Italy). The tip MT1-10 was used to perform the osteotomy. The segmental mandibular

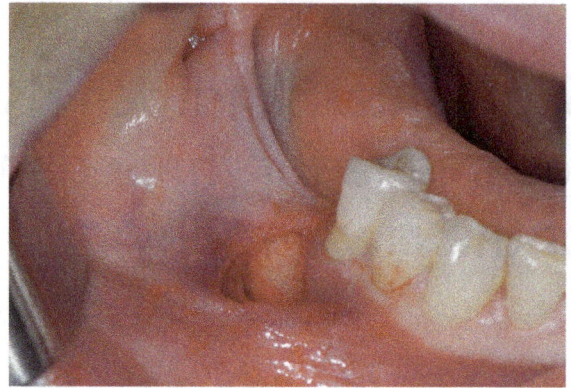

Fig. 1 Tunnel technique

sandwich osteotomy (SMSO) was finished by two (mesial and distal) slightly divergent vertical osteotomies (Fig. 2). The horizontal osteotomy was located at least 2 mm below the ridge bone and approximately 2 mm above the mandibular canal. The vertical mesial osteotomy was made 2 mm distal to the last tooth and 2 mm above the mental foramen. Also, the mesial vertical muco-periosteal incision is necessary to place the incision 2 mm distant from the mental foramen. The bone fragment remains anchored to the lingual and crestal periostea. The entire bone fragment was displaced cranially, and the desirable position was obtained.

The length of the segments was matched to the deficient, resorbed alveolar ridge. The segment was displaced crestally to the desired three-dimensional place and fixed with 0.8 mm thickness, pure titanium, L-Plate with 2.4 mm titanium matrix mandible cortex screws—self-tapping tip (Synthes GmbH Eimattstrasse, Oberdorf, Switzerland; Fig. 3). The gap was filled completely with

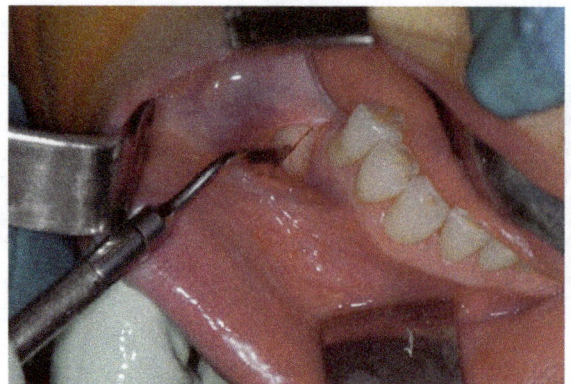

Fig. 2 Mandibular osteotomy by piezosurgery

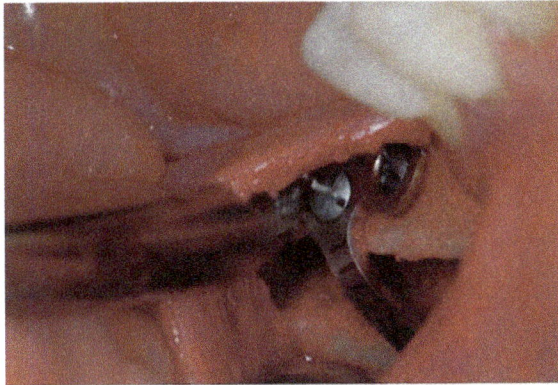

Fig. 3 Mobilised segment moved to the desired three-dimensional position and fixed with plate and screws

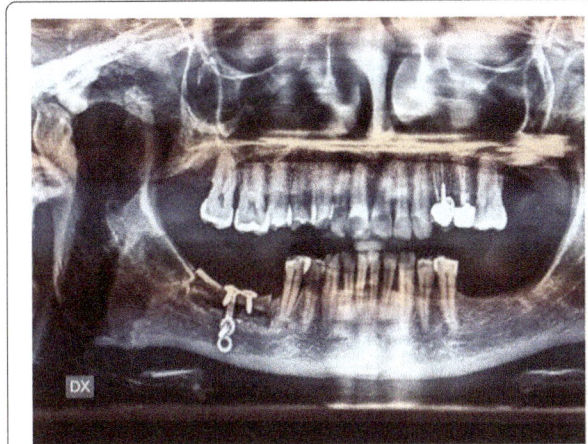

Fig. 5 OPG postoperatively

autologous bone chips harvested from the mandibular ramus by a cortical bone collector (Safescraper Twist, Meta, Italy). No barrier membranes were used to protect the grafts. The vertical incisions were closing with interruptive suturing of the flaps with a resorbable material (Polysorb 3-0, Covidien LLC, MA, USA). In this way, the suture will not fall on the osteotomy line of the jaw; the result will be a better predictability of soft and hard tissue healing (Fig. 4). Orthopantomography (OPG) was performed immediately after the procedure (Fig. 5).

Discussion

The sandwich technique for bone augmentation of the atrophic mandible was first described by Schettler and Holtermann, with promising results. Since then, variations in this surgical procedure have been proposed by several investigators [4–10].

All these authors have proposed the same approach about the flap: paracrestal incision. In order to preserve the blood supply, it is of fundamental importance that the least number possible of the vessels of the soft tissue be damaged. Based on this concept, we believe that changing the flap design can obtain the improvement of the healing of the wound. The sandwich osteotomy with the tunnel technique meets these requests. This is because the incisions were only two and vertical in the buccal side. Another advantage, especially with respect to implants, is that vascularisation is maintained in the bone ridge throughout augmentation intervention; thus, the interface at the implant shoulder in terms of hard-to-soft tissue to implant interface is kept as true to the original as possible.

This technique should be applied in patients with at least 5 mm of minimal crestal amount of bone above the nerve to perform the sandwich osteotomy successfully.

We prefer to obtain not more than 5 mm of the vertical movement for the sandwich graft. Efforts to displace the segment greater than 5 mm not only risk the potential for vascular embarrassment by detaching periosteal blood supply but also can excessively rotate the segment palatally, compromising aesthetic gingival projection.

We observed no signs of impaired sensibility after the sandwich osteotomy technique. Jensen found transient paraesthesia in all patients, lasting up to 6 weeks [7].

Conclusions

In conclusion, segmental mandibular sandwich osteotomy is an easy and safety technique that could be performed in atrophic posterior mandible.

Future studies involving long-term follow-up are needed to evaluate the permanence of these results.

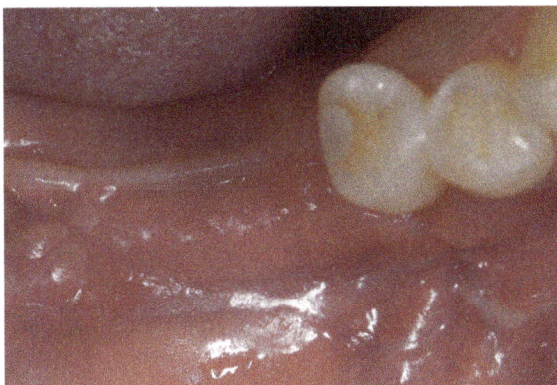

Fig. 4 Wound healing after 2 months

Acknowledgements
None.

Funding
None.

Authors' contributions
All authors were involved with the literature review and performance of the surgery. All authors read and approved the final manuscript.

Competing interests
Mario Santagata, Nicola Sgaramella, Ivo Ferrieri, Giovanni Corvo, Gianpaolo Tartaro and Salvatore D'Amato declare that they have no competing interests.

References

1. Moura LB, Carvalho PH, Xavier CB, Post LK, Torriani MA, Santagata M, Chagas Júnior OL. Autogenous non-vascularized bone graft in segmental mandibular reconstruction: a systematic review. Int J Oral Maxillofac Surg. 2016;45:1388–94.

2. D'Amato S, Tartaro G, Itro A, Nastri L, Santagata M. Block versus particulate/titanium mesh for ridge augmentation for mandibular lateral incisor defects: clinical and histologic analysis. Int J Periodontics Restorative Dent. 2015;35:e1–8.

3. Schettler D, Holtermann W. Clinical and experimental results of a sandwich-technique for mandibular alveolar ridge augmentation. J Maxillofac Surg. 1977;5:199–202.

4. Choi BH, Lee SH, Huh JY, Han SG. Use of the sandwich osteotomy plus an interpositional allograft for vertical augmentation of the alveolar ridge. J Craniomaxillofac Surg. 2004;32:51–4.

5. Egbert M, Stoelinga PJ, Blijdorp PA, de Koomen HA. The "three-piece" osteotomy and interpositional bone graft for augmentation of the atrophic mandible. J Oral Maxillofac Surg. 1986;44:680–7.

6. Frost DE, Gregg JM, Terry BC, Fonseca RJ. Mandibular interpositional and onlay bone grafting for treatment of mandibular bony deficiency in the edentulous patient. J Oral Maxillofac Surg. 1982;40:353–60.

7. Jensen OT. Alveolar segmental "sandwich" osteotomies for posterior edentulous mandibular sites for dental implants. J Oral Maxillofac Surg. 2006;64:471–5.

8. Politi M, Robiony M. Localized alveolar sandwich osteotomy for vertical augmentation of the anterior maxilla. J Oral Maxillofac Surg. 1999;57:1380–2.

9. Stellingsma C, Raghoebar GM, Meijer HJ, Batenburg RH. Reconstruction of the extremely resorbed mandible with interposed bone grafts and placement of endosseous implants. A preliminary report on outcome of treatment and patients' satisfaction. Br J Oral Maxillofac Surg. 1998;36:290–5.

10. Stoelinga PJ, Blijdorp PA, Ross RR, De Koomen HA, Huybers TJ. Augmentation of the atrophic mandible with interposed bone grafts and particulate hydroxylapatite. J Oral Maxillofac Surg. 1986;44:353–60.

12

Narrow implants (2.75 and 3.25 mm diameter) supporting a fixed splinted prostheses in posterior regions of mandible

Tommaso Grandi[1*], Luigi Svezia[1] and Giovanni Grandi[2]

Abstract

Background: Can multiple splinted narrow-diameter implants be used as definitive implants in patients with insufficient bone ridge thickness in posterior regions of the mandible? With this aim, we evaluated their outcomes in this set up to 1 year after loading.

Methods: Forty-two patients with a mean age of 61.3 years old (range 49–73) in need of fixed prosthetic implant-supported rehabilitations in the posterior region of the mandible, presenting a thin alveolar crest, were selected. One hundred twenty-four narrow-diameter implants (2.75 and 3.25 mm diameter) were placed and splinted with a bridge. One implant for each missing tooth was requested to be inserted. Outcomes measured were implant survival, complications, and marginal bone level changes up to 1 year after loading.

Results: At the 12-month follow-up, three implants failed. Two 2.75 mm diameter implants and one 3.2 mm diameter implant failed. The implant survival rate was 97.6%. Peri-implant bone resorption was 0.20 mm (CI 95% 0.14: 0.26) after 6 months and 0.47 mm (CI 95% 0.29; 0.65) after 12 months of loading, not different between 2.75 and 3.25 mm diameter groups ($p = 0.786$). Of the 42 cases, three had an episode of peri-implant mucositis (7.1%).

Conclusions: Within the limits of this study, preliminary short-term data (1 year post-loading) suggested that narrow-diameter implants (2.75 to 3.25 mm) can be successfully used as a minimally invasive alternative to horizontal bone augmentation in the posterior mandible. However, larger and longer follow-ups of 5 years or more are needed.

Keywords: Bone atrophy, Bone resorption, Dental implants, Implant failure, Narrow-diameter implants, Posterior mandible

* Correspondence: t.grandi@grandiclinic.com
[1]Private practice, Via Contrada 323, 41126 Modena, Italy
Full list of author information is available at the end of the article

Background

Historically, implants have been used and documented mainly with diameters between 3.7 and 4.3 mm. Employing these diameters for numerous indications, scientifically substantiated treatment protocols with excellent long-term results have been established [1]. One disadvantage of a standard-diameter implant is the fact that, in clinical use, the available horizontal crestal dimensions of the alveolar ridge are sometimes too small. Although there is some discussion on the amount of bone (buccal and oral) necessary for a successful dental implant, most authors advise at least 1 mm residual bone present adjacent to the implant surface, which consequently requires a horizontal crestal alveolar width of 6 mm for a standard implant. However, the exact threshold for the residual buccal bone thickness has yet not been scientifically clarified and is still under discussion. When inadequate bone width is present for placement of standard-diameter implants, most practitioners have been taught to suggest bone grafting, using either autogenous bone or one of the many available bone substitutes. Bone grafting is a well-documented procedure to restore lost bone volume, but it is associated with increased morbidity and a prolonged treatment time, with the necessary graft-healing period when dentures cannot be worn [2]. While many additive techniques for the reconstruction of missing morphology are employed on a routine basis today, surgical intervention may not always lead to the desired outcome. Physiologically, some patients may be poor candidates for extensive grafting, or they may simply decline such treatment on emotional or financial grounds. Narrow-diameter implants (NDIs) would be beneficial to decrease the rate of augmentations necessary for implant insertion. NDI is an implant with a diameter less than 3.75 mm and is clinically indicated in specific conditions of rehabilitation such as a reduced interradicular bone, thin alveolar crest, or replacing teeth with a small cervical diameter [3]. The availability of residual bone width less than 5 mm is also indicative for the use of NDIs. Several studies have reported the use of narrow-diameter implants in different clinical situations and using different surgical techniques [4–9]. In most cases, satisfactory results have been obtained, achieving medium- and long-term cumulative survival rates equivalent to those obtained in restorations using larger diameter implants (between 94 and 100% survival rates). Until now, the use of NDIs has been restricted to certain defined indications with comparable low occlusal loading like incisors or as retaining elements for overdentures. Posterior regions of the jaws with reduced bone quantity make it challenging to rehabilitate without the use of complex reconstruction techniques.

The aim of this cohort study was to evaluate the outcome of narrow-diameter implants (2.75 and 3.25 mm diameter) used as definitive implants in patients with insufficient bone ridge thickness for placing standard-diameter implants in posterior regions of the mandible. The present study reports the clinical outcome up to 1 year after loading. It is planned to follow up this patients' cohort to the fifth year of function in order to evaluate the success of the procedure over time. The present article is reported according to the STROBE statement for improving the quality of observational studies (http://www.strobe-statement.org).

Methods

The present prospective study was conducted at a private practice (Tommaso Grandi, Modena) in Italy between October 2014 and January 2016.

Any patient with partial edentulism in posterior regions of mandible (premolar/molar areas), requiring one multiple tooth implant-supported restoration (2-, 3-, or 4-unit bridge), having a residual bone height of at least 8 mm and a thickness of at least 4 mm measured on computerized tomography (CT) scans, and who was 18 or older and able to sign an informed consent form, was eligible for inclusion in this trial. Preoperative periapical X-rays were used for initial screening, followed by computer tomography scans to precisely quantify the amount of bone. Patients were not admitted in the study if any of the following exclusion criteria was present: (1) general contraindications to implant surgery, (2) residual bone thickness greater than 5 mm, (3) subjected to irradiation in the head and neck area, (3) treated or under treatment with intravenous amino-bisphosphonates, (4) poor oral hygiene and motivation, (5) untreated periodontitis, (6) uncontrolled diabetes, (7) pregnant or lactating, (8) substance abusers, and (9) lack of opposite occluding dentition in the area intended for implant placement. The principles outlined in the Declaration of Helsinki on clinical research involving human subjects were adhered to. All patients received thorough explanations and signed a written informed consent before being enrolled in the trial. Forty-two patients were consecutively recruited and treated in a private dental practice by one operator (Tommaso Grandi, who performed all the surgical and prosthetic interventions). All patients underwent at least one session of oral hygiene instructions and professionally delivered debridement when required prior to the intervention. Anti-microbial prophylaxis was obtained with 1 g of amoxicillin and clavulanic acid (Augmentin, Roche

S.p.A., Milan, Italy) every 12 h from the day before surgery to the sixth postsurgical day. Patients allergic to penicillin were given clarithromycin 500 mg (Klacid, Abbott srl, Roma, Italy) 1 h before the intervention and 250 mg twice a day for one week. On the day of surgery, patients were treated under local anesthesia. Full-thickness crestal flaps were elevated with a minimal extension to reduce patient discomfort. The implant sites were prepared according to the procedure recommended by the implant manufacturer (JDentalCare, Modena, Italy). Tapered narrow-diameter implants titanium grade 5 (2.75 and 3.25 mm diameter, respectively, JDIcon Ultra S and JDEvolution S, JDental-Care) with internal connection and sandblasted and acid-etched treated surface were used (Fig. 1a, b). No bone flattening was performed. The implants were inserted in the bone without any fenestration/dehiscence. The implant neck was positioned at the coronal marginal crest level. The operator was free to choose implant lengths (8, 10, 11.5, and 13 mm) and diameter (2.75 and 3.25 mm) according to clinical indications. One implant for each missing tooth was requested to be inserted. Healing abutments were attached, and implants were left to a non-submerged healing. Interrupted sutures were placed using a synthetic monofilament thread (Vycril, Ethicon, Johnson & Johnson, Somerville, New Jersey) and were removed after 10 days. After 3 months, all the implants underwent the standard prosthetic protocol and were loaded directly with definitive screw-retained or cemented multiple splinted crowns.

Primary outcome measures were as follows:

- Implant failure: evaluated as implant mobility and removal of stable implants dictated by progressive marginal bone loss or infection. The stability of each implant was measured manually by tightening the abutment screw with a wrench delivering a torque of 20 Ncm. Implant stability assessment was performed at delivery of definitive crowns (3 months after implant placement). After insertion of the definitive restorations, prostheses were not removed to assess clinical mobility of individual implants.
- Complications: any biological and prosthetic complication occurred at the implant site during the entire follow-up time were recorded and reported.

Secondary outcome measures were as follows:

- Peri-implant marginal bone level changes: evaluated on intraoral radiographs taken with the paralleling technique at implant placement, 6 months and 1 year after loading. All measurements were taken by an independent assessor (LS). Radiographs were scanned, digitized in JPG format, converted to TIFF format with a 600 dpi resolution, and stored in a

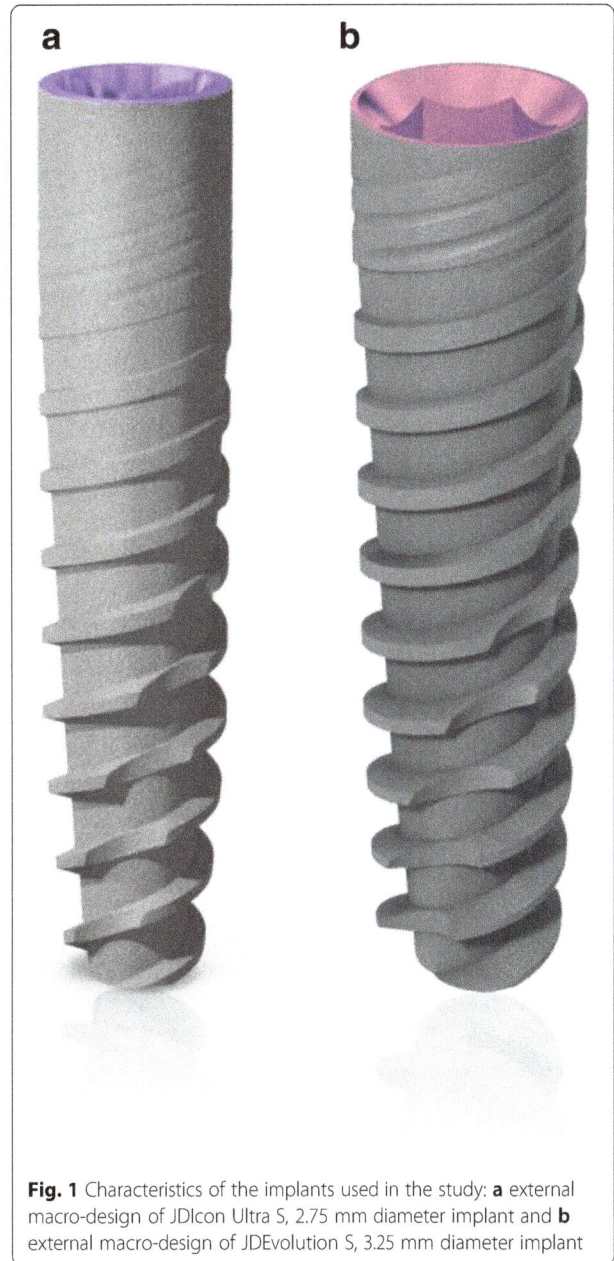

Fig. 1 Characteristics of the implants used in the study: **a** external macro-design of JDIcon Ultra S, 2.75 mm diameter implant and **b** external macro-design of JDEvolution S, 3.25 mm diameter implant

personal computer. Peri-implant marginal bone levels were measured using Image J 1.42 software (National Institute of Mental Health, MD, USA). The software was calibrated for every single image using the known implant diameter. Measurements of the mesial and distal crestal bone levels adjacent to each implant were made to the nearest 0.01 mm and averaged at patient level and then group level. The measurements were taken parallel to the implant axis. Reference points for the linear measurements were the most coronal margin of the implant collar and the most coronal point of bone-to-implant contact.

Statistical analysis was performed using the statistical package StatView (version 5.01.98, SAS Institute Inc., Cary, NC, USA). Significance was considered at $p < 0.05$. The paired-samples t test was used to evaluate the bone level changes. The patient was the statistical unit of the analysis. A medical doctor (GG) with expertise in dental biostatistics analyzed the data.

Results

Forty-eight patients were screened for eligibility, but six subjects were not included for the following reasons: five patients (10.4%) were hesitant to receive implant treatment, and one patient (2.1%) was treated with intravenous amino-bisphosphonates. Forty-two patients were then considered eligible and were consecutively enrolled in the study. All patients were treated according to the allocated intervention, no dropout occurred up to 1 year after loading, and the data of all patients were evaluated in the statistical analysis.

Patients were recruited and operated from October 2014 to January 2016.

Implants and subjects features

The follow-up focused on the time between implant placement and 1 year after loading. One hundred and twenty-four narrow-diameter implants (2.75 and 3.25 mm) inserted in a total of 42 subjects were included. The main baseline patient features are reported in Table 1. Patients were generally healthy, though 19 patients (45.2%) had medication-controlled hypertension and 11 (26.2%) patients had controlled type 2 diabetes. The mean age of the patients at the time of surgery was 61.3 years old (range 49–73). Seating torque values and the dimensions (diameter and length) of the inserted implants are listed in Table 2. Measurements of insertion torque were averaged at patient level and then group level. Average insertion torque was 46.6 Ncm (SD 11.8). Pain and discomfort from the surgical procedure appeared to be within the limits of a flapped implant placement. No incidences of abnormal bleeding or ecchymosis were observed.

Implants failures

After 1 year of function, three implants were lost in three patients (one implant per patient) rendering a survival rate of 97.6%. Two 2.75 mm diameter implants and one 3.2 mm diameter implant failed. The failed implants displayed postoperative pain, edema, and signs of infection with pus. They were mobile 3 weeks after placement in smoker women. They were successfully replaced after 4 months.

Complications

Three patients (7.1%) had an episode of peri-implant mucositis, and they were treated with non-surgical debridement of the affected implants. All permanent bridges remained stable during the 12 months follow-up period.

Marginal bone level changes

The radiographic data are summarized in Tables 3 and 4. The group lost statistically significant marginal peri-implant bone at 6 months (–0.20; 95% C –0.14: –0.26, $p < 0.0001$) and 1-year post-loading (–0.47; 95% CI –0.29: –0.65, $p < 0.0001$), respectively. The marginal bone level changes were not different between the different implant diameters used, 2.75 and 3.25 mm ($p = 0.786$) (Table 4).

Table 1 Features of the subjects included in the study

Number of patients	42
Males (%)	18 (42.9%)
Females (%)	24 (57.1%)
Mean age at insertion (range)	62.6 (49–73)
Smokers (less than 10 cigarettes/die)	12 (28.6%)
Diseases in history	
Controlled diabetes type 2	11 (26.2%)
Hypertension	19 (45.2%)
Site of insertion	
Premolar	81 (65.3%)
Molar	43 (34.7%)
Opposite dentition	
Opposing maxillary complete denture	7 (16.7%)
Opposing fixed rehabilitation and natural teeth	26 (61.9%)
Opposing removable prosthesis and natural teeth	9 (21.4%)

Table 2 Dimensions (diameter and length) and final seating torque of the inserted implants ($n = 124$)

Length (mm)	8	18 (14.5%)
	10	56 (45.2%)
	11.5	43 (34.7%)
	13	7 (5.6%)
Diameter (mm)	2.75	69 (55.6%)
	3.25	55 (44.4%)
Insertion torque (Ncm)	30	21 (16.9%)
	35	16 (12.9%)
	40	10 (8.1%)
	45	11 (8.9%)
	50	32 (25.8%)
	55	7 (5.6%)
	60	16 (12.9%)
	65	5 (4.1%)
	70	6 (4.8%)

Table 3 Comparison of mean bone levels (means ± SD) at different follow-up intervals

Follow-up	Mean bone level (mm) (n = 124)	Time	
		0–6 months (95% CI) (n = 121)	0–12 months (95% CI) (n = 121)
Baseline	0.01 ± 0.06	−0.20 (−0.14; −0.26)	−0.47 (−0.29; −0.65)
6 months	0.21 ± 0.10	p < 0.0001	p < 0.0001
12 months	0.48 ± 0.29		

Figures 2 and 3 show the clinical situations before and after treatment in two patients involved in the study.

Discussion

Dental implants with a reduced diameter are commonly used where bone width is narrow or in cases of restricted mesiodistal anatomy such as laterally maxillary and mandibular incisors. They could also be a viable alternative to bone augmentation especially in challenging situations such as the posterior regions of the mandible. While it has been shown that it is possible to horizontally augment bone in mandible with different procedures, these techniques are associated with significant postoperative morbidity and complications, can be expensive and technique sensitive, and require long treatment periods. Narrow-diameter implants could be simpler, cheaper, and faster alternative to horizontal bone augmentation in the mandible, if they will provide similar success rates. This cohort study was designed to evaluate whether NDIs (2.75 and 3.25 mm diameter) could be used to support partially fixed prostheses in posterior mandibles having insufficient bone ridge thickness for placing standard-diameter implants. At 1-year post loading, implant survival rate was 97.6%, the number of complications was low, and the implants lost an average of 0.47 mm of peri-implant bone. The present data are similar to those observed around other implant systems used in the similar condition. Malo et al. [6] reported a 95.1% survival rate after 11 years of function for narrow-diameter implants (3.3 mm diameter) placed in posterior regions of both jaws. The values for marginal bone resorption recorded in this study at 1, 5, and 10 years (not exceeding 0.2 mm/year of bone loss after the first year) are within the accepted standard success criteria for implants. Regarding the implant failures, the majority occurred in the first 6 months of function, following the pattern for standard-diameter implants. In another retrospective study, Anitua et al. [10] observed a survival rate of 97.3% for 2.5 mm diameter implants used as definitive implants for rehabilitation of missing teeth having a follow-up between 3 and 7 years.

Klein et al., in a recent systematic review, reported that the survival rate of implants with a diameter of < 3 mm was higher than 90% with a follow-up time between 1 and 3 years [3]. In another meta-analysis by Ortega-Oller et al., the majority of the analyzed studies (implants less than 3.3 mm in diameter) have also reported a survival/success rate higher than 90% [11]. However, the results of the meta-analysis have shown higher failure rates for implants with a diameter of < 3.3 mm when compared with implants with a diameter of ≥ 3.3 mm. The authors have related this outcome with the fact that

Table 4 Comparison of mean bone levels (means ± SD) at different follow-up intervals in different implants diameters groups (2.75 and 3.25 mm)

Diameter 2.75 mm				
Follow-up	Mean bone level changes (mm) (n = 69)	0–6 months (95% CI) (n = 67)	0–12 months (95% CI) (n = 67)	p inter-groups
Baseline	0.02 ± 0.07	−0.18 (−0.09; −0.27)	−0.47 (−0.27; −0.67)	p = 0.786
6 months	0.20 ± 0.12	p intra-group		
12 months	0.49 ± 0.30	p < 0.0001	p < 0.0001	
Diameter 3.25 mm				
Follow-up	Mean bone level changes (mm) (n = 55)	0–6 months (95% CI) (n = 54)	0–12 months (95% CI) (n = 54)	
Baseline	0.00 ± 0.11	−0.22 (−0.10; −0.34)	−0.48 (−0.25; −0.71)	
6 months	0.22 ± 0.14	p intra-group		
12 months	0.48 ± 0.33	p = 0.001	p < 0.0001	

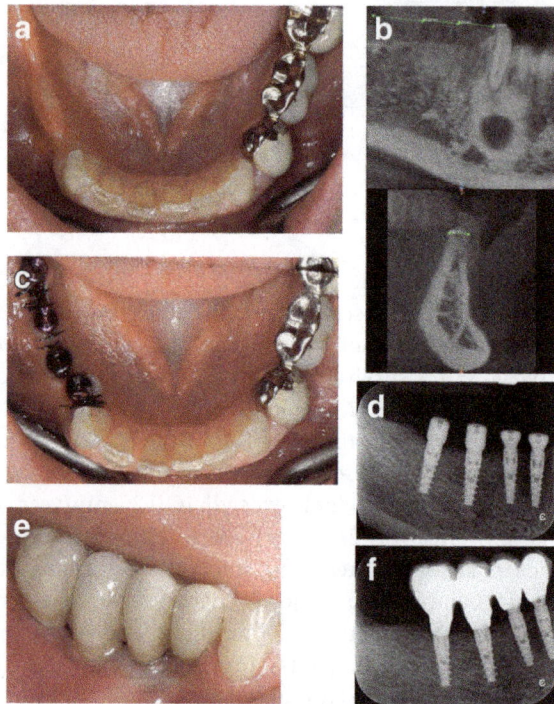

Fig. 2 Case 1: Example of one case involved in the study.
a Preoperative view of a partial edentulism in posterior mandible.
b Preoperative CT scan. The width of the ridge was 4 mm. c Four narrow diameter implants were placed and left to a nonsubmerged healing. d Baseline periapical radiograph. e Buccal vieew of the final metal ceramic restoration. f Periapical radiograph at 1 year after loading

NDIs are usually placed in complicated clinical scenario, and they have a higher possibility of fracture.

On the one hand, due to the small sample size of this study and moreover, the short follow-up (only 1 year after loading), it would be hazardous to conclude that the placement of NDIs to support fixed prostheses in posterior mandible is a predictable treatment modality. In order to draw more reliable conclusions, we need to wait for longer follow-ups, since it may be possible that after several years of function, NDI implants might start to fail due to the reduced available bone-implant contact area or to reduce resistance to fatigue. The placement in the posterior mandible of 2.75 mm diameter implants, as well as 3.25 mm ones, must always be splinted with a bridge, placing one implant for each missing tooth. The placement of a NDI implant in a single molar crown is not recommended. Splinting multiple implants has been reported to minimize the lateral force on the prosthesis, to enhance force distribution, and to reduce the stress on the implants [10]. Thus, splinting of NDI implants would protect the implants from excessive loading and prevent implant/abutment screw fracture. Necessary measures should be taken to minimize off-axis forces like reduction in occlusal table and cusp inclines.

The main limitation of the present study is the small sample size. In addition, a 1-year follow-up is too short to make definitive statements on the predictability of the treatment option tested. Longer follow-up periods and

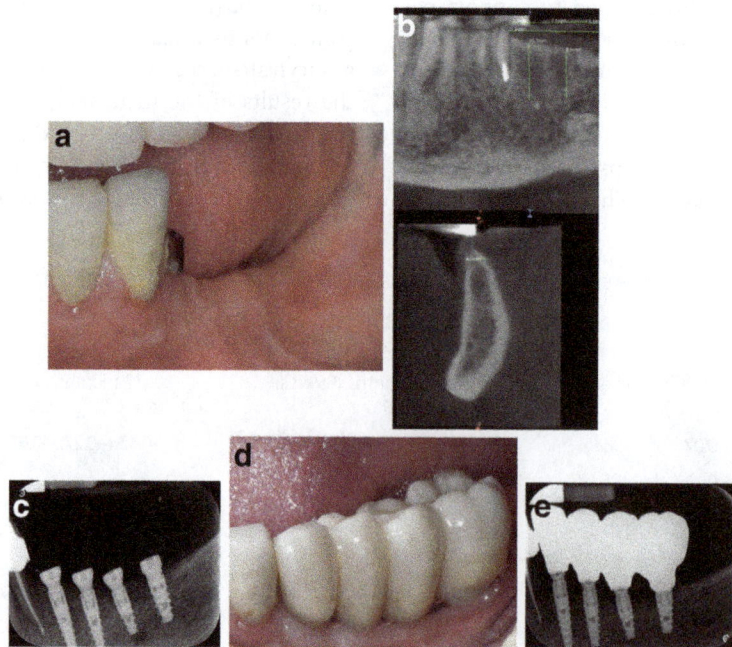

Fig. 3 Example of another case involved in the study. a Preoperative view –premolars and molars are missing in left mandible. b Preoperative CT scan. The width of the ridge was around 4 mm. c Baseline periapical radiograph. Four narrow diameter implants were placed to restore the area. d Buccal view of the final full-contour zirconia restoration. e Periapical radiograph at 1 year after loading

Narrow implants (2.75 and 3.25 mm diameter) supporting a fixed splinted prostheses in posterior...

91

larger sample size are needed, and this trial is currently ongoing.

Conclusions

Within the limits of this prospective cohort study, narrow-diameter implants (2.75 to 3.25 mm) can be successfully used as a minimally invasive alternative to horizontal bone augmentation in posterior mandible up to 1 year of function. This outcome could be related to the fact that these implants have been all splinted to other implants by a fixed prosthesis. These preliminary results must be confirmed by larger and longer follow-ups of 5 years or more.

Authors' contributions
TG contributed to the concept and design, interpretation, study execution, and manuscript draft. LS participated in the study execution and contributed to the revision of the manuscript. GG contributed to the data analysis and interpretation. All authors read and approved the final manuscript.

Competing interests
Tommaso Grandi serves as a consultant for JDentalCare. Luigi Svezia and Giovanni Grandi declare that they have no competing interests.

Author details
[1]Private practice, Via Contrada 323, 41126 Modena, Italy. [2]Department of Obstetrics, Gynecology and Pediatrics, University of Modena and Reggio Emilia, Modena, Italy.

References
1. Esposito M, Grusovin MG, Maghaireh H, Worthington HV. Interventions for replacing missing teeth: different times for loading dental implants (Review). Cochrane Database Syst Rev. 2013;(3):CD003878. https://doi.org/10.1002/14651858.CD003878.pub5.
2. Esposito M, Grusovin MG, Felice P, Karatzopoulos G, Worthington HV, Coulthard P. The efficacy of horizontal and vertical bone augmentation procedures for dental implants—a Cochrane systematic review. Eur J Oral Implantol. 2009;2(3):167–84.
3. Klein MO, Schiegnitz E, Al-Nawas B. Systematic review on success of narrow-diameter dental implants. Int J Oral Maxillofac Implants. 2014;29(Suppl):43–54.
4. Polizzi G, Fabbro S, Furri M, Herrmann I, Squarzoni S. Clinical application of narrow Branemark System implants for single-tooth restorations. Int J Oral Maxillofac Implants. 1999;14:496–503.
5. Anitua E, Errazquin JM, de Pedro J, Barrio P, Begona L, Orive G. Clinical evaluation of Tiny 2.5- and 3.0-mm narrow-diameter implants as definitive implants in different clinical situations: a retrospective cohort study. Eur J Oral Implantol. 2010;3:315–22.
6. Maló P, Nobre M. Implants (3.3 mm diameter) for the rehabilitation of edentulous posterior regions: a retrospective clinical study with up to 11 years of follow-up. Clin Implant Dent Relat Res. 2011;13(2):95–103.
7. Mangano F, Shibli JA, Sammons RL, Veronesi G, Piattelli A, Mangano C. Clinical outcome of narrow-diameter(3.3 mm) locking-taper implants: a prospective study with 1 to 10 years of follow-up. Int J Oral Maxillofac Implants. 2014;29:448–55.
8. Moraguez O, Vailati F, Grutter L, Sailer I, Belser UC. Fourunit fixed dental prostheses replacing the maxillary incisors supported by two narrow-diameter implants—a five-year case series. Clin Oral Implants Res. 2016:1–6. doi:10.1111/clr.12895.
9. Anitua E, Saracho J, Begoña L, Alkhraisat MH. Long-term follow-up of 2.5-mm narrow-diameter implants supporting a fixed prostheses. Clin Implant Dent Relat Res. 2016;18(4):769–77.
10. Anitua E, Tapia R, Luzuriaga F, Orive G. Influence of implant length, diameter, and geometry on stress distribution: a finite element analysis. Int J Periodontics Restorative Dent. 2010;30:89–95.
11. Ortega-Oller I, Suarez F, Galindo-Moreno P, Torrecillas-Martínez L, Monje A, Catena A, Wang HL. The influence of implant diameter on its survival: a meta-analysis based on prospective clinical trials. J Periodontol. 2014;85:569–80.

13

Six-implant-supported immediate fixed rehabilitation of atrophic edentulous maxillae with tilted distal implants

S. Wentaschek[1]* ⓘ, S. Hartmann[1], C. Walter[2] and W. Wagner[2]

Abstract

Background: The aim of this retrospective study was to evaluate the treatment outcome of six Bredent blueSky™ implants (Bredent GmbH, Senden, Germany) immediately loaded with a fixed full-arch prosthesis (two tilted posterior and four axial frontal and premolar implants).

Methods: All 10 patients with atrophic edentulous maxillae being treated with a standardized procedure from 09/2009 to 01/2013, who had a follow-up of at least 3 years, were included. Sixty implants were placed to support 10 screwed prostheses. Twenty-one of them were inserted in fresh extraction sockets. Lab-side-prepared provisional fixed prostheses were placed at the day of implantation. Periotest (PT) values and implant stability quotient (ISQ) were measured after implant surgery and after 3 months of healing in all patients.

Results: The analyzed implants were in function in mean 64 ± 13 months (range 42 to 84 months). One axial and two tilted implants failed in three patients. The mean PT values decreased, and ISQ increased significantly after the first 3 months at the osseointegrated tilted and axial implants. With an area under the curve of 0.503 and 0.506 in the receiver operating characteristic, the PT values and the ISQ were unspecific parameters and unsuitable as a predictor for the risk of non-osseointegration.

Conclusions: Within the limits of this small group (*n* = 10 patients/60 implants), the failure rate of the analyzed implant system (*n* = 3 respective 5% implant loss) seems to be comparable with other immediate-loading protocols. The failure rate of tilted implants in the atrophic upper jaw was quite high, but the aimed treatment concept could be achieved in every patient. The rehabilitation of the posterior region in edentulous maxilla remains a challenge.

Keywords: Tilted implants, Edentulous maxilla, Full-arch prostheses, Immediate loading, Implant stability quotient, Periotest

Background

For a few years, there has been a trend towards minimally invasive implant treatment concepts avoiding bone augmentation even in very atrophic edentulous jaws. These concepts aim to make an implant treatment with a shorter duration, with less inconvenience such as swelling or pain and possibly also economically more attractive [1]. If the implant treatment is less invasive, because of the possible smaller surgical risks and lower costs, implant therapy can be provided for a larger number of patients. Minimally invasive mainly means the adaptation of the implant dimension or position to the existing anatomy to avoid bone augmentation procedures [1]. One possible strategy to avoid augmentations in the distal atrophic maxilla is to insert short implants. In recent reviews, implants of less than 10 mm are not inferior to longer implants relating to bone loss or survival rate [2–4]. But also for the insertion of short implants, the bone height in the atrophic posterior maxilla is often not enough [5].

An alternative to short implants are longer tilted implants [6] with a possibly higher primary stability combined with the posterior position of the implant shoulder [7–9]. These characteristics seem to make them especially suitable for immediate loading in the edentulous jaws [10] as it is often performed [5]. This treatment concept with

---
* Correspondence: stefan.wentaschek@unimedizin-mainz.de
[1]Department of Prosthetic Dentistry, University Medical Center of the Johannes Gutenberg-University Mainz, Augustusplatz 2, 55131 Mainz, Germany
Full list of author information is available at the end of the article

loading on the same day appears to achieve high patient satisfaction [1], but there are also some disadvantages. Tilted implants might be more difficult to insert and need technical angulated abutments. To position the implants in an optimal position parallel to the anterior sinus wall, a computer-guided implant planning and navigated insertion is more often needed.

Different implant systems have been investigated using the concept of tilted implants [11], but due to the different geometric properties and prosthetic components, they may behave differently, so that all systems used for this concept must prove their suitability. Because this implant type was previously rarely investigated in the concept of immediate loading [12], the aim of this retrospective study is to evaluate the success rate of Bredent blueSky™ implants (Bredent GmbH, Senden, Germany) in immediate full-arch loading with tilted posterior implants using minimal invasive surgery. In addition to the osseointegration and bone loss, the stability parameters' implant stability quotient (ISQ; measured by resonance frequency analysis (RFA)) and Periotest (PT) values were compared between tilted and axial implants and their changes after osseointegration were recorded. The suitability of the chosen combination of implants, abutments, and materials for the provisional restorations after use in a clinical setting should be examined.

Methods
Patients
In a retrospective study, all patients with immediately loaded implants in an edentulous maxillae with limited posterior ridge dimensions that received an equal concept were included if they had a follow-up of at least 3 years. The concept contained immediate loading with distal tilted implants and six implants per edentulous maxillae of a single implant system (blueSky™ implants, Bredent GmbH, Senden, Germany), and it includes an equal lab-side-prepared provisional fixed prosthesis.

All patients have received implant stability parameter measurements that were routinely collected at immediate loading directly after implant insertion and after first removal of the provisional restoration 3 months after surgery. The ISQ after RFA and PT values were measured.

The retrospective data analysis was conducted in accordance with the Helsinki Declaration of 1975, as revised in 2008, and all patients signed an informed consent. After consulting the local ethic committee, the decision was that due to the retrospective character of this study with no additional data acquisition, no ethical approval is needed according to the hospital laws of the appropriate state (Landeskrankenhausgesetz Rhineland Palatinate, Germany).

Selection criteria
Patients who were treated with this concept had to have the desire and the indication for an implant-supported full-arch prosthesis and concerns regarding bone-grafting procedures. They had to be physically and psychologically capable of undergoing conventional implant surgery. They had to have a reduced bone volume in the molar region of the maxilla that would not allow placing dental implants of at least 6 mm in length without bone augmentation. But placement of tilted implants in the area of the premolars with an implant length of at least 10 mm had to be possible so that the implant was surrounded by bone. All patients had to be treated by the same maxillofacial surgeon and the same prosthodontist.

The exclusion criteria were an active infection or inflammation at the intended implants sites; major systemic disease, e.g., uncontrolled diabetes mellitus, radiation, or chemotherapy within 5 years prior to the surgery; bone-physiology-changing drugs such as bisphosphonates, severe bruxism, or clenching habit; and poor oral hygiene.

Presurgical phase
The patients were screened with preliminary panoramic radiographs, and since all the implants were 3D planned (SKYplanX™ program, Bredent GmbH, Senden, Germany) and inserted with a guiding template, a cone-beam CT (CBCT) was obtained eventually (KaVo 3D eXam™ unit, KaVo Dental GmbH, Biberach/Riss, Germany).

Surgical procedure
The drillings were performed using a 3D-planned surgical template with different metal sleeves corresponding to the diameter of the drills (Fig. 1). Implants were inserted torque controlled under vision without the surgical template. Primary implant stability was assessed immediately

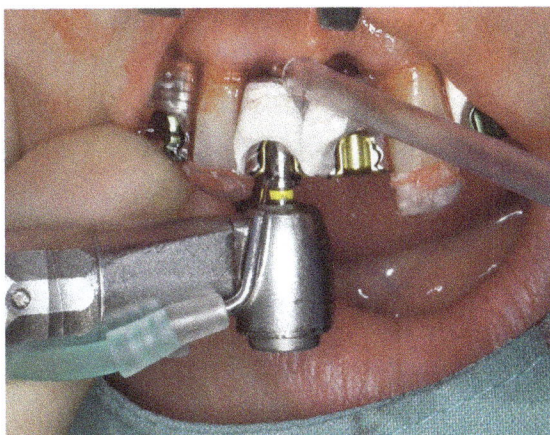

Fig. 1 Preparation of implant cavity through corresponding metal sleeves after extraction of the central incisors using a surgical template supported by hopeless remaining teeth

following implant insertion by PT (Medizintechnik Gulden, Modautal, Germany) and RFA (Osstell, Gothenburg, Sweden).

Prosthetic procedure
Immediate implant loading
Definitive titanium abutments (0°, 17.5°, 35°; fast & fixed abutments, Bredent, Senden, Germany) were attached to the implants. The abutment screws were tightened with a torque of 25 N cm. On these abutments, impression copings for closed trays were seated and an impression and a provisional inter-jaw relationship recording with a silicone were performed.

After cast making, temporary resin prostheses using a composite veneering system (visio.lign, Bredent, Senden, Germany) were prepared in the laboratory (Fig. 2). These temporary restorations were perforated in five of the six implant regions. After the temporary prosthetic titanium cylinders (Bredent, Senden, Germany) were attached on the abutments and the resin superstructures were placed over the cylinders, the superstructure perforations were filled with self-curing resin (Qu-resin™; Bredent, Senden, Germany) (Fig. 3). The superstructure was removed, completed, and relined. The provisional restoration was inserted, the screw holes were sealed, and the denture was adjusted on the occlusal plane. All provisional prostheses were inserted on the same day of implant insertion. With the provisional restorations, no further distal tooth was replaced than that under which the distal implant was positioned. Therefore, the distal cantilever extensions of the provisional prosthesis have not exceeded the width of a half molar.

Post-surgical phase
Three months post-surgery, the temporary restorations were removed for the first time (Fig. 4), ISQ and PT

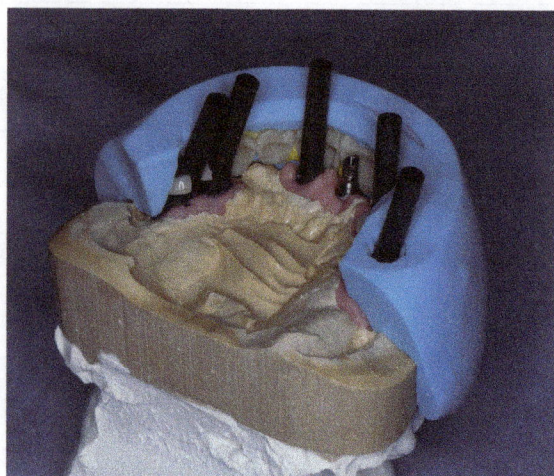

Fig. 3 Fill-in of the occlusal perforations with self-curing resin to connect the prostheses to the temporary titanium cylinders

values were measured, and the final prosthetic protocol was performed if all implants were osseointegrated.

Changes in marginal bone level were measured using the routinely made digital panoramic radiographs if these were available. The measurement tool was calibrated with the known respective implant length. To evaluate the bone loss, the difference was formed between the bone level at follow-up examination (Fig. 5) and at implant placement which is the baseline.

Success criteria
An implant was considered as successful if it fulfilled its function without pain or discomfort or clinically detectable mobility and if no peri-implant radiolucency or peri-implant infection was detectable.

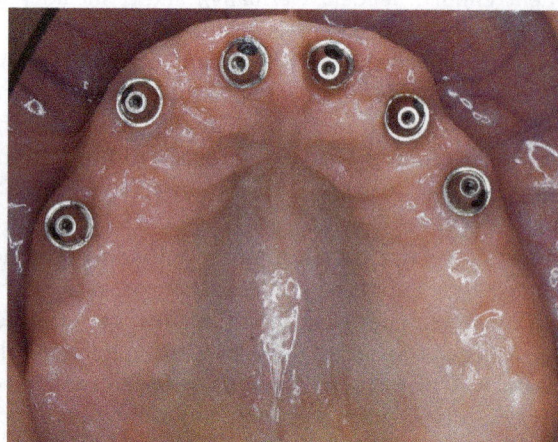

Fig. 2 Preparation of the composite veneers for making the temporary restoration

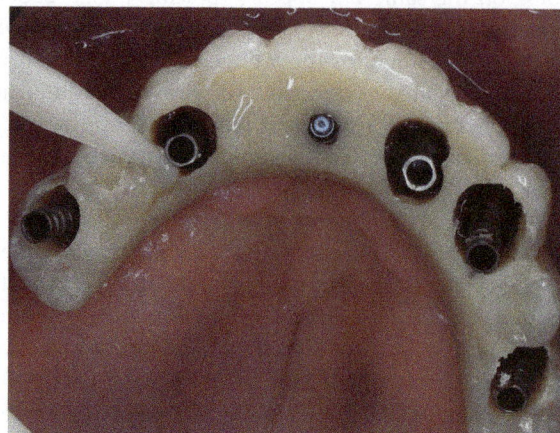

Fig. 4 Occlusal view of implant-abutments 3 months post-surgery at the first removal of the temporary restoration

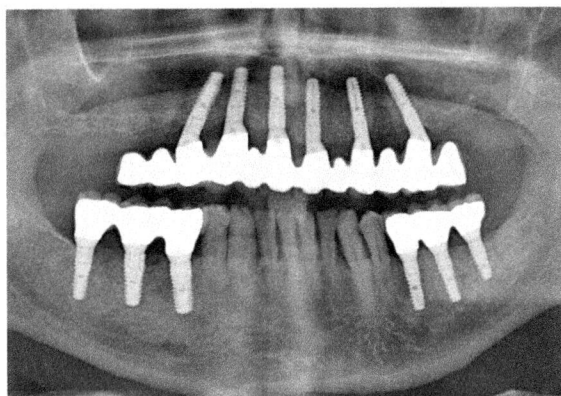

Fig. 5 One-year post-surgery panoramic radiograph with final restoration

Table 1 Diameters and lengths of immediately loaded implants

	Diameter	Length			
		10 mm	12 mm	14 mm	16 mm
Axial	3.5	3	13	3	–
	4.0	2	7	12	–
Tilted	3.5	–	2	4	–
	4.0	1	4	8	1

Data analysis

Descriptive statistics, including mean values and standard deviations, were calculated for the continuous parameters using SPSS software (ver. 17.0; SPSS Inc., Munich, Germany).

The measured values were tested for normal distribution with the Kolmogorov-Smirnov goodness-of-fit test. t test or nonparametric test was used for the evaluation of differences between dependent or independent samples.

The null hypothesis was that there is a significant difference between measured parameters between tilted and axially inserted implants. The alternative hypothesis was that the differences would be purely random. A significance level of 5% was determined as statistically significant.

To assess the suitability of the two stability parameters ISQ and PT values as potential predictors for the risk of non-osseointegration of immediately loaded splinted maxillary implants in this collective, sensitivity values were plotted against complementary specificity values in receiver operating characteristic (ROC) curves [13, 14]. The area under the curve (AUC) of the ROC analysis is a measure for the quality of the parameter analyzed as a prognostic test. An area of 1 represents a perfect test; an area of 0.5 represents an ineffective test.

Results

Ten patients with a mean age at implant insertion of 64 ± 11.3 years (range 38 to 81 years; six women, four men) were included. Sixty titanium screw implants (Table 1) were inserted and immediately loaded between 09/2009 and 01/2013.

Seven patients had remaining teeth until implant surgery (two patients with 4, four patients with 7, and one patient with 12 teeth). Twenty-one (35%) of the 60 immediately loaded implants where inserted in fresh

extraction sockets. Six implants in each patient were splinted by the provisional prosthesis on the day of surgery. The opposing dentition was natural teeth (n = 4 patients), implant-supported fixed prostheses (n = 4 patients), or natural teeth combined with additional implants (n = 2 patients). All patients analyzed showed at least opposite dentition with at least the first molar of the mandible replaced on both sides.

Osseointegration

Three of 60 immediately loaded implants (5%) in three patients were not osseointegrated after first removal of the temporary restorations 3 months after surgery (1 implant among the 40 axial implants [2.5%] and 2 implants among the 20 tilted implants [10%]).

The lost axial implant (12 × 4 mm, ISQ 68, PT value −2) was inserted in a fresh extraction socket in the patient with the most remaining teeth before implant surgery. In this patient, the temporary restoration broke two times.

The two non-osseointegrated tilted implants were both 14 × 4 mm. One was inserted in a maxilla which was edentulous for several years (ISQ 68, PT value −4). The other tilted implant was inserted in a maxilla with seven remaining teeth (ISQ of 49 and a PT value of +1). This implant was located with its apical half in the extraction socket of an immediately extracted canine. All failed implants were immediately replaced with implants of a larger diameter or length. All replaced implants healed load free and transmucosal. In both cases of the two non-osseointegrated tilted implants, the provisional prostheses were shortened but a cantilever extension of one molar width was left since the other implants were osseointegrated at this time. The final prosthesis procedure for the three patients with initial failures started 6 months after the first implant insertion, but the patients were functionally restored with a fixed prosthesis over the entire time.

After the temporary restoration with a fixed prosthesis, all 10 patients selected a fixed final restoration. These consisted of a cast metal framework with a full ceramic veneering including the replacement of at least the second premolars. They were made after a new impression on the abutment level (Figs. 6 and 7). The neck of the 20 tilted distal implants was positioned in region 4

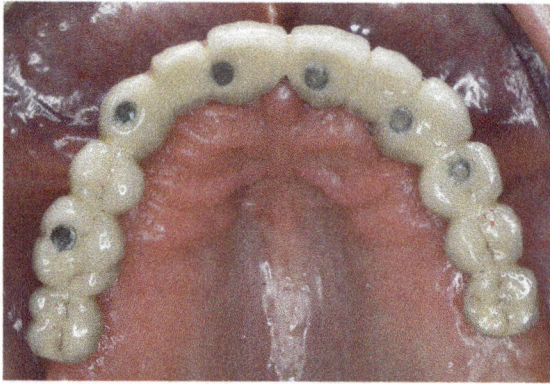

Fig. 6 Occlusal view of the final restoration. In this case, with the longest cantilever extension on a final restoration within this collective

(n = 5 implants), region 5 (n = 11 implants), and region 6 (n = 4 implants). The length of the distal cantilevers had a mean of 7.5 ± 4.1 mm (range 2.0 to 15.5) and replaced a premolar (n = 5), a molar (n = 5), or two premolars (n = 3). Seven times the distal cantilevers did not exceed the tooth under which the distal implant was positioned, leading to very small cantilevers in a range from 2 to 3.5 mm.

The follow-up was 64 ± 13 months (range 42 to 84 months; seven patients ≥5 years, two patients ≥4 years, one patient = 3.5 years) (Table 2).

Except the three failures after the first 3 months, no more failures were recorded and no technical complications occurred at the final restorations. The overall cumulative implant survival rate is 95% (Table 2).

Implant stability parameters

The mean PT value for osseointegrated implants after 3 months (n = 57) was significantly lower (p < 0.001), and their ISQ significantly higher (p < 0.001) than their means at baseline. Separated into axial (n = 39) and

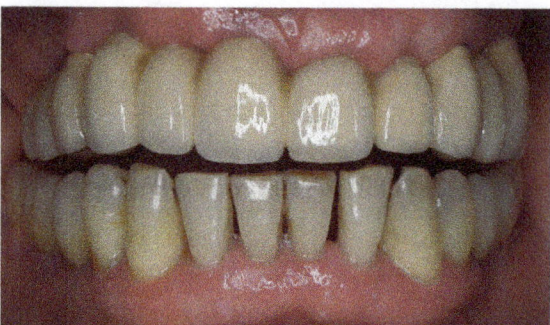

Fig. 7 Vestibular view of the final restoration

tilted (n = 18) implants, the differences were also significant (p < 0.005) (Tables 3 and 4).

Neither the PT value nor the ISQ differed statistically significantly between the axial and tilted implants neither at the baseline examination or after 3 months.

The AUC of the intraoperative-measured PT values was 0.503, with a 95% confidence interval of 0.130–0.876 (p = 0.986). The ISQ-AUC was 0.506, with a 95% confidence interval of 0.148–0.864 (p = 0.973).

Marginal bone loss

Bone loss was measured at all 57 osseointegrated implants after 1 year (Table 5) with no statistical significance regarding the implant site (mesial/distal) and the implant inclination (axial/tilted). In 51 implants, an additional bone loss was measured. In contrast to the radiological examination after 1 year, the second radiological examination was not obtained at an identical period. These control radiographs were made at a mean of 55 ± 14 months (range 40 to 84 months; one patient after 7 years, two patients after 5.5 years, one patient after 4.5 years, two patients after 4 years, three patients after 3.5 years) after loading with no statistical significance regarding the implant site and the implant inclination.

Discussion

The overall implant survival rate of 95% is slightly lower than the reported mean survival rates of the concept of tilted implants and immediate loading in edentulous jaws [11] but still close to them and maybe more comparable to investigations in which implants were also immediately loaded in the edentulous maxilla which were partly placed in fresh extraction sites [15, 16]. Nevertheless, what is remarkable is the two lost tilted implants (n = 2 of 20). In some reviews, there seems hardly to be a difference in the survival rate between axial and tilted implants [5, 11]. The potentially higher implant loss rate in this study might be due to the limited number of tilted implants.

In 30% of the patients (n = 3 of 10), one implant failed. There might be some reasons which could be responsible:

In the present study, one implant failed with a low primary stability. That confirms the assumption that a high primary stability is an important precondition for immediate loading [10]. However, the two other lost implants had high stability parameters. As shown by the low AUC values, the ISQ and PT values were unspecific parameters and unsuitable as a predictor for the risk of non-osseointegration in this collective, and this is in line with other studies [17, 18].

Table 2 Life table of implants

Period	# of implants	# of failures	Survival rate (%)	Cumulative survival rate (%)
0 to 3 months	60	3	95	95
3 to 6 months	57	0	100	95
6 to 9 months	57	0	100	95
9 to 12 month	57	0	100	95
1 year	57	0	100	95
2 years	57	0	100	95
3 years	57	0	100	95
4 years	51	0	100	95
5+ years	40	0	100	95

Another failure occurred in a situation where the provisional prostheses broke twice so that this implant might have been overloaded. Two of the failed three implants were completely or partially inserted in fresh extraction sockets, and studies have shown that this is an additional risk for implant failure in immediate loading in edentulous maxillae [16, 19].

That we have not found a significant difference in bone loss between straight and tilted implants is in line with the literature [5, 20]. In both reviews, the differences in bone loss after 12 months are in a range below a tenths of a millimeter and most probably not clinically relevant. It should be taken into account that the level of evidence of most studies is rather low due to the lack of randomized studies and the non-systematic use of a standardized technique to obtain a reproducible bone loss measurement [5, 11, 20]. This is a limit of the present study as well with a single cohort and measurements on digital panoramic radiographs and with irregular time intervals of the second measurement. This could explain that in some cases, even a bone growth was measured (up to 0.4 mm). Another limit of this study is the rather small patient group.

Between baseline and first removal of the temporary restoration after 3 months, the mean ISQ increased and the mean PT value decreased significantly in the axial and tilted implants. This is in contrast to some other studies which evaluated no significant differences of

stability parameters between primary and secondary stability with immediate loading in edentulous maxilla [16, 21, 22].

The present study shows that immediate splinted loading on six implants with tilted distal implants is a potential predictable treatment modality for edentulous maxilla even if extraction of remaining teeth and simultaneous implant placement is performed or if very limited bone is available in very atrophic jaws. Immediate implant placement and fractures of provisional prostheses seem to increase the risk of implant failure.

Immediate loading in edentulous maxilla with tilted implants could have a higher risk of initial implant failure, but treatment is less time consuming, less invasive, and in case of immediate implantation may be more comfortable and enhance or restore life quality. If a patient is informed in detail, this protocol seems to have an adequate success probability and treatment of choice for specific situations and patient's need.

Conclusions

Within the limits of this small group ($n = 10$ patients/60 implants), the failure rate of the analyzed implant system ($n = 3$ respective 5% implant loss) seems to be comparable with other immediate-loading protocols. On the other side, the implant loss rate of tilted implants ($n = 2$ of 20) in the atrophic upper jaw was quite high, but still,

Table 3 Mean Periotest values (PT) of survived axial and tilted implants

Collective	PT value		P
	At insertion	3 months	
Total ($n = 57$)	−1.8 ± 2.4 Range −8 to 1	−3.5 ± 1.6 Range −7 to −1	<0.001
Axial ($n = 39$)	−2.0 ± 2.5 Range −8 to 1	−3.4 ± 1.5 Range −6 to −1	<0.005
Tilted ($n = 18$)	−1.4 ± 2.1 Range −6 to 1	−3.6 ± 1.7 Range −6 to −1	<0.005

Table 4 Mean implant stability quotients (ISQ) of survived axial and tilted implants

Collective	ISQ		P
	At insertion	3 months	
Total ($n = 57$)	61.3 ± 7.8 Range 44 to 73	70.8 ± 5.5 Range 56 to 85	<0.001
Axial ($n = 39$)	61.6 ± 7.5 Range 49 to 73	70.7 ± 5.4 Range 56 to 85	<0.001
Tilted ($n = 18$)	60.6 ± 8.7 Range 44 to 72	71.1 ± 5.9 Range 62 to 83	<0.001

Table 5 Marginal bone loss measured in mm

Collective	Mesial		Distal	
	1 year	55 months (40–84)	1 year	55 months (40–84)
Total	−0.57 ± 0.46 Range −1.3 to 0.1 (*n* = 57)	−0.81 ± 0.67 Range −2.6 to 0.2 (*n* = 51)	−0.43 ± 0.41 Range −1.6 to 0.1 (*n* = 57)	−0.81 ± 0.74 Range −3.1 to 0.4 (*n* = 51)
Axial	−0.57 ± 0.46 Range −1.3 to 0.3 (*n* = 39)	−0.90 ± 0.68 Range −2.6 to 0.2 (*n* = 35)	−0.41 ± 0.41 Range −1.6 to 0.1 (*n* = 39)	−0.80 ± 0.76 Range −2.6 to 0.4 (*n* = 35)
Tilted	−0.56 ± 0.46 Range −1.3 to 0.1 (*n* = 18)	−0.62 ± 0.64 Range −2.1 to 0.1 (*n* = 16)	−0.51 ± 0.41 Range −1.0 to 0.1 (*n* = 18)	−0.81 ± 0.72 Range −3.1 to 0.0 (*n* = 16)

the aimed treatment concept could be achieved in every patient. The analyzed combination of implants, abutments, and materials for the provisional restorations seems to be suitable in the here chosen clinical setting for immediate loading, in part even in combination with immediate implantation.

Abbreviations
AUC: Area under the curve; ISQ: Implant stability quotient; PT: Periotest; ROC: Receiver operating characteristic

Acknowledgements
The authors would like to thank Bredent Medical (Senden, Germany) for providing the 3D-planning system and supporting the treatment nonfinancially.

Authors' contributions
SW and WW designed and performed the investigation. All prosthetic treatments were performed by SW, and all surgical treatments were performed by WW. SW and SH acquired and analyzed the data, and CW and WW helped to interpret them. SH, CW, and WW helped to draft the manuscript, and all authors have read and approved the final manuscript.

Competing interests
Stefan Wentaschek, Sinsa Hartmann, Christian Walter, and Wilfried Wagner declare that they have no competing interests.

Author details
[1]Department of Prosthetic Dentistry, University Medical Center of the Johannes Gutenberg-University Mainz, Augustusplatz 2, 55131 Mainz, Germany. [2]Department of Oral and Maxillofacial Surgery - Plastic Surgery, University Medical Center of the Johannes Gutenberg-University Mainz, Augustusplatz 2, 55131 Mainz, Germany.

References
1. Pommer B, Mailath-Pokorny G, Haas R, Busenlechner D, Furhauser R, Watzek G. Patients' preferences towards minimally invasive treatment alternatives for implant rehabilitation of edentulous jaws. Eur J Oral Implantol. 2014; 7(Suppl 2):S91–109.
2. Monje A, Suarez F, Galindo-Moreno P, Garcia-Nogales A, Fu JH, Wang HL. A systematic review on marginal bone loss around short dental implants (<10 mm) for implant-supported fixed prostheses. Clin Oral Implants Res. 2014; 25(10):1119–24.
3. Monje A, Fu JH, Chan HL, Suarez F, Galindo-Moreno P, Catena A, et al. Do implant length and width matter for short dental implants (<10 mm)? A meta-analysis of prospective studies. J Periodontol. 2013;84(12):1783–91.
4. Monje A, Chan HL, Fu JH, Suarez F, Galindo-Moreno P, Wang HL. Are short dental implants (<10 mm) effective? a meta-analysis on prospective clinical trials. J Periodontol. 2013;84(7):895–904.
5. Del Fabbro M, Ceresoli V. The fate of marginal bone around axial vs. tilted implants: a systematic review. Eur J Oral Implantol. 2014;7(Suppl 2):S171–89.
6. Mattsson T, Kondell PA, Gynther GW, Fredholm U, Bolin A. Implant treatment without bone grafting in severely resorbed edentulous maxillae. J Oral Maxillofac Surg. 1999;57(3):281–7.
7. Krekmanov L, Kahn M, Rangert B, Lindstrom H. Tilting of posterior mandibular and maxillary implants for improved prosthesis support. Int J Oral Maxillofac Implants. 2000;15(3):405–14.
8. Malo P, Rangert B, Nobre M. All-on-4 immediate-function concept with Branemark System implants for completely edentulous maxillae: a 1-year retrospective clinical study. Clin Implant Dent Relat Res. 2005;7(Suppl 1): S88–94.
9. Hong J, Lim YJ, Park SO. Quantitative biomechanical analysis of the influence of the cortical bone and implant length on primary stability. Clin Oral Implants Res. 2012;23(10):1193–7.
10. Papaspyridakos P, Chen CJ, Chuang SK, Weber HP. Implant loading protocols for edentulous patients with fixed prostheses: a systematic review and meta-analysis. Int J Oral Maxillofac Implants. 2014;29(Suppl 29):256–70.
11. Chrcanovic BR, Albrektsson T, Wennerberg A. Tilted versus axially placed dental implants: a meta-analysis. J Dent. 2014;43(2):149–70.
12. Bayer G, Kistler F, Kistler S, Adler S, Neugebauer J. Sofortversorgung mit reduzierter Implantatanzahl: Wissenschaftliche Konzeption und klinische Ergebnisse. Berlin: Quintessenz; 2011.
13. Hanley JA. Receiver operating characteristic (ROC) methodology: the state of the art. Crit Rev Diagn Imaging. 1989;29(3):307–35.
14. Atieh MA, Alsabeeha NH, Payne AG, de Silva RK, Schwass DS, Duncan WJ. The prognostic accuracy of resonance frequency analysis in predicting failure risk of immediately restored implants. Clin Oral Implants Res. 2014; 25(1):29–35.
15. Tealdo T, Bevilacqua M, Pera F, Menini M, Ravera G, Drago C, et al. Immediate function with fixed implant-supported maxillary dentures: a 12-month pilot study. J Prosthet Dent. 2008;99(5):351–60.
16. Andersson P, Degasperi W, Verrocchi D, Sennerby L. A retrospective study on immediate placement of Neoss implants with early loading of full-arch bridges. Clin Implant Dent Relat Res. 2013;2013(3). Epub ahead of print.
17. Atieh MA, Alsabeeha NH, Payne AG. Can resonance frequency analysis predict failure risk of immediately loaded implants? Int J Prosthodont. 2012; 25(4):326–39.
18. Wentaschek S, Scheller H, Schmidtmann I, Hartmann S, Weyhrauch M, Weibrich G, et al. Sensitivity and specificity of stability criteria for immediately loaded splinted maxillary implants. Clin Implant Dent Relat Res. 2014;2014(23). Epub ahead of print.
19. Covani U, Orlando B, D'Ambrosio A, Sabattini VB, Barone A. Immediate rehabilitation of completely edentulous jaws with fixed prostheses supported by implants placed into fresh extraction sockets and in healed sites: a 4-year clinical evaluation. Implant Dent. 2012;21(4):272–9.
20. Monje A, Chan HL, Suarez F, Galindo-Moreno P, Wang HL. Marginal bone loss around tilted implants in comparison to straight implants: a meta-analysis. Int J Oral Maxillofac Implants. 2012;27(6):1576–83.
21. Calandriello R, Tomatis M. Simplified treatment of the atrophic posterior maxilla via immediate/early function and tilted implants: a prospective 1-year clinical study. Clin Implant Dent Relat Res. 2005;7(Suppl 1):S1–12.

14

Early marginal bone stability of dental implants placed in a transalveolarly augmented maxillary sinus: a controlled retrospective study of surface modification with calcium ions

Eduardo Anitua[1,2,3,5*] iD, Laura Piñas[4] and Mohammad Hamdan Alkhraisat[2,3]

Abstract

Background: Recently, components of the extracellular cellular matrix have been assessed to enhance the biological response to dental implants. This study aims to assess the effect of surface modification with calcium ions on the early marginal bone loss of dental implants placed in a transalveolarly augmented maxillary sinus.

Methods: A retrospective study of transalveolar sinus floor augmentation was conducted in a single private dental clinic. The predictor variable was the surface of the dental implant. The primary outcome was the marginal bone loss. The secondary outcomes were the intraoperative complications and the dental implant failure. Descriptive analysis was performed for patients' demographic data and implant details.

Results: Fifty-one patients with a mean age of 58 ± 11 years had a mean follow-up time of 13 months. Thirty-four dental implants had a Ca^{2+}-modified hydrophilic surface, and 31 had no Ca^2 (control). The experimental group showed a statistically significant lower marginal bone loss (0.36 ± 0.42 vs 0.61 ± 0.39 mm). However, there were no statistically significant differences in the implant survival. No implant failed in the experimental group while two implants failed in the control group.

Conclusions: The modification of an acid-etched surface with calcium ions seems to reduce the marginal bone remodeling around the dental implants, placed after transalveolar sinus floor elevation.

Keywords: Calcium, Dental implant, Implant surface, Marginal bone loss, Osseointegration

Background

Dental implants are nowadays the treatment of choice to replace missing teeth due to their high predictability and long-term success [1]. This success is the outcome of several cellular and molecular events that take place at the implant-bone interface. Although the process of osseointegration is not fully understood, research is ongoing to enhance and accelerate this process. Moderately rough implant surface has enhanced implant osseointegration and has increased the implant secondary stability [2, 3]. Recently, elements of the extracellular cellular matrix have been introduced to bio-activate the dental implant surface [4, 5].

Calcium is one of these elements that has been studied to enhance the osseointegration process [6, 7]. Recently, Favero et al. have compared modifications of an acid-etched surface with calcium ions (UnicCa®) against a surface modified by a nanometer-scale Discrete Crystalline Deposition (DCD™) of Calcium Phosphate [8]. The patterns of sequential healing have been similar for the two surfaces, although the UnicCa® surface showed a statistically significant higher new bone formation at 2 and 4 weeks. Moreover, the osseointegration process of UnicCa® and the

* Correspondence: eduardo@fundacioneduardoanitua.org
[1]Private practice in oral implantology, Clínica Eduardo Anitua, Vitoria, Spain
[2]University Institute for Regenerative Medicine and Oral Implantology - UIRMI (UPV/EHU-Fundación Eduardo Anitua), Vitoria, Spain
Full list of author information is available at the end of the article

SLActive® surfaces has been very similar without statistically significant differences [9].

A research is needed to study if these enhancements to the dental implant surface would improve the outcome of dental implants. It has been reported that 40% of the implant failures occur during the period of osseointegration (early failures) [10]. The presence of low-density bone is a challenging situation to achieve the success of dental implants and requires specific treatment plan and surgical protocol to minimize the risk of implant failure [11, 12]. The rehabilitation of posterior maxilla with an implant-supported prosthesis could be complicated by the presence of low-density bone [13].

For that, the aim of this study is to evaluate the early survival of UnicCa® dental implants placed in transalveolarly augmented maxillary sinus. The null hypothesis of the study is that the UnicCa® surface does not enhance implant survival nor the marginal bone stability. The principal outcome has been the marginal bone stability and as secondary outcome the implant survival.

Methods

The manuscript was written following STROBE (Strengthening the Reporting of Observational studies in Epidemiology) guidelines. All described data and treatments were obtained from a single dental clinic in Vitoria, Spain. The time period of the study was between December 2014 and April 2016. Patients' records were retrospectively reviewed to identify patients that fulfilled the following inclusion criteria:

- Male and female patients older than 18 years old.
- Transalveolar sinus floor augmentation.
- The insertion of dental implants.

Patients/implants were excluded if not completed with all these criteria. Patients with incomplete data were also excluded. An exemption from IRB approval of the study protocol was granted by the author's institution as it was a retrospective study, and the evaluated medical devise had already been approved for clinical use. This study was performed following the Helsinki declaration regarding the investigation with human subjects.

The principal outcome was the marginal bone loss. The experimental group was composed of the dental implants with Ca^{2+} ions (UnicCa® surface), and the control group was composed of the implants having the same surface as the UnicCa® but without the calcium ion modification (known as Optima® surface). The surface is acid-etched to generate a multi-scale roughness at the different parts of the implant (neck, valleys, and threads) in adaptation to the different biological needs: homogenous and attenuated roughness at the neck to avoid the risk of bacterial colonization, micro-roughness at the valleys to enhance the

osseointegration, and micro-roughness + pores at the threads to enhance anchorage.

Outcome assessment

Data about patients' age and sex were collected. Cone-beam CT scans were visualized in BTI Scan III (Biotechnology Institute, Vitoria, Spain) to measure the residual bone height and the bone density at the surgical site. The sequence of bone drilling was determined according to the bone density [14].

Implant survival determined whether the implant was still physically in the mouth or lost at the time of evaluation. To assess the marginal bone stability, the distance between the uppermost point of the implant platform and the most coronal bone-implant contact was measured mesial and distal to the implant by a computer software (Sidexis, Sirona, USA). Implant length was used to calibrate the linear measurements on the radiograph.

Surgical procedure

The plasma rich in growth factors (PRGF) was prepared using the Endoret® system following the manufacturer instructions (BTI Biotechnology Institute, Vitoria, Spain). The technique for transalveolar sinus floor elevation is explained elsewhere [15]. Briefly, conventional drills working at low speed (150 rpm) without irrigation was used to prepare the implant site. A frontal cutting drill was then introduced to prepare the last 1 mm of the implant alveolus. When a window (half of the sinus floor) was created, a well-retracted fibrin plug was introduced. The sinus floor could be opened further, if it was needed. A blunt hand instrument was introduced to push apically the fibrin membrane and to elevate the Schneiderian membrane, simultaneously. The area below the Schneiderian membrane was grafted by PRGF clot. Before implant insertion, the implant socket was irrigated with PRGF. The implants were inserted by a surgical motor at a torque value of 25 N cm. Then, the implant was completed seated with a calibrated torque wrench.

After completing the surgical and prosthetic phases, the patient was reviewed at 6 and 12 months during the observation period of the study.

Statistical analysis

Data collection and analysis were performed by an independent examiner (other than restorative dentist and surgeon). A descriptive analysis of the implant location, length, diameter, bone grafting, and marginal bone loss was performed by considering the implant as the statistical unit of analysis. Shapiro-Wilk test was selected as normality test. Mann-Whitney test was applied to compare the follow-up time, insertion torque, and proximal bone loss between the study groups. Patients' age, sex, and medical history were also analyzed. The

Early marginal bone stability of dental implants placed in a transalveolarly augmented maxillary...

101

bone type was compared with Fischer's exact test and the number of implant failures by χ^2 test.

The statistical significance level was 5% ($p < 0.05$). SPSS v15.0 for Windows statistical software package (SPSS Inc., Chicago, IL, USA) was used.

Results and discussion

In this study, 51 patients participated with 65 dental implants. The mean age of the patients was 58 ± 11 years (range 38 to 72 years) at the time of surgery, and 28 were females.

The experimental group had 34 Ca^{2+}-modified dental implants, and the control group had 31 dental implants (without surface modification with calcium ions).

Tables 1 and 2 show the diameters and lengths of the placed dental implants in the experimental and control groups, respectively. Figure 1 shows the anatomical position of the dental implants in the study groups. The residual alveolar bone was of type II (12 implants), type III (16 implants), and type IV (6 implants) in the experimental group. Table 3 shows the bone type in the control group that had significantly more bone of better quality. Dental implants were placed at a mean insertion torque > 30 N cm in both groups (Table 3). The healing time was 4 months. They were mainly supporting fixed screw-retained prostheses, and delayed implant loading was performed.

No intraoperative complications were recorded. During the follow-up period (13 months), no implant failure was encountered in the experimental group. The control group had two implant failures. However, these differences were not statistically significant (Table 3). The mesial and distal bone loss in the experimental group was 0.3 ± 0.5 and 0.5 ± 7 mm, respectively. The proximal bone loss was significantly lower in the experimental group (Table 3).

The results of this study do not support the acceptance of the null hypothesis. The modification of an acid-etched surface with calcium ions (UnicCa®) has enhanced the marginal bone stability.

Maxillary sinus floor elevation using the transalveolar approach may be a valid and less invasive supplement to the lateral window technique [16, 17]. A prerequisite for using this technique is that primary implant stability could be achieved. Implant's primary stability is the result of quantity and quality of hosting bone, the design

Table 1 Length and diameter of the dental implants in the experimental group

		Diameter (mm)					Total
		4.25	5.00	5.50	6.00	6.25	
Length (mm)	5.5	1	3	3	0	0	7
	6.5	0	5	12	4	2	23
	7.5	0	2	1	0	1	4
Total		1	10	16	4	3	34

Table 2 Length and diameter of the dental implants in the control group

		Diameter (mm)					Total
		4.25	5.00	5.50	6.00	6.25	
Length (mm)	5.5	0	1	1	0	0	2
	6.5	0	2	6	0	4	12
	7.5	0	1	10	1	2	14
	8.5	0	0	2	1	0	3
Total		0	4	19	2	6	31

of the implant, and the drilling technique [18]. Implant macro-design is a parameter that significantly influences implant primary stability. Ca^{2+}-modified dental implants were placed following the same surgical procedure described by Anitua et al. [15] to place the same dental implant but without Ca^{2+}. For that, no statistically significant differences in primary stability were found between the two dental implants.

Unlike Ca^{2+}-modified dental implants, two early implant losses were observed for the same dental implants but without Ca^{2+}. Moderately rough implant surface has enhanced implant osseointegration and has increased the implant secondary stability [2, 3, 19]. Hydrophilic moderately rough surfaces showed faster osseointegration compared to those with hydrophobic characteristics [20, 21]. Ca^{2+} ions have been shown to protect the hydrophilic implant surface against aging and the formation of carbon-rich species [4, 6].

Upon exposure to blood plasma, Ca^{2+}-modified surface has induced surface clot formation, platelet adsorption, and activation [6]. By using a peri-implant gap model in

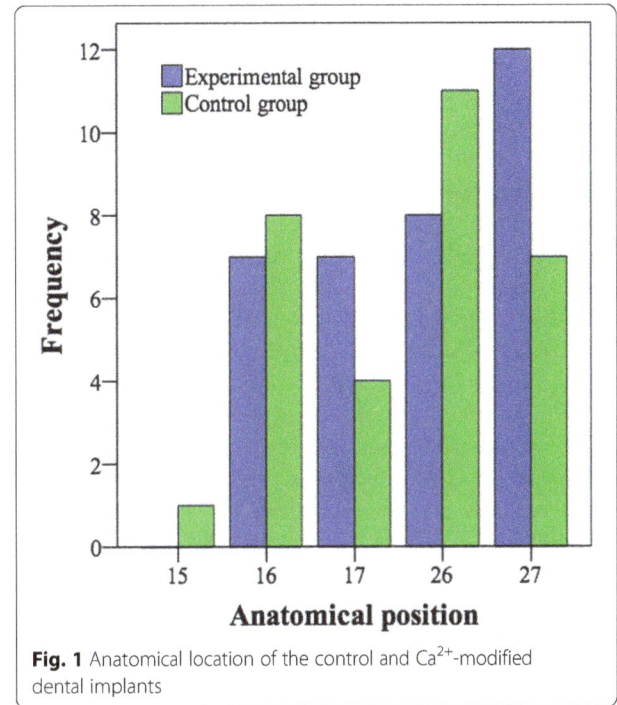

Fig. 1 Anatomical location of the control and Ca^{2+}-modified dental implants

Table 3 Outcomes of experimental and control groups

Variable		Experimental	Control	$P < 0.05$
Number of implants		34	31	
Bone type	II	35.3%	74.2%	Yes[a]
	III	47.1%	22.6%	
	IV	17.6%	3.2%	
Follow-up time (months)		13 ± 1[d]	13 ± 2[d]	No[b]
Insertion torque (N cm)		36 ± 15[d]	30 ± 15[d]	No[b]
Implant failure		0	2	No[c]
Proximal bone loss (mm)		0.36 ± 0.42[d]	0.61 ± 0.39[d]	Yes[b]

[a]Fischer's exact test
[b]Mann-Whitney test
[c]χ^2 test
[d]Mean ± standard deviation

rabbit, Ca^{2+}-modified surface has significantly improved peri-implant bone volume and density at 2 weeks and bone-to-implant contact at 8 weeks [6]. Ca^{2+}-modified surface presented a significantly more new bone formation at 2 and 4 weeks compared to a surface modified by nanometer-scale discrete crystalline deposition of calcium phosphate [8].

In this study, the modifications of an acid-etched surface with calcium ions have significantly decreased the marginal bone loss. Preservation of the crestal bone has been higher in Ca^{2+}-modified implants compared to unmodified implants. One of the criteria of dental implant success as defined by Buser et al. [22] and modified by Albrektsson et al. [23] is the absence of persistent peri-implant bone resorption greater than 1.5 mm during the first year of loading and 0.2 mm per year during the following years. Östman et al. have documented the outcomes of dental implants modified with nanometer-scale discrete crystalline deposition of calcium phosphate [24]. The dental implants have been immediately loaded by the fixed prostheses in both maxillary and mandibular regions. The average marginal bone resorption was 0.37 ± 0.39 mm during the first year in function. This outcome might be related to the implant surface modification.

This study was limited by the retrospective design, data dependency on the accuracy of the patients' record, and the short follow-up. Further prospective controlled studies with a long-term follow-up are required. The use of panoramic radiographs could be a source of error in measurement that was reduced by performing a 1:1 calibration of the radiograph. This would render the measurements sufficiently accurate for clinical use [25].

Conclusions

The modification of an acid-etched surface with calcium ions (UnicCa®) seems to enhance the marginal bone stability of dental implants, placed after transalveolar sinus floor elevation.

Abbreviations
PRGF: Plasma rich in growth factors; STROBE: Strengthening the Reporting of Observational studies in Epidemiology

Acknowledgements
Not applicable

Funding
No funding was received for this study.

Authors' contributions
EA, LP, and MHA was responsible for the concept/design of the study. EA, LP, and MHA collected the data. LP and MHA interpreted and analyzed the data. LP and MHA drafted the article. EA, LP, and MHA critically revised and aproved the article. All authors read and approved the final manuscript.

Competing interests
Eduardo Anitua is the Scientific Director of BTI Biotechnology Institute (Vitoria, Spain). He is the head of the Foundation Eduardo Anitua, Vitoria, Spain. Laura Piñas has no conflict of interest. Mohammad Hamdan Alkhraisat is a scientist at BTI Biotechnology Institute (Vitoria, Spain).

Author details
[1]Private practice in oral implantology, Clínica Eduardo Anitua, Vitoria, Spain. [2]University Institute for Regenerative Medicine and Oral Implantology - UIRMI (UPV/EHU-Fundación Eduardo Anitua), Vitoria, Spain. [3]BTI Biotechnology Institute, Vitoria, Spain. [4]Universidad Europea de Madrid, Madrid, Spain. [5]Eduardo Anitua Foundation, C/Jose Maria Cagigal 19, 01007 Vitoria, Spain.

References
1. Moraschini V, Poubel LA, Ferreira VF, Barboza Edos S. Evaluation of survival and success rates of dental implants reported in longitudinal studies with a follow-up period of at least 10 years: a systematic review. Int J Oral Maxillofac Surg. 2015;44:377–88.
2. Berglundh T, Abrahamsson I, Lang NP, Lindhe J. De novo alveolar bone formation adjacent to endosseous implants. Clin Oral Implants Res. 2003;14: 251–62.
3. Buser D, Schenk RK, Steinemann S, Fiorellini JP, Fox CH, Stich H. Influence of surface characteristics on bone integration of titanium implants. A histomorphometric study in miniature pigs. J Biomed Mater Res. 1991;25:889–902.
4. Anitua E, Tejero R, Alkhraisat MH, Orive G. Platelet-rich plasma to improve the bio-functionality of biomaterials. BioDrugs. 2013;27:97–111.
5. Tejero R, Anitua E, Orive G. Toward the biomimetic implant surface: biopolymers on titanium-based implants for bone regeneration. Prog Polym Sci. 2014;39:1406–47.
6. Anitua E, Prado R, Orive G, Tejero R. Effects of calcium-modified titanium implant surfaces on platelet activation, clot formation, and osseointegration. J Biomed Mater Res A. 2015;103:969–80.
7. Mendes VC, Moineddin R, Davies JE. The effect of discrete calcium phosphate nanocrystals on bone-bonding to titanium surfaces. Biomaterials. 2007;28:4748–55.
8. Favero R, Botticelli D, Antunes AA, Martinez Sanchez R, Caroprese M, Salata LA. Sequential healing at calcium- versus calcium phosphate-modified titanium implant surfaces: an experimental study in dogs. Clin Implant Dent Relat Res. 2016;18:369–78.
9. Favero R, Lang NP, Salata LA, Neto EC, Caroprese M, Botticelli D. Sequential healing events of osseointegration at UnicCa® and SLActive® implant surfaces: an experimental study in the dog. Clin Oral Implants Res. 2016;27:203–10.
10. Esposito M, Hirsch JM, Lekholm U, Thomsen P. Biological factors contributing to failures of osseointegrated oral implants. (II). Etiopathogenesis. Eur J Oral Sci. 1998;106:721–64.
11. Bahat O. Branemark system implants in the posterior maxilla: clinical study of 660 implants followed for 5 to 12 years. Int J Oral Maxillofac Implants. 2000;15:646–53.

Early marginal bone stability of dental implants placed in a transalveolarly augmented maxillary...

103

12. Friberg B, Sennerby L, Meredith N, Lekholm U. A comparison between cutting torque and resonance frequency measurements of maxillary implants. A 20-month clinical study. Int J Oral Maxillofac Surg. 1999;28:297–303.

13. Jaffin RA, Berman CL. The excessive loss of Branemark fixtures in type IV bone: a 5-year analysis. J Periodontol. 1991;62:2–4.

14. Anitua E, Alkhraisat MH, Pinas L, Orive G. Efficacy of biologically guided implant site preparation to obtain adequate primary implant stability. Ann Anat. 2015;199:9–15.

15. Anitua E, Alkhraist MH, Piñas L, Orive G. Association of transalveolar sinus floor elevation, platelet rich plasma, and short implants for the treatment of atrophied posterior maxilla. Clin Oral Implants Res. 2015;26:69–75.

16. Del Fabbro M, Corbella S, Weinstein T, Ceresoli V, Taschieri S. Implant survival rates after osteotome-mediated maxillary sinus augmentation: a systematic review. Clin Implant Dent Relat Res. 2012;14(Suppl 1):e159–68.

17. Peleg M, Garg AK, Mazor Z. Predictability of simultaneous implant placement in the severely atrophic posterior maxilla: a 9-year longitudinal experience study of 2132 implants placed into 731 human sinus grafts. Int J Oral Maxillofac Implants. 2006;21:94–102.

18. Rabel A, Kohler SG, Schmidt-Westhausen AM. Clinical study on the primary stability of two dental implant systems with resonance frequency analysis. Clin Oral Investig. 2007;11:257–65.

19. Wennerberg A, Albrektsson T, Andersson B, Krol JJ. A histomorphometric and removal torque study of screw-shaped titanium implants with three different surface topographies. Clin Oral Implants Res. 1995;6:24–30.

20. Bosshardt DD, Salvi GE, Huynh-Ba G, Ivanovski S, Donos N, Lang NP. The role of bone debris in early healing adjacent to hydrophilic and hydrophobic implant surfaces in man. Clin Oral Implants Res. 2011;22:357–64.

21. Lang NP, Salvi GE, Huynh-Ba G, Ivanovski S, Donos N, Bosshardt DD. Early osseointegration to hydrophilic and hydrophobic implant surfaces in humans. Clin Oral Implants Res. 2011;22:349–56.

22. Buser D, Weber HP, Bragger U, Balsiger C. Tissue integration of one-stage implants: three-year results of a prospective longitudinal study with hollow cylinder and hollow screw implants. Quintessence Int. 1994;25:679–86.

23. Albrektsson T, Zarb GA. Determinants of correct clinical reporting. Int J Prosthodont. 1998;11:517–21.

24. Ostman PO, Wennerberg A, Albrektsson T. Immediate occlusal loading of NanoTite PREVAIL implants: a prospective 1-year clinical and radiographic study. Clin Implant Dent Relat Res. 2010;12:39–47.

25. Schulze R, Krummenauer F, Schalldach F, d'Hoedt B. Precision and accuracy of measurements in digital panoramic radiography. Dentomaxillofac Radiol. 2000;29:52–6.

15

Platelet-rich fibrin prepared from stored whole-blood samples

Kazushige Isobe[1], Masashi Suzuki[1], Taisuke Watanabe[1], Yutaka Kitamura[1], Taiji Suzuki[1], Hideo Kawabata[1], Masayuki Nakamura[1], Toshimitsu Okudera[1], Hajime Okudera[1], Kohya Uematsu[2], Koh Nakata[3], Takaaki Tanaka[4] and Tomoyuki Kawase[5*] (iD)

Abstract

Background: In regenerative therapy, self-clotted platelet concentrates, such as platelet-rich fibrin (PRF), are generally prepared on-site and are immediately used for treatment. If blood samples or prepared clots can be preserved for several days, their clinical applicability will expand. Here, we prepared PRF from stored whole-blood samples and examined their characteristics.

Methods: Blood samples were collected from non-smoking, healthy male donors (aged 27–67 years, $N = 6$), and PRF clots were prepared immediately or after storage for 1–2 days. Fibrin fiber was examined by scanning electron microscopy. Bioactivity was evaluated by means of a bioassay system involving human periosteal cells, whereas PDGF-BB concentrations were determined by an enzyme-linked immunosorbent assay.

Results: Addition of optimal amounts of a 10% $CaCl_2$ solution restored the coagulative ability of whole-blood samples that contained an anticoagulant (acid citrate dextrose) and were stored for up to 2 days at ambient temperature. In PRF clots prepared from the stored whole-blood samples, the thickness and cross-links of fibrin fibers were almost identical to those of freshly prepared PRF clots. PDGF-BB concentrations in the PRF extract were significantly lower in stored whole-blood samples than in fresh samples; however, both extracts had similar stimulatory effects on periosteal-cell proliferation.

Conclusions: Quality of PRF clots prepared from stored whole-blood samples is not reduced significantly and can be ensured for use in regenerative therapy. Therefore, the proposed method enables a more flexible treatment schedule and choice of a more suitable platelet concentrate immediately before treatment, not after blood collection.

Keywords: Platelet-rich fibrin, Coagulation, Fibrin fiber, Anticoagulant, Calcium chloride

Background

Blood preservation is generally and widely used in the fields of blood transfusion and surgery for either autologous or allogeneic blood [1–3]. In case of small lots of blood-derived materials used in regenerative therapy, such as platelet concentrates, it is generally accepted that autologous blood samples should be collected on-site and immediately centrifuged for processing [4]. Accordingly, it is officially recommended to use thus prepared materials immediately. The advantages of this preparation protocol are the zero cost of preservation and no risk of degradation and contamination.

In Niigata University Hospital, when relatively severe surgical operations (e.g., large bone defects that require hospitalization for alveolar ridge augmentation and sinus floor elevation) are planned, relatively large volumes of blood samples are usually collected the day before the operation, and platelet-rich plasma (PRP) is prepared and stored at ambient temperature until use [5]. Nevertheless, there are no established methods for preparation of self-clotted platelet concentrates from stored whole-blood (WB) samples. This may be another reason why platelet-rich fibrin (PRF) should be prepared on-site and used immediately.

* Correspondence: kawase@dent.niigata-u.ac.jp
[5]Division of Oral Bioengineering, Institute of Medicine and Dentistry, Niigata University, Niigata, Japan
Full list of author information is available at the end of the article

On the other hand, if PRF can be prepared from stored WB samples on the next day or later without significant reduction in the bioactivity, clinical applications of PRF will expand. In this study, we developed a method for preparation of PRF from stored WB samples by adding $CaCl_2$ and evaluated the quality in terms of suitability for regenerative therapy. As a result, we successfully validated the method and ensured the quality of PRF prepared from stored WB samples.

Methods

Blood collection, preservation, and PRF preparation

The study design and consent forms for all procedures performed on the study subjects were approved by the ethics committee for human subjects at Niigata University School of Medicine in accordance with the Helsinki Declaration of 1975 as revised in 2008.

With informed consent, blood samples (~9.0 mL per tube) were collected from six non-smoking, healthy, male volunteers (27 to 67 years old) using 21-gauge needles equipped with conventional vacuum plain glass tube (Plain BD Vacutainer Tube; Becton, Dickinson and Company, Franklin Lakes, NJ, USA) as described previously [6–8]. For preparation of control PRF by the conventional method, the anticoagulant was not added. Blood samples were immediately centrifuged or stored by gentle mixing using a tube rotator at ambient temperature (18–22 °C).

The blood samples collected with the anticoagulant and stored for up to 2 days were centrifuged by means of a Medifuge centrifugation system (Silfradent S.r.l., Santa Sofia, Italy). After elimination of the red blood cell fractions, the resulting PRF clots, more specifically termed as concentrated growth factors (CGF) [9], were stored at −80 °C until measurement of growth factor concentration.

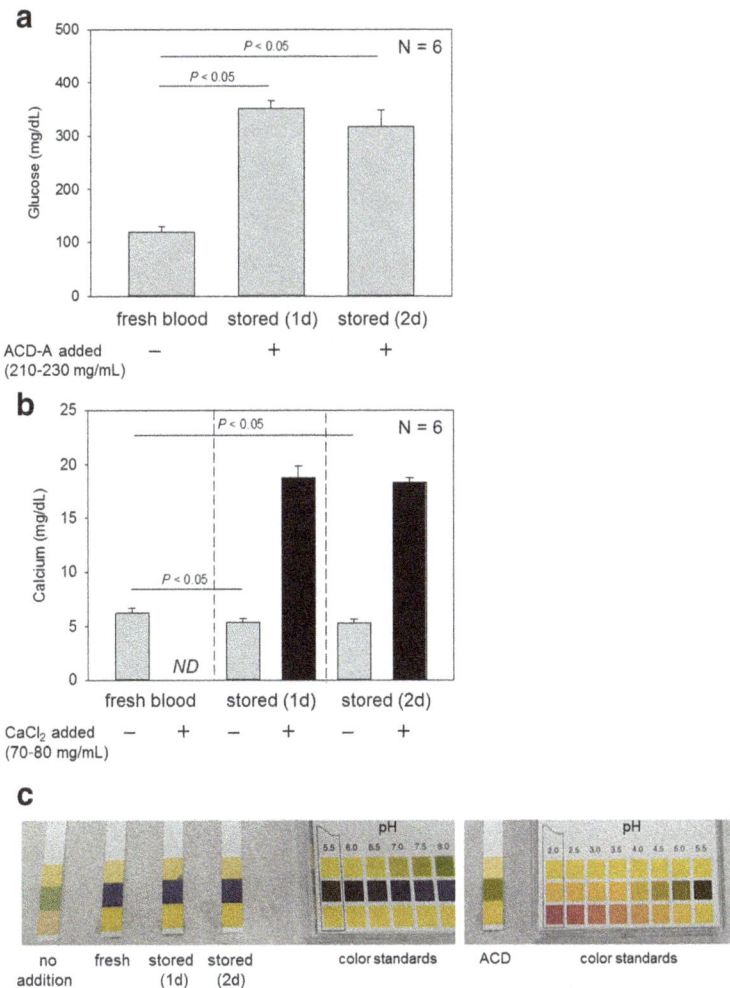

Fig. 1 Glucose levels (a), calcium levels (b), and pH (c) of stored WB samples. Supernatant serum fractions were examined. Plasma fractions prepared by quick centrifugation were used to determine calcium levels in fresh and stored WB samples that were not added $CaCl_2$. $N = 6$

For preparation of platelet-poor plasma (PPP), blood samples (~9.0 mL) were collected from the same volunteers by means of plastic vacuum blood collection tubes (Neotube®; NIPRO, Osaka, Japan) equipped with 21-gauge needles, in the presence of 1.0 mL acid citrate dextrose solution-A formulation (ACD-A; Terumo, Tokyo, Japan), an anticoagulant [8, 10]. The blood samples were centrifuged on a KS-5000 centrifuge (Kubota, Tokyo, Japan) equipped with a swing rotor at 1700 rpm (530g) and 3000 rpm (1660g) for the first and second spin (8 min), respectively. The resulting supernatant fractions were collected as PPP preparations. To form fibrin clots, bovine thrombin (Liquid Thrombin MOCHIDA softbottle, Mochida Pharmaceutical Co., Ltd., Tokyo, Japan) was added to PPP at a final volume percentage of 2.5%.

Determination of glucose, calcium, and pH

WB samples were quickly centrifuged at 1500 rpm for 3 min to prepare plasma fraction, which were subjected to determine total free calcium levels using a commercial kit based on MXB method (Calcium E-test WAKO; Wako Pure Chemicals, Osaka, Japan).

Stored WB samples were then mixed intermittently with 200 μL (20 μL × 10 times) of 10% CaCl$_2$ solution and centrifuged by a Medifuge centrifugation system to prepare PRF. When lower amounts of CaCl$_2$ were added, PRF clots were less reproducibly prepared. When higher amounts of CaCl$_2$ were added intermittently, or when the optimal amount of CaCl$_2$ were added at once, PRF clots were never prepared (Kawase, unpublished observations).

The supernatant serum fractions were subjected to determine calcium and glucose levels as described above and using a commercial kit based on GOD method (Glucose CII-test WAKO; Wako Pure Chemicals). The serum fractions were also used to determine pH levels by pH indicators (MColorHast; EMD Millipore Corp., Billerica, MA, USA).

A bioassay on human periosteal cells

The frozen PRF samples were minced with scissors and homogenized using a disposable homogenizer (Bio-Masher II, Nippi, Tokyo, Japan). After high-speed centrifugation (7340g), supernatants (PRF extracts) were collected and used for the bioassay described below and for measurement of growth factor levels.

Because alveolar periosteum strongly contributes to regeneration of periodontal skeletal tissue [11], we used human alveolar bone-derived periosteal cells for evaluation of the potency and efficacy of PRF preparations. The periosteal cells were obtained and expanded as described elsewhere [8, 12]. With informed consent,

human periosteum tissue segments were aseptically excised from the periodontal tissue on the healthy buccal side of the retromolar region of the mandibles of two non-smoking female volunteers (age = 19 and 29). Small periosteum pieces were expanded to form multilayered cellular periosteal sheets (∅ 30–40 mm), and then these sheets were enzymatically digested with 0.05% trypsin plus 0.52 mM EDTA (Invitrogen, Carlsbad, CA, USA) to release single cells. After expansion in monolayer cultures, the cells were seeded at a density of 0.4×10^4 per well in 24-well plates and treated with PRF extracts (0, 0.5, 1, 2, or 4%) for 72 h in DMEM containing 1% of fetal bovine serum (Invitrogen, Carlsbad, CA, USA). Six different lots of PRF extracts were used for each experiment. At the end of the incubation periods, the cells were harvested using 0.05% trypsin plus 0.53 mM EDTA and immediately counted on an automated cell counter (Moxi-z; ORLFO Technologies, Ketchum, ID, USA) ($N = 6$) [13].

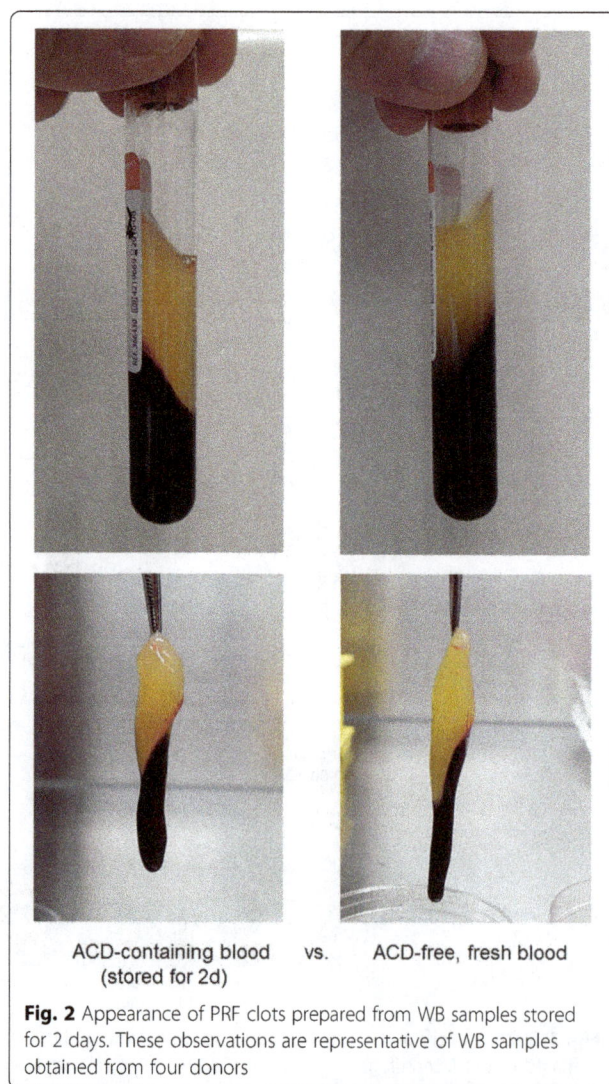

ACD-containing blood   vs.   ACD-free, fresh blood
(stored for 2d)

Fig. 2 Appearance of PRF clots prepared from WB samples stored for 2 days. These observations are representative of WB samples obtained from four donors

Quantification of a growth factor by an enzyme-linked immunosorbent assay (ELISA)

PRF extracts prepared as described above were subjected to measurement of PDGF-BB levels using the Human PDGF-BB Quantikine ELISA Kit (R&D Systems, Inc., Minneapolis, MN, USA) as described previously [8].

Scanning electron microscopy (SEM)

The PRF clots that were compressed in a stainless-steel compressor were fixed with 2.5% neutralized glutaraldehyde, dehydrated with a series of ethanol solutions and t-butanol, freeze-dried, and then examined under a scanning electron microscope (TM-1000, Hitachi, Tokyo, Japan) with an accelerating voltage of 15 kV, as described elsewhere [7, 14].

Statistical analysis

The data were expressed as mean ± standard deviation (SD). For multigroup comparisons, statistical analyses were conducted to compare the mean values by one-way analysis of variance (ANOVA) followed by Tukey's multiple-comparison test (SigmaPlot 12.5; Systat Software, Inc., San Jose, CA, USA). Differences with P values <0.05 were considered significant.

Results

Glucose and calcium contents and pH of WB or serum samples after centrifugation are shown in Fig. 1. Because glucose is contained in the ACD-A solution, glucose levels in the stored WB and serum samples (see Fig. 4c) after centrifugation were significantly greater than those of freshly collected WB samples. Total free calcium levels, including calcium chelated by citrate, in WB samples decreased significantly during storage and were significantly increased by addition of a 10% $CaCl_2$ solution. The pH levels of freshly collected WB samples were 6.0–6.5, and similar pH was observed in stored WB samples. Addition of the ACD-A solution (~10%) did not significantly decrease the pH of the stored WB samples. For reference, pH of ACD-A solution was 4.5–5.0.

The appearance of PRF clots prepared from freshly collected WB samples and WB samples stored for 2 days are shown in Fig. 2. There were no visual differences between these two PRF preparations. Microstructure of fibrin clots formed from fresh and 2-day-old WB samples is shown in Fig. 3. As for thickness and cross-links of fibrin fibers, no substantial differences were observed. For reference, fibrin clots that were prepared from PPP and bovine thrombin were composed of apparently thinner fibrin fibers as compared with PRF clots from either fresh or stored WB samples.

The biological activity was tested on human periosteal cells. The effects of PRF extracts on the cell proliferation are shown in Fig. 4a. PRF extracts (0–4%) prepared from fresh, 1-day-old, and 2-day-old WB samples exerted similar stimulatory effects on the proliferation of

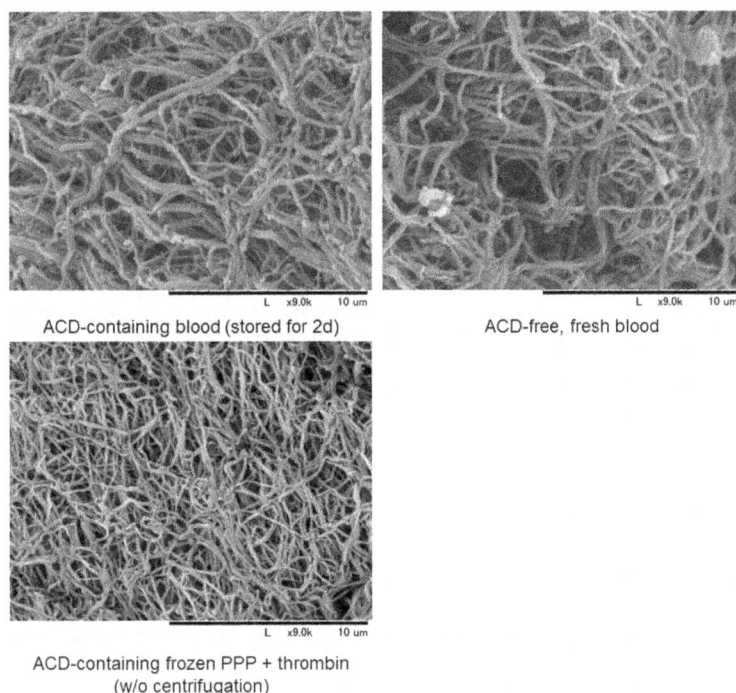

ACD-containing blood (stored for 2d)

ACD-free, fresh blood

ACD-containing frozen PPP + thrombin
(w/o centrifugation)

Fig. 3 SEM examination of fibrin fibers formed in self-clotted PRF and thrombin-stimulated PPP clots. PRF was prepared from fresh and 2-day-old WB samples. Similar observations were obtained from WB samples collected from three other donors. *Scale bars* = 10 μm

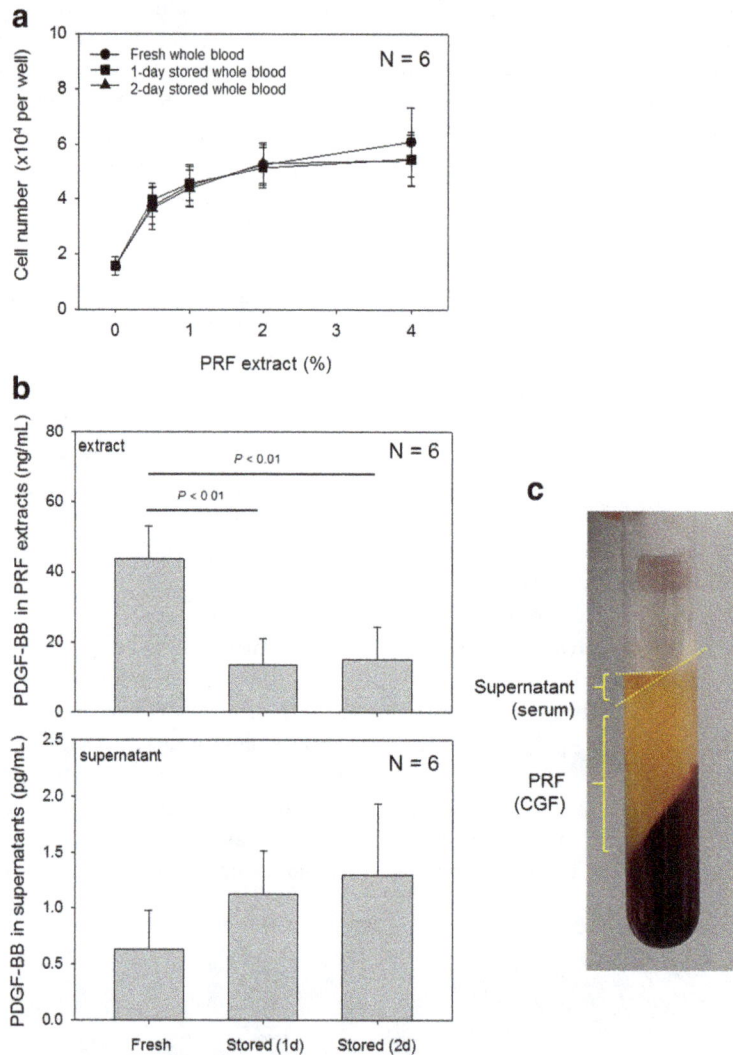

Fig. 4 Bioactivities and PDGF-BB concentrations in PRF extracts and the supernatant serum fraction. **a** PRF extracts were added to periosteal cell cultures and incubated for 3 days to evaluate their effects on cell proliferation. No significant differences were observed among three groups. **b** PRF extracts were subjected to measurement of PDGF-BB levels using an ELISA kit. No significant differences were observed in the supernatant among three groups. N = 6. **c** Representative localization of supernatant serum fraction of PRF preparation just after centrifugation

periosteal cells. PDGF-BB concentrations in PRF extracts prepared from fresh and stored WB samples are shown in Fig. 4b. PRF extracts and the supernatant serum fraction (see Fig. 4c) were subjected to measurement of PDGF-BB levels. The concentration of this representative growth factor of platelet concentrates [4] was significantly reduced in PRF extracts by storage. In contrast, PDGF-BB levels noticeably (but not significantly) increased in the supernatants.

Discussion

Platelet preservation is restricted to 3 and 5 days in Japan and worldwide, respectively. This limit is based on the fact that platelets are sensitive to changes in temperature and pH: when samples are stored at 2 to 6 °C, platelets become

unsuitable for production of platelet concentrates [3]. Preservation of platelet concentrates results in a drop of pH below 6.0 depending on the platelet count [15], and pH below 6.2 correlates with decreased in vivo efficacy of platelets [16]. Furthermore, it was recently demonstrated that growth factors in PRP degrade in the course of storage at 22 °C [17].

On the other hand, in general, WB can be stored in the presence of ACD or citrate phosphate and dextrose (CPD) at room temperature for a relatively long period (3 weeks or longer) before it is processed into blood components [1]. The WB storage has also been supported by recent developments in oxygen-permeable plastic bags. Nevertheless, out of concern about bacterial contamination, the maximal storage period is restricted to 8 h in some countries [3]. To minimize and prevent bacterial proliferation, it is recommended to maintain white blood cells in WB samples during the initial 16 to 20 h of storage to digest bacteria during storage [18, 19].

Here, it is worth discussing which functional states of platelets are expected to be maintained during storage for subsequent preparation of platelet concentrates (to be used for regenerative therapy). There is no doubt that the functional states observed in freshly isolated platelets are the best for preparation of platelet concentrates and for their best clinical performance. Nevertheless, given that platelet concentrates are expected to provide significant amounts of growth factors and fibrin(ogen) at implantation sites, stored platelets are not necessarily expected to function as fully as fresh ones (e.g., in terms of aggregation). Rather, stored platelets are expected not to lose growth factors during the storage period, while coagulation factors, especially those involved in the endogenous coagulation cascade, should maintain their activities to convert and polymerize fibrinogen to form well cross-linked fibrin fibers.

Considering the current status of clinical use of platelet concentrates in the fields of periodontology and oral surgery, in this study, we used 10-mL glass tubes that are not oxygen-permeable instead of oxygen-permeable plastic bags for storage of large volumes of WB or platelets. We advanced a working hypothesis that the storage of WB samples in glass tubes would result in a more rapid and substantial pH drop and inactivation of several enzymes involved in coagulation. This study revealed that addition of an optimal amount of a $CaCl_2$ solution successfully restored the coagulation ability of the anticoagulant-supplemented WB samples. The fibrin fibers prepared from the stored WB samples were almost identical to those of fresh WB samples. PDGF-BB concentrations were significantly lower in PRF extracts prepared from stored WB samples than in those of fresh WB samples. This effect can be explained by a growth factor release from platelets after stimulation by calcium ions or maybe (less likely) by degradation of PDGF-BB. Nonetheless, the bioactivities did not significantly worsen during the short storage.

In general, autologous platelet concentrates are prepared and immediately used for regenerative therapy in dental clinics at present. Our method should expand the clinical applicability of platelet concentrates, especially PRF preparations, and make the treatment schedule more flexible.

Conclusions

The self-clotted types of platelet concentrates (PRF) can be prepared from ACD-containing stored WB by addition of $CaCl_2$ without a significant reduction in their bioactivity and without other specific reagents or devices. This approach should contribute to dissemination of PRF therapy.

Abbreviations
ACD: Acid citrate dextrose solution; CGF: Concentrated growth factors; CPD: Citrate phosphate and dextrose; EDTA: Ethylenediaminetetraacetic acid; PDGF: Platelet-derived growth factor; PPP: Platelet-poor plasma; PRF: Platelet-rich fibrin; PRP: Platelet-rich plasma; SEM: Scanning electron microscope; WB: Whole blood

Authors' contributions
KI, MS, TW, YK, and TK conceived and designed the study, performed the experiments, and wrote the manuscript. TS, HK, MN, TO, KU, and TT performed the experiments and data analysis. HO and KN participated in the manuscript preparation. All authors read and approved the final version of the manuscript.

Author details
[1]Tokyo Plastic Dental Society, Kita-ku, Tokyo, Japan. [2]Division of Oral Implantology, Niigata University Medical and Dental Hospital, Niigata, Japan. [3]Bioscience Medical Research Center, Niigata University Medical and Dental Hospital, Niigata, Japan. [4]Department of Materials Science and Technology, Niigata University, Niigata, Japan. [5]Division of Oral Bioengineering, Institute of Medicine and Dentistry, Niigata University, Niigata, Japan.

References
1. Hess J. Conventional blood banking and blood component storage regulation: opportunities for improvement. Blood Transfus. 2010;8 Suppl 3: s9–s15.
2. World Health Organization. Manual on the management, maintenance and use of blood cold chain equipment. http://www.who.int/bloodsafety/Manual_on_Management,Maintenance_and_Use_of_Blood_Cold_Chain_Equipment.pdf. Accessed 26 Nov 2016.
3. van der Meer PF, de Wildt-Eggen J. The effect of whole-blood storage time on the number of white cells and platelets in whole blood and in white cell-reduced red cells. Transfusion. 2006;46:589–94.
4. Kawase T. Platelet-rich plasma and its derivatives as promising bioactive materials for regenerative medicine: basic principles and concepts underlying recent advances. Odontology. 2015;103:126–35.
5. Nagata M, Hoshina H, Li M, Arasawa M, Uematsu K, Ogawa S, Yamada K, Kawase T, Suzuki K, Ogose A, Fuse I, Okuda K, Uoshima K, Nakata K, Yoshie H, Takagi R. A clinical study of alveolar bone tissue engineering with cultured autogenous periosteal cells: coordinated activation of bone formation and resorption. Bone. 2012;50:1123–9.
6. Kobayashi M, Kawase T, Okuda K, Wolff LF, Yoshie H. In vitro immunological and biological evaluations of the angiogenic potential of platelet-rich fibrin preparations: a standardized comparison with PRP preparations. Int J Implant Dent. 2015;1:31.
7. Kobayashi M, Kawase T, Horimizu M, Okuda K, Wolff LF, Yoshie H. A proposed protocol for the standardized preparation of PRF membranes for clinical use. Biologicals. 2012;40:323–9.
8. Masuki H, Okudera T, Watanebe T, Suzuki M, Nishiyama K, Okudera H, Nakata K, Uematsu K, Su CY, Kawase T. Growth factor and pro-inflammatory cytokine contents in platelet-rich plasma (PRP), plasma rich in growth factors (PRGF), advanced platelet-rich fibrin (A-PRF), and concentrated growth factors (CGF). Int J Implant Dent. 2016;2:19.
9. Corigliano M, Sacco L, Baldoni E. CGF-una proposta terapeutica per la medicina rigenerativa. Odontoiatria. 2010;1:69–81.
10. Kawase T, Okuda K, Wolff LF, Yoshie H. Platelet-rich plasma-derived fibrin clot formation stimulates collagen synthesis in periodontal ligament and osteoblastic cells in vitro. J Periodontol. 2003;74:858–64.
11. Duan X, Bradbury SR, Olsen BR, Berendsen AD. Matrix Biol. 2016;52-54:127–40.
12. Kawase T, Okuda K, Kogami H, Nakayama H, Nagata M, Nakata K, Yoshie H. Characterization of human cultured periosteal sheets expressing bone-forming potential: in vitro and in vivo animal studies. J Tissue Eng Regen Med. 2009;3:218–29.
13. Kawase T, Hayama K, Tsuchimochi M, Nagata M, Okuda K, Yoshie H, Burns DM, Nakata K. Evaluating the safety of somatic periosteal cells by flow-cytometric analysis monitoring the history of DNA damage. Biopreserv Biobank. 2016;14:129–37.
14. Horimizu M, Kawase T, Nakajima Y, Okuda K, Nagata M, Wolff LF, Yoshie H.

An improved freeze-dried PRP-coated biodegradable material suitable for connective tissue regenerative therapy. Cryobiology. 2013;66:223–32.

15. de Wildt-Eggen J, Schrijver JG, Bouter-Valk HJ, Fijnheer R, Bins M, van Prooijen HC. Improvement of platelet storage conditions by using new polyolefin containers. Transfusion. 1997;37:476–81.

16. Murphy S, Rebulla P, Bertolini F, Holme S, Moroff G, Snyder E, Stromberg R. In vitro assessment of the quality of stored platelet concentrates. The BEST (Biomedical Excellence for Safer Transfusion) Task Force of the International Society of Blood Transfusion. Transfus Med Rev. 1994;8:29–36.

17. Sonker A, Dubey A. Determining the effect of preparation and storage: an effort to streamline platelet components as a source of growth factors for clinical application. Transfus Med Hemother. 2015;42:174–80.

18. Hogman CF, Gong J, Hambraeus A, Johansson CS, Eriksson L. The role of white cells in the transmission of Yersinia enterocolitica in blood components. Transfusion. 1992;32:654–7.

19. Pietersz RN, Reesink HW, Pauw W, Dekker WJ, Buisman L. Prevention of Yersinia enterocolitica growth in red-blood-cell concentrates. Lancet. 1992; 340:755–6.

16

The zygomatic implant perforated (ZIP) flap: a new technique for combined surgical reconstruction and rapid fixed dental rehabilitation following low-level maxillectomy

C. J. Butterworth* and S. N. Rogers

Abstract

This aim of this report is to describe the development and evolution of a new surgical technique for the immediate surgical reconstruction and rapid post-operative prosthodontic rehabilitation with a fixed dental prosthesis following low-level maxillectomy for malignant disease.

The technique involves the use of a zygomatic oncology implant perforated micro-vascular soft tissue flap (ZIP flap) for the primary management of maxillary malignancy with surgical closure of the resultant maxillary defect and the installation of osseointegrated support for a zygomatic implant-supported maxillary fixed dental prosthesis.

The use of this technique facilitates extremely rapid oral and dental rehabilitation within a few weeks of resective surgery, providing rapid return to function and restoring appearance following low-level maxillary resection, even in cases where radiotherapy is required as an adjuvant treatment post-operatively. The ZIP flap technique has been adopted as a standard procedure in the unit for the management of low-level maxillary malignancy, and this report provides a detailed step-by-step approach to treatment and discusses modifications developed over the treatment of an initial cohort of patients.

Keywords: Low-level maxillectomy, Zygomatic implants, Zygomatic oncology implant, Fixed dental prosthesis, ZIP flap, Micro-vascular reconstruction, Radiotherapy, Early implant loading, Oral cancer rehabilitation

Background

The surgical management and prosthodontic rehabilitation of the maxillectomy patient is complex with a variety of options available to the head and neck cancer team ranging from simple prosthodontic obturation [1] to reconstruction using pre-fabricated or digitally planned composite flaps [2] with or without the placement of osseointegrated implants [3]. The primary aims of treatment include effective eradication of the primary tumour, closure of the resulting maxillary defect, preservation of facial form, and ideally, the restoration of the resected maxillary dentition. Whilst the techniques for surgical closure of the low-level maxillectomy defect are well established, it can be challenging to subsequently achieve effective dental rehabilitation. The use of an obturator is not without its difficulties in terms of fit, retention and comfort, as well as preventing the transgress of fluid from the mouth to the nose. Providing and maintaining an effective obturator is demanding on both the patient and prosthodontist. Although some patients are able to tolerate the use of a removable denture following treatment, depending on retention, many are unable due to the change in the oral anatomy, oral dryness and the fragility of the irradiated tissues. Sealing the defect and providing bone and soft tissue through the use of free tissue transfer has both advantages and disadvantages. Following free tissue transfer providing secondary rehabilitation might be delayed or not possible. The

---
* Correspondence: c.butterworth@liv.ac.uk
Department of Oral & Maxillofacial Surgery, University Hospital Aintree, Lower Lane, Liverpool L9 7AL, UK

situation is made worse by the frequent requirement for post-operative radiotherapy, which ideally should start as soon as feasible following tumour ablation.

The development of highly specialised tools such as zygomatic, oncology and co-axis implants (Southern Implants Ltd., South Africa) have provided a platform for effective maxillary dental rehabilitation in a rapid manner following maxillary resective surgery. Boyes-Varley et al. (2007) [4] successfully demonstrated the use of early loading in this cancer setting utilising oncology zygomatic and dental implants together with prosthetic obturation. Whilst implant survival was not a problem, the amount of prosthodontic maintenance was significant and most likely related to the complex issues around establishing and maintaining an oro-nasal seal in a changing maxillectomy cavity. The technique presented here incorporates an early loading zygomatic and oncology implant protocol for maxillectomy patients together with microvascular free-flap closure of the resultant defect with a fascio-cutaneous flap and early delivery of a fixed dental prosthesis within a few weeks following surgery.

Case presentation

A 66-year-old male patient presented with an enlarging mass in the left maxilla (Fig. 1). The mass had been present for a few weeks. An incisional biopsy revealed squamous cell carcinoma. Staging scans were undertaken (Fig. 2) which demonstrated a T4N0M0 maxillary alveolus tumour in close proximity to the left orbital floor with obliteration of the maxillary antrum and destruction of the lateral maxillary wall (Fig. 3). The patient was partially dentate in both jaws with no significant dental pathology (Fig. 4).

The findings were discussed with the patient together with the treatment options for this malignant tumour requiring a low-level Brown class 2b maxillectomy [5]. The patient preference was not to have prosthodontic

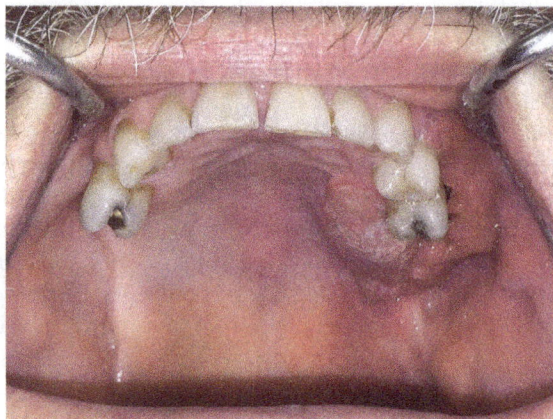

Fig. 2 Staging MRI scan showing destructive lesion left maxilla

obturation but rather reconstruction using microvascular free tissue transfer. In view of the unilateral low-level nature of the tumour, a soft tissue reconstruction combined with primary insertion of zygomatic implants to support a subsequent fixed dental prosthesis on a shortened dental arch concept was considered the best

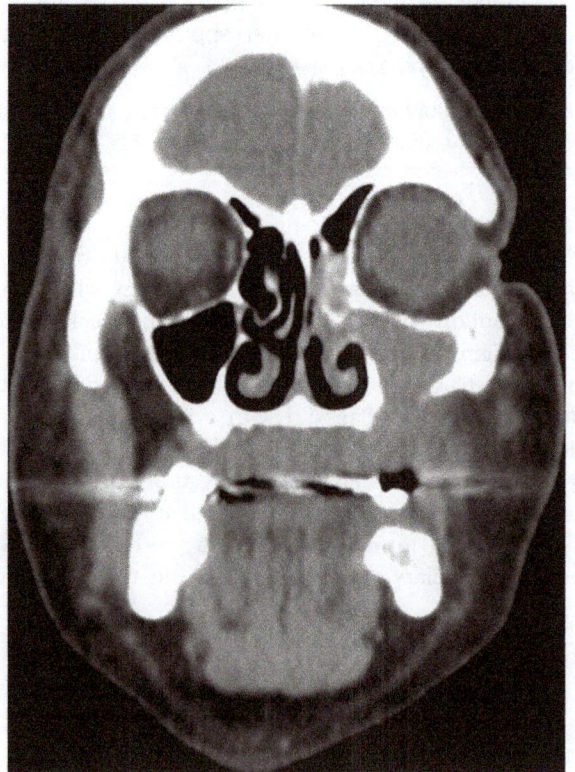

Fig. 1 Clinical view of left-sided maxillary tumour at presentation

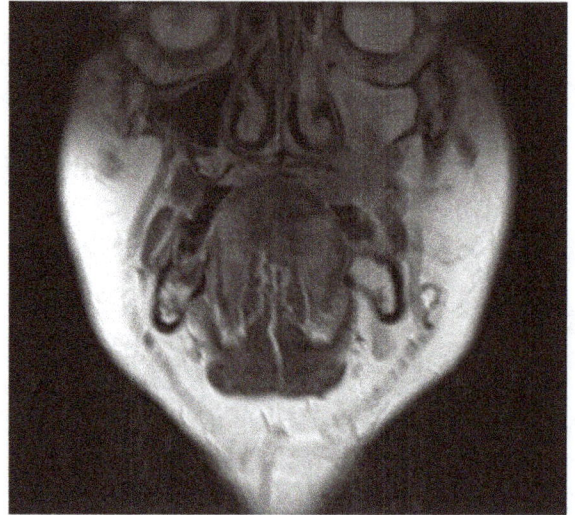

Fig. 3 Staging CT scan confirming maxillary destruction but preservation of the orbital floor

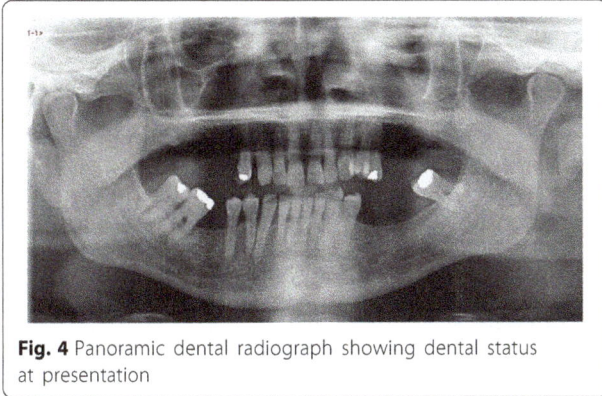

Fig. 4 Panoramic dental radiograph showing dental status at presentation

option. The remaining molar teeth were planned for extraction based on the potential need for post-operative radiotherapy and likelihood of trismus post-operatively. The remaining maxillary teeth on the non-defect right-hand side were planned for extraction to allow either the placement of immediate dental implants or the placement of conventional zygomatic implants depending on the state of the socket anatomy post-extraction.

Dental impressions were taken to allow construction of a maxillary complete denture template to both aid the placement of the zygomatic implants on the defect side and to act as an occlusal registration device during surgery. The occlusal vertical dimension was also measured between nasal tip and chin point to allow subsequent registration to occur at the correct level during surgery.

The ZIP flap technique

The patient underwent tracheostomy, a limited left-sided selective neck dissection for node sampling and vessels preparation. The maxillary tumour was excised in a standard manner via an intra-oral approach with preservation of the left orbital floor (Fig. 5). The resection extended to the maxillary alveolar midline in the incisor region with extension posteriorly just into the soft palate. The defect was measured to allow the harvesting of a slightly oversized left fascio-cutaneous radial forearm flap which was carried out in parallel to the implant procedures. Following resection, the amount of bone remaining in the left zygoma was assessed and deemed satisfactory for the placement of two zygomatic oncology implants [6] (Southern Implants Ltd., South Africa) which were subsequently inserted with excellent primary stability (Fig. 6). The remaining maxillary teeth were then carefully extracted although it was not possible to preserve all the labial socket bone which was fused to several of the teeth. It was therefore decided to proceed with an alveoloplasty and insertion of two conventional zygomatic implants (Southern Implants Ltd., South Africa) on the right side which were inserted into the canine and second premolar sites with high primary stability (Fig. 7). Standard implant bridge abutments (AMCZ abutments, Southern Implants, South Africa) were then torqued into place onto all four zygomatic implants with longer 5 mm versions being used on the defect side to facilitate the later flap perforation. The soft tissues of the right maxilla were then closed with multiple resorbable sutures.

The implant positions were then accurately registered by utilising light-cured resin tray material (Individo® Lux, Voco Gmbh, Germany) and abutment level impression copings. The resin material was applied in sections around the impression copings and cured incrementally to ensure a rigid splinting of the impression copings (Fig. 8). Abutment protection caps were then placed over all four abutments prior to the jaw registration procedure which was undertaken using the pre-fabricated

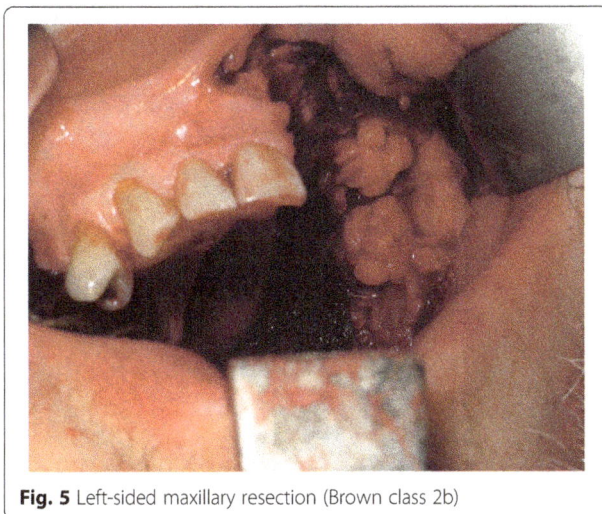

Fig. 5 Left-sided maxillary resection (Brown class 2b)

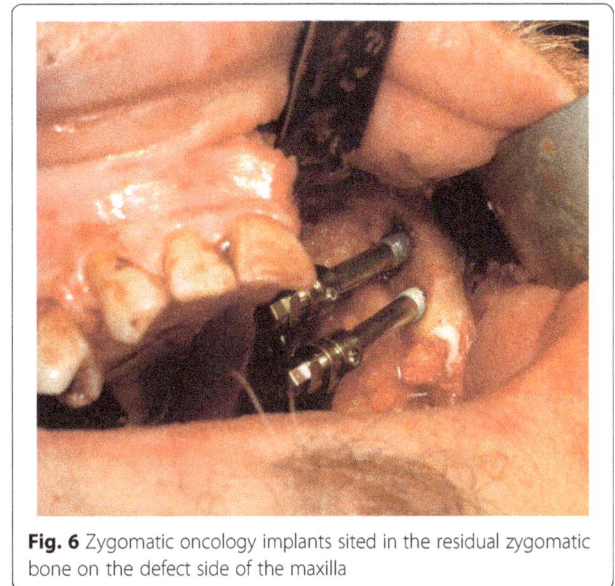

Fig. 6 Zygomatic oncology implants sited in the residual zygomatic bone on the defect side of the maxilla

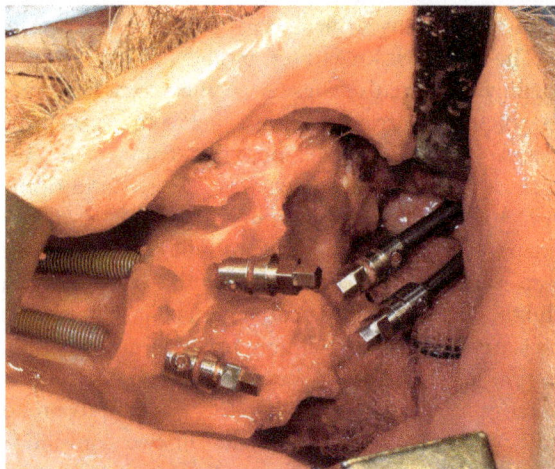

Fig. 7 Conventional zygomatic implant insertion on the non-defect side of the maxilla following extraction of the remaining teeth and an alveoloplasty

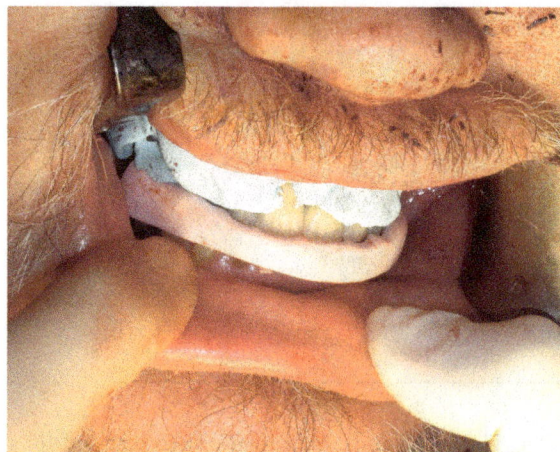

Fig. 9 Inter-occlusal registration using the pre-fabricated maxillary denture prosthesis relined with silicone putty over the implant abutment protection caps

denture appliance relined with silicone putty material (Provil soft putty, Heraeus Kulzer GmbH) (Fig. 9).

The radial forearm free flap (RFFF) was then disconnected from the arm and inset into the maxillary defect after creating a tunnel down into the left neck for the pedicle. The flap was carefully perforated over the zygomatic implant abutment protection caps using a short incision just through the skin layer followed by blunt dissection to allow the abutment and cap to perforate the flap ensuring a tight adaptation of the flap around the abutment (Fig. 10). The flap anastomosis was then completed utilising the operating microscope and the neck and arm wounds closed. The patient recovered well from the surgery and was subsequently discharged at 8 days post-operatively. The tumour and neck dissection specimens were examined and reported as pT4a N0 M0

squamous cell carcinoma of the left maxilla with a 7.2 mm depth of invasion. There was a close anterior mucosal margin of 1.3 mm and the decision was therefore taken for post-operative adjuvant radiotherapy.

Three weeks post-surgery, the patient was seen for review and to try-in the provisional prosthesis. Unfortunately, in the interim, the RFFF had overgrown the zygomatic implants (Fig. 11.) and so, under local anaesthesia, the implants were re-exposed to allow the provisional prosthesis to be tried in. The incisal level of the prosthesis was modified, and the prosthesis was then finalised in the laboratory and fitted 1 week later, 1 month following surgery (Fig. 12). A post-fitting radiograph demonstrated good positioning of the implants and seating of the initial prosthesis (Fig. 13). The patient then completed 6 weeks of radiotherapy (63 Gy in 30

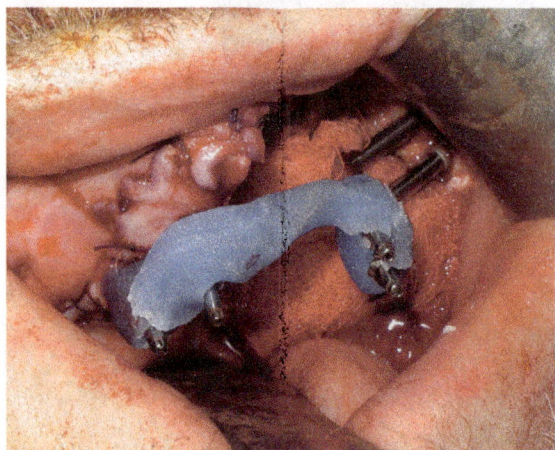

Fig. 8 Abutment level impression utilising light-cured acrylic tray material

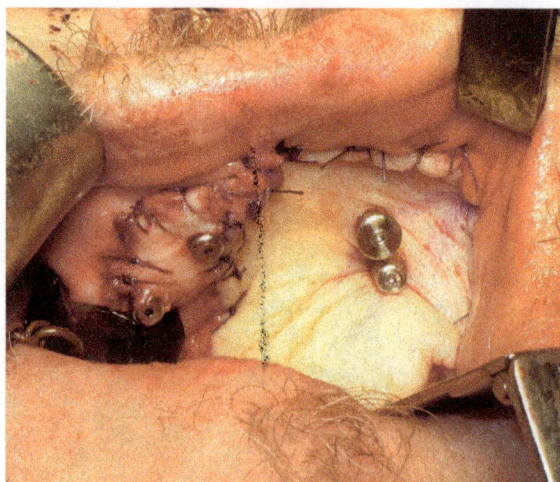

Fig. 10 Radial forearm flap inset and sutured into the maxillary defect and perforated by the zygomatic oncology implant abutments

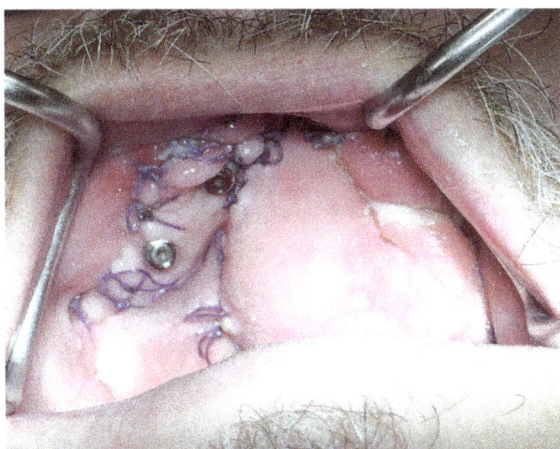

Fig. 11 Intra-oral view of the soft tissue flap at 3 weeks post-operatively with overgrowth of flap over the zygomatic oncology implants

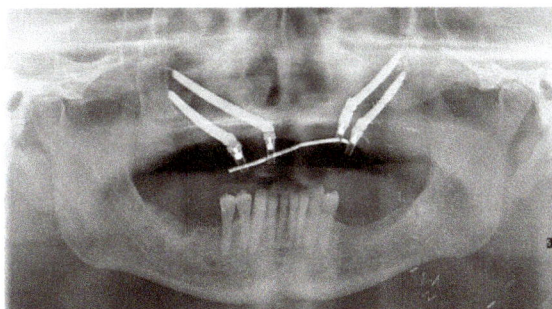

Fig. 13 Panoramic dental radiograph showing the position of the zygomatic implants and the seating of the initial fixed prosthesis

fractions). He subsequently attended with a fracture of the provisional prosthesis 3 weeks after completion of radiotherapy when the bridge was removed for repair. All implants were firmly integrated, the initial oral ulceration was now settling and the flap reconstruction was performing well with no evidence of breakdown or dehiscence (Fig. 14). The bridge was repaired and re-fitted the same day, and arrangements were made for the construction of a new definitive acrylic bridge with a cobalt-chrome framework which was subsequently fitted for the patient. The patient continued to be followed up, and 12 months following surgery completed a quality of life feedback questionnaire [7] where he rated his overall quality of life as "very good" and scored maximally in most domains with the exception of speech and fear of recurrence (Table 1). At 18 months post-surgery, the patient was still disease free with no further incidents of prosthodontic related complications since the definitive bridge was fitted. His facial appearance (Fig. 15) was

symmetrical with no significant distortion despite his previous maxillary resective surgery.

Procedural modifications to the ZIP flap technique

In order to address some of the issues highlighted in this early case, the technique was modified slightly to try and prevent flap overgrowth and prosthesis fracture in the early stages. In order to prevent flap overgrowth over the zygomatic oncology implant abutments, the use of a polythene washer was instituted on subsequent cases treated in the unit. Once the flap was perforated, a 2-mm thick polythene sheet (Centriform Soft Mouthguard material, WHW Plastics Ltd., Hull, UK) was taken and a small disc cut out corresponding to an area of 1–2 cm^2 surrounding the zygomatic oncology implants. Using a 5-mm tissue biopsy punch, holes were cut into the sheet corresponding to the positions of the abutments and the perforated polythene sheet was then placed over the abutments to keep the flap in a superior position during the initial healing phase prior to restoration. The polythene washer was then kept in place using conical abutment protection caps (Fig. 16), and this enabled the prevention of flap tissue overgrowth and retained access to the oncology

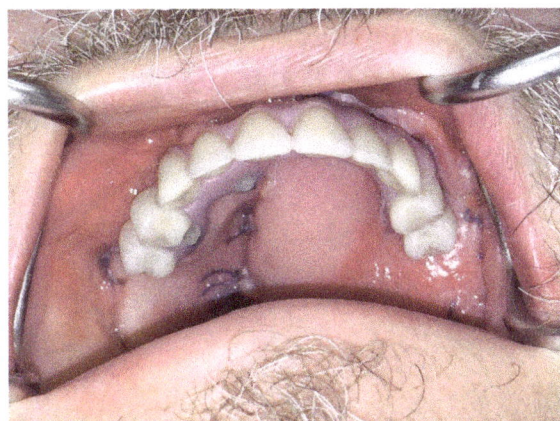

Fig. 12 Provisional acrylic fixed dental prosthesis fitted at 4 weeks post-surgery

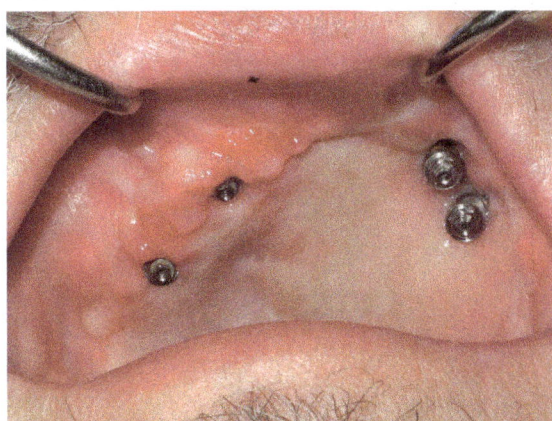

Fig. 14 Intra-oral view of perforated flap 3 weeks following radiotherapy

Table 1 Patient-reported quality of life outcomes following ZIP flap procedure

Domain	Score
Activity	100 ("I am as active as I have ever been")
Anxiety	100 ("I am not anxious about my cancer")
Appearance	75 ("The change in my appearance is minor")
Chewing	100 ("I can chew as well as ever")
Fear	75 ("I have a little fear, with occasional thoughts but they don't really bother me")
Intimacy	100 ("I have no problems with intimacy as a result of my cancer")
Mood	100 ("My mood is excellent and unaffected by my cancer")
Pain	100 ("I have no pain")
Recreation	100 ("There are no limitations to recreation at home or away from home")
Saliva	100 ("My saliva is of normal consistency")
Speech	75 ("I have difficulty saying some words but I can be understood over the phone")
Shoulder	100 ("I have no problem with my shoulder")
Swallowing	100 ("I can swallow as well as ever")
Taste	100 ("I can taste food normally")
Overall QOL	Very good
Most important aspect	Fear of recurrence

implants for subsequent restoration (Fig. 17). In view of the fracture of the interim prosthesis reported in this case, the technique was modified with a definitive cobalt chrome framework being constructed within the first 2 weeks post-surgery with one visit for try-in of the framework and tooth set-up being scheduled to allow any modifications required to either incisal level, occlusion and overall soft tissue fit to be completed. This try in visit occurred at 2–3 weeks post-surgery with the final fit occurring 1 week later. This has prevented further issues for all subsequent patients.

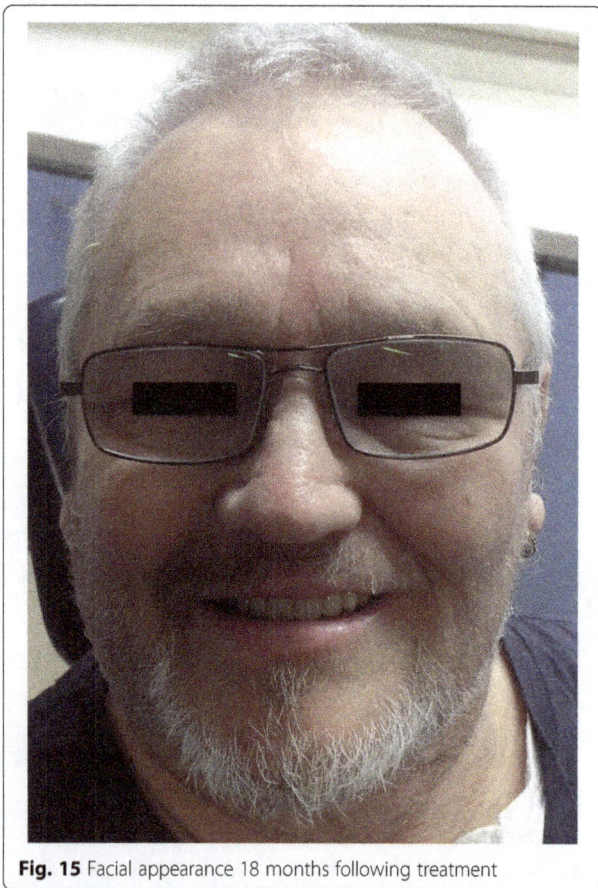

Fig. 15 Facial appearance 18 months following treatment

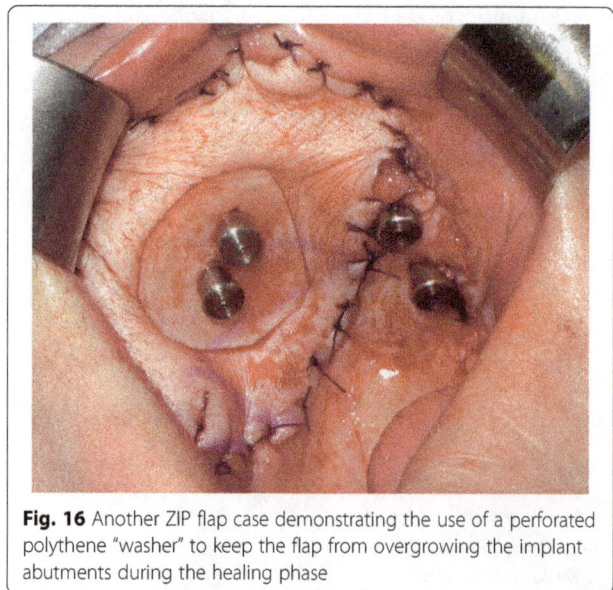

Fig. 16 Another ZIP flap case demonstrating the use of a perforated polythene "washer" to keep the flap from overgrowing the implant abutments during the healing phase

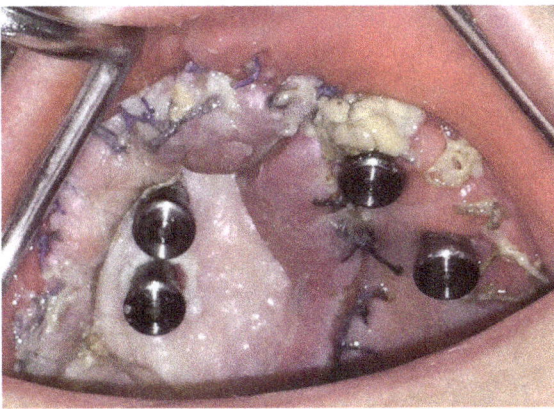

Fig. 17 The appearance of the case shown in Fig. 16 with the polythene "washer" removed at 2 weeks post-surgery, providing access to the zygomatic oncology implants

Discussion

In order to reduce intra-operative time, the soft tissue free flap is harvested at the same time as the implant placement and prosthodontic procedures. On raising a skin island, it is appropriate to make it a little over-sized for the required defect to ensure that tension and possible dehiscence at the surgical margins during healing is reduced.

In low-level maxillectomy (Brown class II), the need for bony reconstruction is questionable depending on the horizontal component. With the preservation of the orbital floor, zygomatic prominence and some bony support for the nose, facial appearance, in the experience of the authors and, as demonstrated by this case, is not significantly worsened despite low-level removal of the maxilla. The key issues in these low level defects are adequate clearance of tumour, dealing with the oro-nasal communication and reconstruction of the dentition. Whilst prosthodontic obturation can deal with these aspects in a simple manner, the stability of the obturator prosthesis and its ability to completely seal the oro-nasal defect has limitations. In addition, these prostheses require a significant amount of adjustments, clinic visits and on-going maintenance. The soft lining materials perish, discolour and harbour surface biofilm often resulting in some mal-odour and the need for regular replacement. For many patients, there is a psychological impact of retaining the maxillectomy defect and high anxiety related to the insertion and removal of the prosthesis as well as concerns relating to the handicap they would experience to speech, and eating should their prosthesis fracture or fail in some way. The use of implants to retain maxillary obturators certainly improves their stability and retention, but efficacy of the oro-nasal seal still requires regular maintenance and patients still often dislike the hygiene aspects of looking after the defect and their implant supra-structure within the defect.

The use of soft tissue flaps to close a typical hemi-maxillectomy defect is an effective way of dealing with the oro-nasal communication, but in isolation, this technique works against dental rehabilitation as the bulk of the flap provides a very poor moveable foundation for a subsequent removable prosthesis. The move towards the use of composite reconstruction (especially the fibula flap) has been facilitated by the use of digital planning in which dental implants can be inserted into the fibula flap at the time of harvest and inset facilitated by the use of stereolithographic guides. However, this procedure is not widely applicable for all patients due to financial, technological and medical restrictions and is not currently able to provide patients with an early loaded fixed dental prosthesis especially when post-operative radiotherapy is being utilised. Many older patients presenting with maxillary malignant tumours also have significant peripheral vascular disease and other significant medical co-morbidities which may prevent the harvest of a vascularised composite flap.

In contrast, the use of a soft tissue flap such as the RFFF or antero-lateral thigh flap can often be safely employed in elderly patients with peripheral vascular disease without unduly lengthening the operation too significantly with two-team operating. In addition, the predictability of these flaps with their excellent pedicle lengths is ideal for closure of the resulting oro-nasal surgical defect. The use of a slightly oversized graft is recommended to ensure that any tension on the wound peripheries is kept to a minimum during the healing phase. In addition, for those patients undergoing post-operative radiotherapy, a degree of shrinkage and tightening of the flap tissues is to be expected.

Immediate/early loading of zygomatic [8] and dental implants [9] have been well demonstrated already within the literature with very high implant survival rates. In the oncology setting, Boyes-Varley et al. [4] lost no zygomatic/oncology implants in their series of 20 patients restored with implant-retained obturators, 6 of whom received radiotherapy post-operatively. The case reported has been followed up for 18 months so far without evidence of zygomatic implant failure despite the use of radiotherapy. A recent review of conventional zygomatic implant surgery demonstrated that the incidence of failure after the 6-month stage was extremely low [8] although for zygomatic oncology implants, this data is not yet fully reported in the literature with the only data available on zygomatic oncology implants being limited to the work of Boyes-Valey [4], Pellegrino [10] and the authors themselves [6]. The removal of teeth at primary cancer surgery to facilitate placement of implants on the non-defect side requires careful consideration; where teeth are of poor prognosis with poor bone support, it is easier to extract, perform localised osteoplasty prior to the insertion of a conventional zygomatic implant with its inherent excellent stability and ability to be loaded early in the post-operative period. Where teeth have excellent bone support but additional implants are required to facilitate the construction of a fixed prosthesis, then careful extraction of selected teeth with the immediate installation of a root form implant can be utilised with good success as long as high primary stability is achieved at these sites.

Whilst technically, it would be possible to construct and fit the prosthesis on the same day or even a week later, the need for microvascular flap monitoring in the immediate post-operative period, together with the significant recovery period required by the patient following surgery has lead the authors to delay the fitting of the prosthesis at the 4 to 6-week period post-operatively. In terms of ongoing clinical implant follow-up, no attempt was made at peri-implant probing for the oncology zygomatic implants perforating the soft-tissue flap as it was deemed important not to disturb the soft tissue seal of the skin flap around the implant abutments. No discharge or suppuration was noted during follow-up in this case. Periodontal probing around the conventionally placed zygomatic implants was undertaken periodically during follow up and remained within normal limits.

The use of a soft tissue rather than composite reconstruction may also facilitate a shorter hospital stay and allow adjuvant radiotherapy to be delivered in a more rapid timescale with possible impact on overall cure rates of this very debilitating tumour. The initial experiences with this procedure in over ten cases have been extremely positive with excellent appreciation by patients who value being provided with a fixed dental prosthesis so quickly after major surgery.

Conclusions

The ZIP flap technique represents an innovative approach to the management of patients presenting with low-level malignant maxillary tumours. It provides effective closure of the resulting maxillary defect restoring speech and swallowing functions and also establishing a high-quality fixed dental rehabilitation in a rapid timescale, thus facilitating a more timely return to function and restored facial appearance. This approach has now been adopted routinely in the unit and it is hoped that a cases series will be presented in due course with more detailed patient outcomes. Further work on the long-term results of the ZIP flap procedure is required together with an ongoing appreciation of the important case selection factors for this treatment protocol.

Authors' contributions
CB devised the treatment concept and undertook all implant surgeries and prosthodontics. SR undertook all surgical resections and free flap reconstructions.

CB and SR both wrote the manuscript and reviewed the available literature. Both authors read and approved the final manuscript.

Competing interests
Chris Butterworth and Simon Rogers declare that they have no competing interests.

References
1. Okay DJ, Genden E, Buchbinder D, Urken M. Prosthodontic guidelines for surgical reconstruction of the maxilla: a classification system of defects. J Prosthet Dent. 2001;86(4):352–63.
2. Rohner D, Bucher P, Hammer B. Prefabricated fibular flaps for reconstruction of defects of the maxillofacial skeleton: planning, technique, and long-term experience. Int J Oral Maxillofac Implants. 2013;28(5):e221–9.
3. Runyan CM, Sharma V, Staffenberg DA, Levine JP, Brecht LE, Wexler LH, et al. Jaw in a day: state of the art in maxillary reconstruction. J Craniofac Surg. 2016; 27(8):2101–4.
4. Boyes-Varley JG, Howes DG, Davidge-Pitts KD, Brånemark I, McAlpine JA. A protocol for maxillary reconstruction following oncology resection using zygomatic implants. Int J Prosthodont. 2007;20(5):521–31.
5. Brown JS, Shaw RJ. Reconstruction of the maxilla and midface: introducing a new classification. Lancet Oncol. 2010;11(10):1001–8.
6. Dattani A, Richardson D, Butterworth CJ. A novel report on the use of an oncology zygomatic implant-retained maxillary obturator in a paediatric patient. Int J Implant Dent. 2017;3(1):9.
7. Rogers SN, Gwanne S, Lowe D, Humphris G, Yueh B, Weymuller EA Jr. The addition of mood and anxiety domains to the University of Washington quality of life scale. Head Neck. 2002;24(6):521–9.
8. Chrcanovic BR, Albrektsson T, Wennerberg A. Survival and complications of zygomatic implants: an updated systematic review. J Oral Maxillofac Surg. 2016;74(10):1949–64.
9. Engelhardt S, Papacosta P, Rathe F, Özen J, Jansen JA, Junker R. Annual failure rates and marginal bone-level changes of immediate compared to conventional loading of dental implants. A systematic review of the literature and meta-analysis. Clin Oral Implants Res. 2015;26(6):671–87.
10. Pellegrino G, Tarsitano A, Basile F, Pizzigallo A, Marchetti C. Computer-aided rehabilitation of maxillary oncological defects using zygomatic implants: a defect-based classification. J Oral Maxillofac Surg. 2015;73(12):2446. e1-.e11

17

Alveolar ridge preservation with autologous particulated dentin

Silvio Valdec[1*], Pavla Pasic[1], Alex Soltermann[2], Daniel Thoma[3], Bernd Stadlinger[1] and Martin Rücker[1]

Abstract

Introduction: Ridge preservation can be performed with autologous bone, alloplastic bone substitute material or a combination of both. Dentin is similar to bone in its chemical composition. In its use as bone substitute material, it undergoes a remodelling process and transforms to bone. The presented case report introduces a technique in which the extraction socket is augmented with autologous, particulated dentin.

Material and methods: The fractured, non-savable mesial incisor of the upper jaw was carefully extracted in axial direction. After the extraction, the tooth was cleared from remaining periodontal tissue. The vital pulp tissue or a root canal filling, enamel and cementum were also removed. Following the particulation of the remaining dentin in a bone mill, the dentin particles were immediately filled orthotope into the alveolar socket. The soft tissue closure was performed with a free gingival graft of the palate.

Results: After an observation period of 4 months, an implant was placed in the augmented area, which osseointegrated successfully and could be restored prosthodontically in the following. The results of this method showed a functional and aesthetic success.

Conclusion: The pre-implantological, autologous ridge preservation with dentin could be performed successfully. For the establishment of dentin as augmentation material for jaw augmentation procedures, a prospective, clinical trial is now necessary.

Keywords: Alveolar ridge preservation, Particulated dentin, Autologous augmentation, Bone augmentation, Bone substitute

Background

Subsequent to tooth extraction, a resorption of the host bone as defined by atrophy of the alveolar ridge can be observed. Sutton et al. classified the different degrees of alveolar ridge atrophy [32]. Bone resorption especially occurs in the frontal and premolar area of the jaw in the region of the thin buccal lamella. This may lead to a change in contour [11, 28]. Physiological reason for this atrophy is the periodontal ligament blending into the bone. Overall, a total clinically relevant loss of bone height of approximately 2–5 mm in the first 6 months can be observed in the vertical dimension [10, 20]. After 12 months, the alveolar ridge may lose up to 50% of its width. With regard to dental implants, this implicates that an implant insertion in a sufficient bone bed will often not be possible. In order to prevent this bone atrophy, different methods of alveolar ridge preservation have been described. The augmentation of extraction sockets with deproteinized bovine bone is clinically well established and has analysed in various studies [17, 18, 31]. Systematic reviews showed a preservation of the bone contour for this method [6, 15].

Today, clinical techniques like the socket-shield technique are performed [9]. Applying this technique, a vestibular slice of the tooth root is left in the alveolar socket during tooth extraction. The reason is to prevent the resorption of the vestibular bony lamella. Studies show the osseointegration of implants having been inserted in such areas, thus indicating the biocompatibility of autologous tooth material [8, 13, 16]. The application of autologous dentin as a bone

* Correspondence: silvio.valdec@zzm.uzh.ch
[1]Clinic of Cranio-Maxillofacial and Oral Surgery, Center of Dental Medicine, University of Zurich, University Hospital Zurich, Plattenstrasse 11, 8032 Zürich, Switzerland
Full list of author information is available at the end of the article

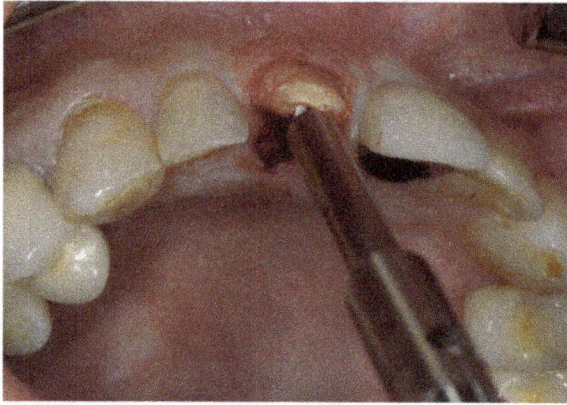

Fig. 1 Extraction with the benex system

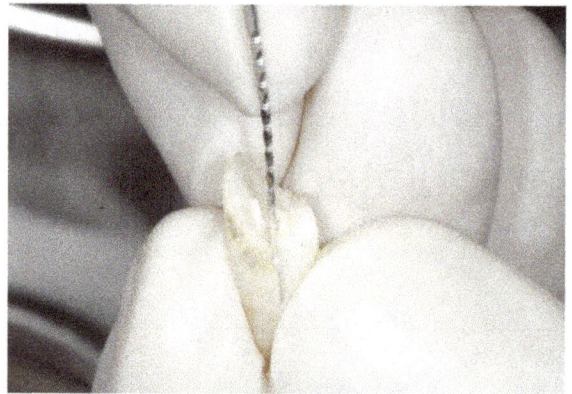

Fig. 3 Removal of the pulp

substitute for alveolar augmentation may serve as an alternative to the usage of xenogeny biomaterials. The chemical properties of dentin show a close relationship to bone and demonstrated a good osseous regeneration in an animal model [9].

Aim of this case series is to demonstrate the augmentation with autologous dentin as an interesting alternative to the application of xenogeny grafts.

Material and methods
Clinical technique

Four patients between 36 and 65 years of age are presented in this case series. There was no financial compensation. All four patients suffered from a trauma, causing damage to one or two teeth of the anterior maxilla. The frontal tooth/teeth has/had to be extracted. The pulp of the extracted teeth of three patients and the root canal filling of one patient had to be removed. All patients were informed on the operative procedure and possible risks and signed an informed consent. Treatment options were discussed.

After mouth rinsing with a chlorhexidine solution (Chlorhexamed® FORTE 0.2%, GlaxoSmithKline Consumer Healthcare GmbH & Co.KG, Bühl, Germany), local anaesthesia (4% Ubistesin® with 1: 200,000 adrenaline, 3M Espe AG, Seefeld, Germany) was applied. The tooth extraction was performed carefully using a special extraction-system (Benex II extraction-system, Helmut Zepf medical technology GmbH, Seitigen-Oberflacht, Germany) in order to preserve bone and soft tissue (Figs. 1 and 2).

The clinical and radiographic examination showed healthy periodontal structures; the buccal wall was intact without fenestration with a minimal thickness of 1 mm; the discrepancy between the buccal height of the socket and the palatal height was not more than 3 mm; and the socket was within the bony envelope in all four cases.

The root surface was carefully cleaned from periodontal tissue. The pulp was removed, using a root canal instrument (K-file, Dema Dent AG, Bassersdorf, Switzerland). Layers of enamel and cementum were removed, using a rotating instrument (Diamond polisher, Rodent AG, Montlingen, Switzerland) (Figs. 3 and 4).

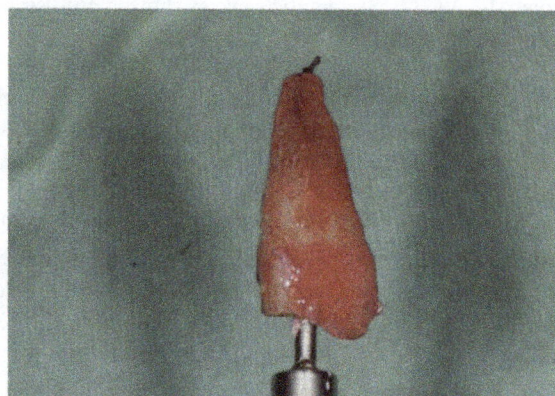

Fig. 2 The remaining root of tooth 11

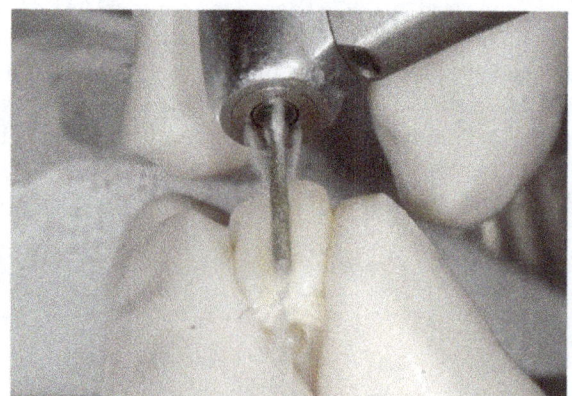

Fig. 4 Removal of enamel and the cementum

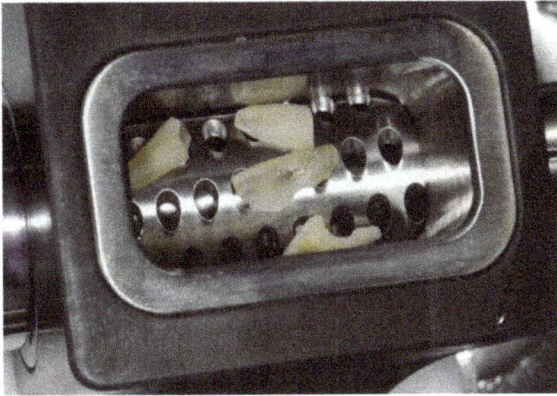

Fig. 5 Autologous dentin in a bone mill

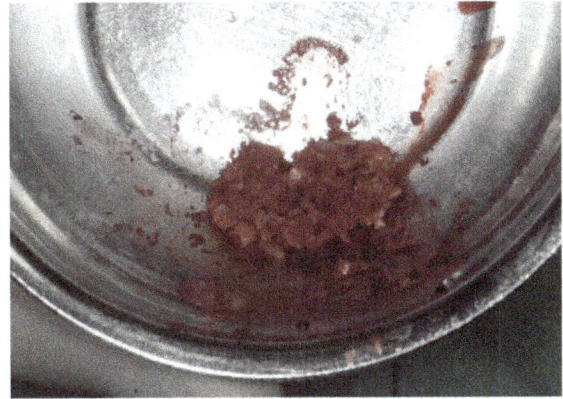

Fig. 7 Autologous, particulated dentin mixed with blood from the operating site

Subsequently, the remaining dentin was cut into pieces (Bone rongeur forceps, Carl Martin BmbH, Solingen, Germany). These pieces of dentin were grinded using a bone mill (USTOMED INSTRUMENTE, Ulrich Storz GmbH & Co., Tuttingen, Germany) in order to achieve a particle size between 0.25 and 2 mm (Figs. 5 and 6).

The autologous, particulated dentin was mixed with autogenous blood from the operating site (Fig. 7) and carefully inserted into the alveolar socket under controlled pressure to the level of the palatal/vestibular bone plate (Fig. 8).

An autologous soft tissue graft was harvested from the patient's palate using a soft tissue punch (Biopsy Punch, kai Europe GmbH, Solingen, Germany) (Fig. 9). The graft had a comparable dimension as the recipient site. The gingival graft was placed on top of the augmentation material, adapted and carefully sutured to the marginal gingiva after the sulcus epithelium was removed with a rotating diamond (Vicryl 6-0, Ermed AG, Schleithem, Switzerland) (Fig. 10).

In order to evaluate the ridge preservation properly, a cone beam computed tomography (CBCT, 3D Accuitomo,

J. Morita Mfg. Corp., Kyoto, Japan) was taken post-surgery with a resolution of 0.25 mm (scan time 17.5 s, 90 kV, 5 mA). The findings were assessed on a computer (HP Compaq 6200 Pro Microtower PC, graphics card: Intel HD Graphics 2000 Dynamic Video Memory Technology, mouse: HP Compaq DC 172B; Hewlett Packard, Palo Alto, CA, USA) with a calibrated monitor (HP Compaq LA 2306x; Hewlett Packard, Palo Alto, CA, USA) using the reconstruction software Morita version I Dixel (J. Morita Mfg. Corp., Kyoto, Japan) (Figs. 11 and 12).

The patients received antibiotics peri-operatively and for 7 days post-surgery (Amoxicillin® 750 mg 1-1-1).

The first follow-up consultation was 7 days post-surgery. The patients did not report any discomfort, and wound healing was regular in all four cases. No clinical signs of significant infection or graft loss were present. The sutures were removed 14 days post-surgery. Consecutive follow-up examinations did not show any complications, and implant placement was performed after 3 to 4 months (Fig. 13a, b).

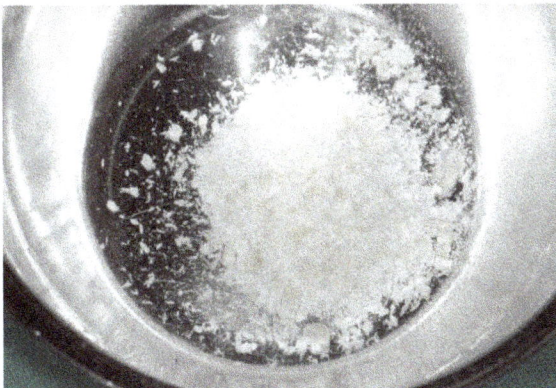

Fig. 6 Autologous dentin with the desired particle size

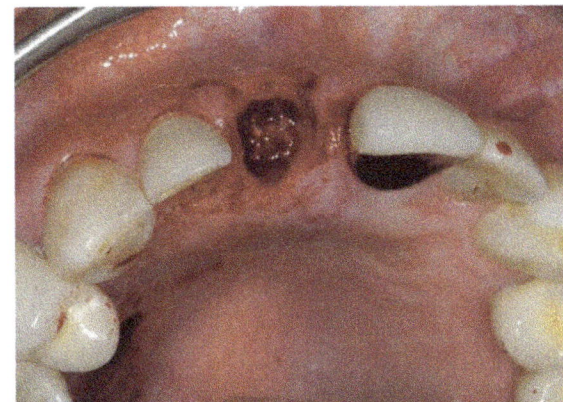

Fig. 8 Autologous, particulated dentin in the alveolar socket

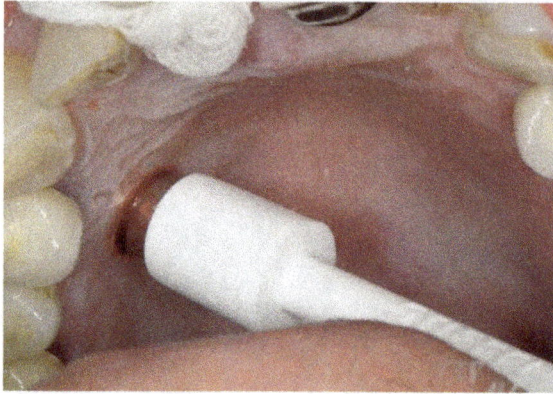

Fig. 9 Soft tissue punch

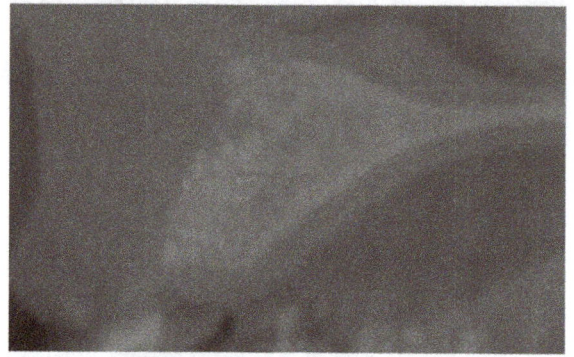

Fig. 11 Sagittal view

The height and width of the ridge were sufficient prior to implant placement, which left at least 2 mm of buccal bone after implant placement.

Case presentation

The 1-year follow-up examination of the presented case showed an implant success, according to the appropriate clinical criteria [2] (Figs. 14, 15 and 16).

The pink esthetic score (PES) was used for the evaluation of reproducible soft tissue around the final implant crown as a parameter for the aesthetic outcome [12]. Seven variables were evaluated comparing the soft tissue around the implant with the neighbouring reference tooth. Using a 0-1-2 scoring system, the mesial papilla, distal papilla, soft tissue level, soft tissue contour, alveolar process deficiency, soft tissue colour and texture were evaluated.

The situation before the extraction of the tooth was scanned with an intraoral scanner (CEREC Omnicam®, Sirona-Dentsply, Bensheim, Germany), also the situation after the finalized prosthodontic restoration. The scans were superimposed, and the difference of the vertical and

horizontal dimensions was calculated with specialized analysis software (Oracheck, Cyfex, Zurich, Switzerland).

Results

Four months post-extraction and augmentation with autologous, particulated dentin, all four patients received an implant placement in the augmented area. In all cases, a CBCT was taken in between the dentin augmentation and the implant placement.

During implant placement, a biopsy of the bone from the augmented area was taken for histological examination (Fig. 17).

The final prosthetic solution demonstrated a functional and esthetical success of the used treatment method (Fig. 18).

In the presented case, a PES of 13 was evaluated, deducting one point for the soft tissue level under critical observation.

A loss of 0.76 mm in the vertical dimension and a loss of 1.1 mm in the horizontal dimension could be observed in the calculation of the superimposed situations before extraction and 1 year after finalized prosthetic restoration (Figs. 19 and 20).

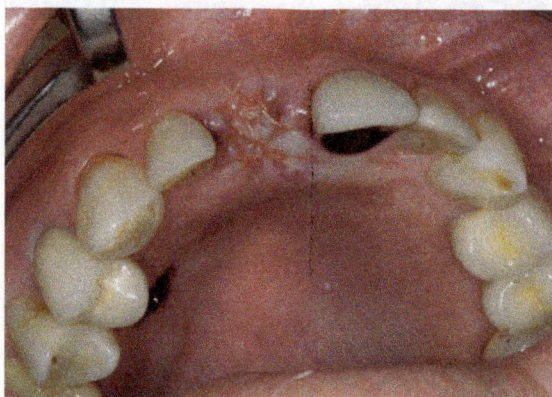

Fig. 10 Soft tissue graft placed on the recipient site

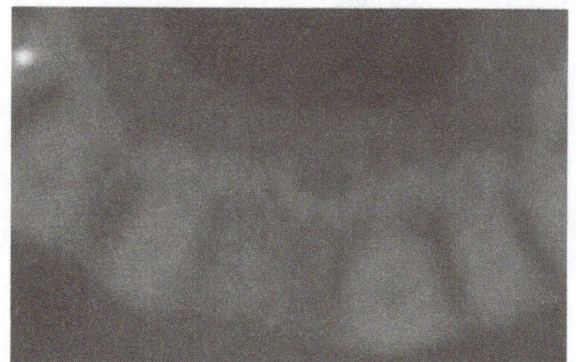

Fig. 12 Axial view

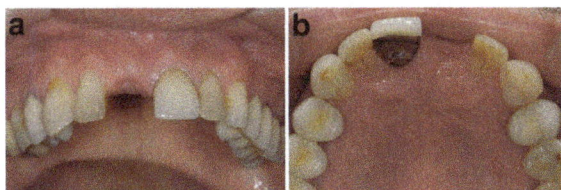

Fig. 13 a, b Clinical situation prior to implant placement

Discussion

The aim of this case series is to demonstrate the efficacy and safety of this novel augmentative procedure for ridge preservation prior to implant therapy. This shall serve as a basis for a prospective study.

In all four cases, patients showed a stable volume of soft and hard tissues after the augmentation with AutoPD and good osseointegration of titanium implants, having been placed in this augmented socket.

The application of autologous bone and xenogeneic biomaterials for alveolar bone augmentation following tooth extraction has been intensively studied. This so called ridge preservation aims at the prevention of bone atrophy. From a biological point of view,

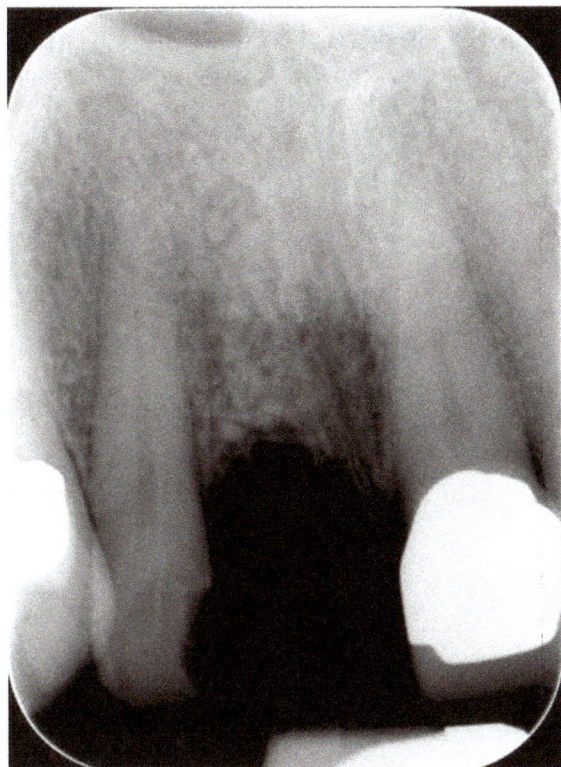

Fig. 15 Single tooth X-ray, showing a constant bone level 7 months after implant placement

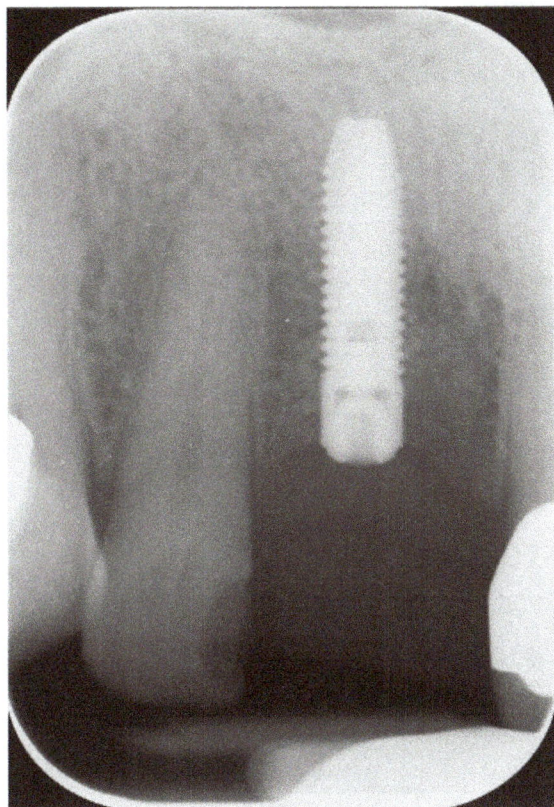

Fig. 14 Single tooth X-ray immediately after the augmentation using autogenous dentin

autologous bone is still considered to be the optimal augmentation material due to its osteogenic, osteoinductive and osteoconductive properties [1, 34]. However, especially in small defects, possible donor-site morbidity, limited graft volume availability and additional length of operation for harvesting autologous bone led to the increasing usage of xenogeneic biomaterials such as demineralized bovine bone substitute (DBBS—Bio-Oss©). These kind of non-resorbable biomaterials have great potential in maintaining the dimension of the contour of the ridge by serving as a framework for new bone formation [7]. Although DBBS shows great osteoconductive potential and has been proven to be as effective as autologous bone alone or in combination with autologous bone, it has a slow and incomplete resorption rate [4, 14, 22, 24].

In addition, the use of DBBS increases treatment cost and may be incompatible to some patients. Regarding these factors of influence, it is of interest to test alternative bone substitute materials.

In traumatology, many studies showed that replanted teeth with a devitalized periodontal tissue will ankylose and dentin will be replaced by bone [1, 3].

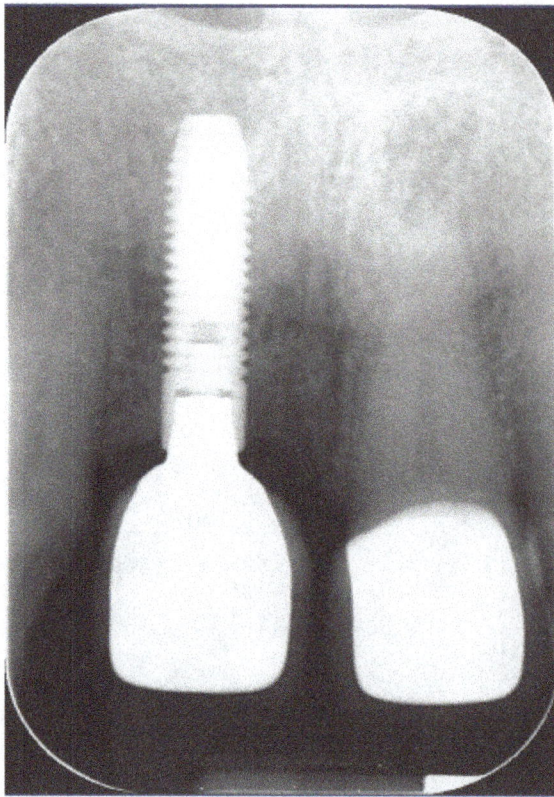

Fig. 16 Single tooth X-ray, 1 year post-implantation, showing the finalized crown

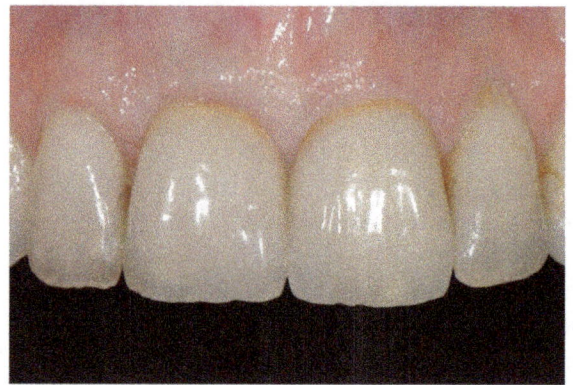

Fig. 18 Finalized prosthetic restoration after 1 year

It is well known that dentin and bone have a similar organic and inorganic structure [21]. Recent studies have focused on dentin as a potential bone substitute in different models of alveolar defects. It could be shown that dentin, being used either as a block graft or in particulated form, is involved in bone remodelling, expressing osteoconductive and even osteoinductive properties [3, 5, 9, 26, 29, 30]. In vivo studies in mice showed that dentin scaffolds performed similar with regard to the inflammatory response and neovascularization compared to isogenic bone [9]. Both materials induced an acute short-term inflammatory response with increased leukocyte-endothelial cell interaction, a process often observed after the implantation of biomaterials [19, 27]. Additionally, in vitro studies showed

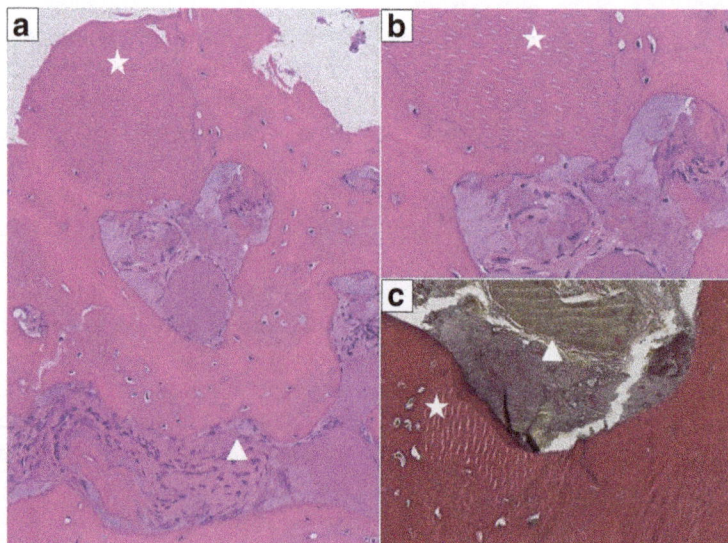

Fig. 17 Histology of dentin augmentation. a *Asterisk* denotes incorporated dentin particle, surrounded by vital woven bone. *Triangle* shows reactive process in the bone marrow lacunae with osteoblast rimming. No signs of necrosis or infection (H&E stain, ×100 magnification). b Larger magnification at ×200. c EvG (Elastica van Gieson) stain, ×200

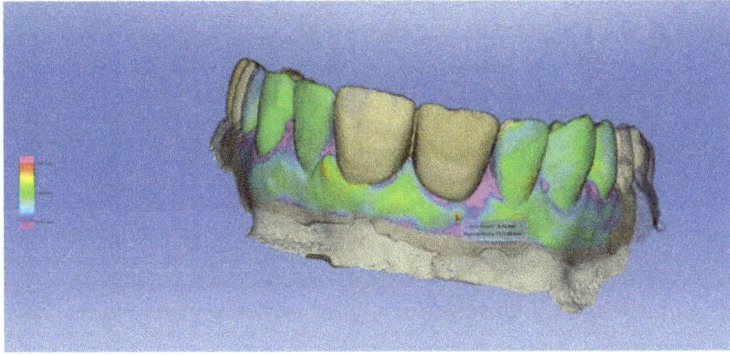

Fig. 19 Colour-coded superimposition of intraoral scans before extraction and after definitive prosthetic restoration

that protein extracts from dentin affect proliferation and differentiation of osteoprogenitor cells. Results suggested that TGFβ and perhaps other factors in dentin can regulate cell behaviour and, therefore, can influence development, remodelling and regeneration of mineralized tissues [33].

In humans, particulated tooth material has been used for sinus augmentation in order to enhance implant therapy. Preliminary results from five patients histologically showed an osteoconductive osteogenesis with partial resorption of tooth components [25].

In the present case series, all patients underwent socket preservation with AutoPD. In all cases, one or two upper frontal central incisors were extracted. The teeth were immediately removed of the pulp or root canal filling, enamel and cementum. AutoPD enriched by autogenous blood was inserted into the alveolar socket without a further chemical modification or sterilization process during the same operation. In a recent study, Pang et al. used a demineralized autologous dentin matrix for socket preservation, however 2 to 4 weeks after tooth extraction. Additionally, the

dentin matrix was sterilized before the augmentation process [23]. This procedure should potentially reduce the risk of inflammation but demands a second surgical intervention. It is currently unknown, whether such a procedure is necessary.

In the present experimental treatment concept, it has to be emphasized that the extraction was performed as atraumatic as possible. In all cases, the buccal lamella was intact prior to augmentation of AutoPD and a flapless approach had been chosen. After augmentation, the socket was covered by a patch, harvested from the palate with the punch technique. Wound healing was uneventful for all patients. In one case, a histological probe has been gained after 4 months during implant placement. The histological examination showed evidence of remodelling processes between dentin and bone without any signs of inflammation.

Conclusion

Within the limits of this case series, it has been shown that particulated dentin of autologous teeth may serve as an alternative to autologous bone for alveolar ridge

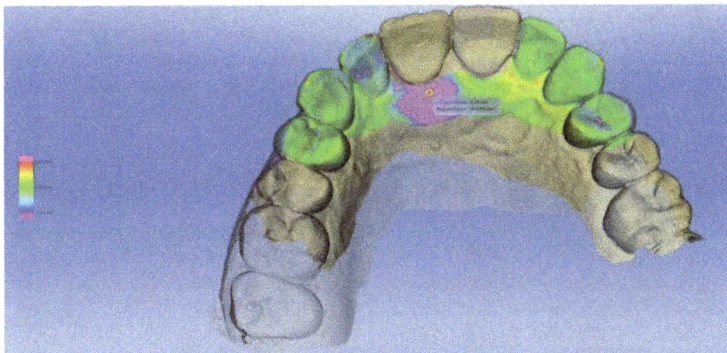

Fig. 20 Colour-coded superimposition of intraoral scans before extraction and after definitive prosthetic restoration

preservation prior to implant therapy. However, randomized studies on this treatment option are necessary.

Acknowledgements
We would like to express our thanks to Dr. Gabriel Bosch for the superimposition, calculation and illustration of the intraoral scans.

Authors' contributions
SV, BS and MR created the conception and study design. MR performed the surgical and DT the prosthodontic treatment. SV, PP and DT performed the data collection and AS the histological examination. SV, BS and AS analysed and interpreted the data. SV drafted the manuscript and PP helped hereby. BS and MR revised the manuscript. All authors read and approved the final manuscript.

Competing interests
This research did not receive any specific grant from funding agencies in the public, commercial, or not-for-profit sectors. Silvio Valdec, Pavla Pasic, Alex Soltermann, Daniel Thoma, Bernd Stadlinger and Martin Rücker declare that they have no competing interests.

Author details
[1]Clinic of Cranio-Maxillofacial and Oral Surgery, Center of Dental Medicine, University of Zurich, University Hospital Zurich, Plattenstrasse 11, 8032 Zürich, Switzerland. [2]Institute of Surgical Pathology, University Hospital Zurich, Zurich, Switzerland. [3]Clinic of Fixed and Removable Prosthodontics and Dental Material Science, Center of Dental Medicine, University of Zurich, Zurich, Switzerland.

References
1. Al-Asfour A, Andersson L, Kamal M, Joseph B. New bone formation around xenogenic dentin grafts to rabbit tibia marrow. Dent Traumatol. 2013;29(6): 455–60. doi:10.1111/edt.12045.
2. Albrektsson T, Zarb G, Worthington P, Eriksson AR. The long-term efficacy of currently used dental implants: a review and proposed criteria of success. Int J Oral Maxillofac Implants. 1986;1(1):11–25.
3. Andersson L. Dentin xenografts to experimental bone defects in rabbit tibia are ankylosed and undergo osseous replacement. Dent Traumatol. 2010; 26(5):398–402. doi:10.1111/j.1600-9657.2010.00912.x.
4. Andersson L, Blomlof L, Lindskog S, Feiglin B, Hammarstrom L. Tooth ankylosis. Clinical, radiographic and histological assessments. Int J Oral Surg. 1984;13(5):423–31.
5. Atiya BK, Shanmuhasuntharam P, Huat S, Abdulrazzak S, Oon H. Liquid nitrogen-treated autogenous dentin as bone substitute: an experimental study in a rabbit model. Int J Oral Maxillofac Implants. 2014;29(2):e165–170. doi:10.11607/jomi.te54.
6. Avila-Ortiz G, Elangovan S, Kramer KW, Blanchette D, Dawson DV. Effect of alveolar ridge preservation after tooth extraction: a systematic review and meta-analysis. J Dent Res. 2014;93(10):950–8. doi:10.1177/0022034514541127.
7. Baldini N, De Sanctis M, Ferrari M. Deproteinized bovine bone in periodontal and implant surgery. Dent Mater. 2011;27(1):61–70. doi:10.1016/j.dental.2010.10.017.
8. Baumer D, Zuhr O, Rebele S, Schneider D, Schupbach P, Hurzeler M. The socket-shield technique: first histological, clinical, and volumetrical observations after separation of the buccal tooth segment - a pilot study. Clin Implant Dent Relat Res. 2015;17(1):71–82. doi:10.1111/cid.12076.
9. Bormann KH, Suarez-Cunqueiro MM, Sinikovic B, Kampmann A, von See C, Binger T, Winkler M, Gellrich NC, Tavassol F, Rucker M. Dentin as a suitable bone substitute comparable to ss-TCP—an experimental study in mice. Microvasc Res. 2012;84(2):116–22. doi:10.1016/j.mvr.2012.06.004.
10. Camargo PM, Lekovic V, Weinlaender M, Klokkevold PR, Kenney EB, Dimitrijevic B, Nedic M, Jancovic S, Orsini M. Influence of bioactive glass on changes in alveolar process dimensions after exodontia. Oral Surg Oral Med Oral Pathol Oral Radiol Endod. 2000;90(5):581–6. doi:10.1067/moe.2000.110035.
11. Cardaropoli G, Araujo M, Lindhe J. Dynamics of bone tissue formation in tooth extraction sites. An experimental study in dogs. J Clin Periodontol. 2003;30(9):809–18.
12. Furhauser R, Florescu D, Benesch T, Haas R, Mailath G, Watzek G. Evaluation of soft tissue around single-tooth implant crowns: the pink esthetic score. Clin Oral Implants Res. 2005;16(6):639–44. doi:10.1111/j.1600-0501.2005.01193.x.
13. Guirado JL, Troiano M, Lopez-Lopez PJ, Ramirez-Fernandez MP, de Val JE, Marin JM, Gehrke SA. Different configuration of socket shield technique in peri-implant bone preservation: an experimental study in dog mandible. Ann Anat. 2016. doi:10.1016/j.aanat.2016.06.008.
14. Hallman M, Lundgren S, Sennerby L. Histologic analysis of clinical biopsies taken 6 months and 3 years after maxillary sinus floor augmentation with 80% bovine hydroxyapatite and 20% autogenous bone mixed with fibrin glue. Clin Implant Dent Relat Res. 2001;3(2):87–96.
15. Hammerle CH, Araujo MG, Simion M. Evidence-based knowledge on the biology and treatment of extraction sockets. Clin Oral Implants Res. 2012;23 Suppl 5:80–2. doi:10.1111/j.1600-0501.2011.02370.x.
16. Hurzeler MB, Zuhr O, Schupbach P, Rebele SF, Emmanouilidis N, Fickl S. The socket-shield technique: a proof-of-principle report. J Clin Periodontol. 2010; 37(9):855–62. doi:10.1111/j.1600-051X.2010.01595.x.
17. Jung RE, Philipp A, Annen BM, Signorelli L, Thoma DS, Hammerle CH, Attin T, Schmidlin P. Radiographic evaluation of different techniques for ridge preservation after tooth extraction: a randomized controlled clinical trial. J Clin Periodontol. 2013;40(1):90–8. doi:10.1111/jcpe.12027.
18. Kotsakis GA, Salama M, Chrepa V, Hinrichs JE, Gaillard P. A randomized, blinded, controlled clinical study of particulate anorganic bovine bone mineral and calcium phosphosilicate putty bone substitutes for socket preservation. Int J Oral Maxillofac Implants. 2014;29(1):141–51. doi:10.11607/jomi.3230.
19. Laschke MW, Haufel JM, Thorlacius H, Menger MD. New experimental approach to study host tissue response to surgical mesh materials in vivo. J Biomed Mater Res A. 2005;74(4):696–704. doi:10.1002/jbm.a.30371.
20. Lekovic V, Kenney EB, Weinlaender M, Han T, Klokkevold P, Nedic M, Orsini M. A bone regenerative approach to alveolar ridge maintenance following tooth extraction. Report of 10 cases. J Periodontol. 1997;68(6):563–70. doi:10.1902/jop.1997.68.6.563.
21. Linde A. Dentin matrix proteins: composition and possible functions in calcification. Anat Rec. 1989;224(2):154–66. doi:10.1002/ar.1092240206.
22. Liu X, Li Q, Wang F, Wang Z. Maxillary sinus floor augmentation and dental implant placement using dentin matrix protein-1 gene-modified bone marrow stromal cells mixed with deproteinized boving bone: a comparative study in beagles. Arch Oral Biol. 2016;64:102–8. doi:10.1016/j.archoralbio.2016.01.004.
23. Pang KM, Um IW, Kim YK, Woo JM, Kim SM, Lee JH. Autogenous demineralized dentin matrix from extracted tooth for the augmentation of alveolar bone defect: a prospective randomized clinical trial in comparison with anorganic bovine bone. Clin Oral Implants Res. 2016. doi:10.1111/clr.12885.
24. Pjetursson BE, Tan WC, Zwahlen M, Lang NP. A systematic review of the success of sinus floor elevation and survival of implants inserted in combination with sinus floor elevation. J Clin Periodontol. 2008;35(8 Suppl): 216–40. doi:10.1111/j.1600-051X.2008.01272.x.
25. Pohl V, Schuh C, Fischer MB, Haas R. A new method using autogenous impacted third molars for sinus augmentation to enhance implant treatment: case series with preliminary results of an open, prospective longitudinal study. Int J Oral Maxillofac Implants. 2016;31(3):622–30. doi:10.11607/jomi.4172.
26. Qin X, Raj RM, Liao XF, Shi W, Ma B, Gong SQ, Chen WM, Zhou B. Using rigidly fixed autogenous tooth graft to repair bone defect: an animal model. Dent Traumatol. 2014;30(5):380–4. doi:10.1111/edt.12101.
27. Rucker M, Laschke MW, Junker D, Carvalho C, Tavassol F, Mulhaupt R, Gellrich NC, Menger MD. Vascularization and biocompatibility of scaffolds consisting of different calcium phosphate compounds. J Biomed Mater Res A. 2008;86(4):1002–11. doi:10.1002/jbm.a.31722.
28. Schropp L, Wenzel A, Kostopoulos L, Karring T. Bone healing and soft tissue contour changes following single-tooth extraction: a clinical and radiographic 12-month prospective study. Int J Periodontics Restorative Dent. 2003;23(4):313–23.
29. Schwarz F, Golubovic V, Becker K, Mihatovic I. Extracted tooth roots used for lateral alveolar ridge augmentation: a proof-of-concept study. J Clin Periodontol. 2016;43(4):345–53. doi:10.1111/jcpe.12481.
30. Schwarz F, Golubovic V, Mihatovic I, Becker J. Periodontally diseased tooth

roots used for lateral alveolar ridge augmentation. A proof-of-concept study. J Clin Periodontol. 2016;43(9):797–803. doi:10.1111/jcpe.12579.

31. Sculean A, Berakdar M, Chiantella GC, Donos N, Arweiler NB, Brecx M. Healing of intrabony defects following treatment with a bovine-derived xenograft and collagen membrane. A controlled clinical study. J Clin Periodontol. 2003;30(1):73–80.

32. Sutton DN, Lewis BR, Patel M, Cawood JI. Changes in facial form relative to progressive atrophy of the edentulous jaws. Int J Oral Maxillofac Surg. 2004; 33(7):676–82. doi:10.1016/S0901-5027(03)00132-2.

33. Takata T, D'Errico JA, Atkins KB, Berry JE, Strayhorn C, Taichman RS, Somerman MJ. Protein extracts of dentin affect proliferation and differentiation of osteoprogenitor cells in vitro. J Periodontol. 1998; 69(11):1247–55. doi:10.1902/jop.1998.69.11.1247.

34. Yildirim M, Spiekermann H, Handt S, Edelhoff D. Maxillary sinus augmentation with the xenograft Bio-Oss and autogenous intraoral bone for qualitative improvement of the implant site: a histologic and histomorphometric clinical study in humans. Int J Oral Maxillofac Implants. 2001;16(1):23–33.

18

Implant decontamination with phosphoric acid during surgical peri-implantitis treatment

Diederik F. M. Hentenaar[1], Yvonne C. M. De Waal[2], Hans Strooker[2], Henny J. A. Meijer[1,2], Arie-Jan Van Winkelhoff[2,3] and Gerry M. Raghoebar[1*]

Abstract

Background: Peri-implantitis is known as an infectious disease that affects the peri-implant soft and hard tissue. Today, scientific literature provides very little evidence for an effective intervention protocol for treatment of peri-implantitis. The aim of the present randomized controlled trial is to evaluate the microbiological and clinical effectiveness of phosphoric acid as a decontaminating agent of the implant surface during surgical peri-implantitis treatment.

Methods: Peri-implantitis lesions were treated with resective surgical treatment aimed at peri-implant granulation tissue removal, bone recontouring, and pocket elimination. Fifty-three implant surfaces in 28 patients were mechanically cleaned and treated with either 35% phosphoric etching gel (test group) or sterile saline (control group). Microbiological samples were obtained during surgery; clinical parameters were recorded at baseline and at 3 months after treatment. Data were analyzed using multi-variable linear regression analysis and multilevel statistics.

Results: Significant immediate reductions in total anaerobic bacterial counts on the implant surface were found in both groups. Immediate reduction was greater when phosphoric acid was used. The difference in log-transformed mean anaerobic counts between both procedures was not statistical significant ($p = 0.108$), but there were significantly less culture-positive implants after the decontamination procedure in the phosphoric acid group ($p = 0.042$). At 3 months post-surgery, 75% of the implants in the control group and 63.3% of the implants in the test group showed disease resolution. However, no significant differences in clinical and microbiological outcomes between both groups were found.

Conclusions: The application of 35% phosphoric acid after mechanical debridement is superior to mechanical debridement combined with sterile saline rinsing for decontamination of the implant surface during surgical peri-implantitis treatment. However, phosphoric acid as implant surface decontaminant does not seem to enhance clinical outcomes on a 3-month follow-up.

Keywords: Peri-implantitis, Decontamination, Dental implants, Surgery, Microbiology

* Correspondence: g.m.raghoebar@umcg.nl
[1]Department of Oral and Maxillofacial Surgery, University of Groningen, University Medical Center Groningen, PO Box 30.001, 9700 RB Groningen, The Netherlands
Full list of author information is available at the end of the article

Background

Triggered host defense responses initiate inflammation of the peri-implant soft tissue (peri-implant mucositis), which can lead to loss of peri-implant supporting bone (peri-implantitis), and eventually, result in implant failure [1]. An increasing prevalence of peri-implantitis has been described in recent literature [2], with current incidence ranging from 1 to 47%. A non-linear, accelerating pattern of progress is suggested for the majority of cases, with an occurring onset within 3 years of function [3]. As for periodontal disease, the presence of microorganisms is an important factor for the development of an inflammatory response in peri-implant tissue [4]. In order to effectively treat the peri-implant inflammation, disruption of microbial adhesion and reduction of biofilm accumulation on the implant surface is probably of eminent importance.

A number of mechanical interventions (e.g., abrasive air powder, teflon curettes, ultrasonic devices) and chemical agents (e.g., chlorhexidine, hydrogen peroxide) solely or in combination have been described as methods for implant surface decontamination in both in vivo and in vitro studies, in both a surgical and non-surgical setting ([5–12]). According to different reviews on in vivo and in vitro mechanical debridement [13–17], a gold standard mechanical debridement regimen still does not exists. Possibly, the implant surface roughness and screw-shaped design of dental implants may compromise an effective mechanical intervention. Therefore, the additional use of chemical agents for implant decontamination may be advocated.

Antimicrobial solutions have been studied in different clinical studies [9, 10, 18, 19]. No superior clinical effectiveness has been shown in a single study for a specific chemical decontamination protocol (for reviews see [17, 20, 21]). However, studies using acids at low pH (<2) have shown potentially beneficial antiseptic effects [22–29]. Especially, results on decontamination with phosphoric acid might be promising. Wiltfang et al. [27] showed that surface decontamination with phosphoric acid (pH 1) in a surgical treatment protocol resulted in complete elimination of the bacterial microflora. Also, results of a short-term clinical trial by Strooker et al. [26] showed an instant greater reduction of colony-forming units on the implant surface when using phosphoric etching gel (pH 1). In addition, animal studies [30, 31] showed re-osseointegration and direct bone-to-implant contact when acids were used. Therefore, phosphoric acids might be considered a potentially feasible decontaminating agent.

Thus far, the use of phosphoric acid etching gel as decontaminating agent has not been evaluated in a randomized controlled trial. The aim of the present randomized controlled trial is to evaluate the short-term microbiological and clinical effectiveness of 35% phosphoric etching gel as a decontaminating agent of the implant surface during resective surgical treatment of peri-implantitis.

Methods

Trial design

The present study is a double-blind randomized controlled trial evaluating the effect of 35% phosphoric etching gel (test group) compared to the effect of saline (control group) for implant surface decontamination combined with mechanical debridement during surgical peri-implantitis treatment. Patients were randomly assigned to the test or control group using a one-to-one allocation ratio. The study has been conducted in full accordance with the World Medical Association Declaration of Helsinki (version 2008) and was approved by the Institutional Review Board of the University Medical Center Groningen, the Netherlands (METc2013.005). Written informed consent was obtained from all participants before entering the trial. Clinical trial registration was done at the Netherlands National Trial Register (http://www.trialregister.nl, trial number NTR5185). The CONSORT guidelines for reporting a clinical trial were followed.

Participants

Patients participating in this study were consecutively selected from the patient populations of the Center of Dentistry and Oral Hygiene and the Department of Oral and Maxillofacial Surgery of the University Medical Center Groningen, Groningen, The Netherlands, from October 2012 to April 2014.

Adult patients with at least one endosseous implant with clinical and radiographical signs of peri-implantitis were included. Peri-implantitis was defined as a loss of marginal bone ≥2 mm in combination with bleeding and/or suppuration on probing and a peri-implant probing depth ≥5 mm [32]. Implants had to be in function for at least 2 years.

Exclusion criteria were:

- Contraindications for the surgical procedures;
- A history of local radiotherapy to the head and neck region;
- Pregnancy and lactation;
- Uncontrolled diabetes;
- Systemic use of antibiotics within 3 months before inclusion;
- Long-term use of anti-inflammatory drugs;
- Incapability of performing basal oral hygiene measures as a result of physical or mental disorders;
- Uncontrolled periodontitis (PPD >5 mm);

- Implants with bone loss exceeding two thirds of the length of the implant or implants with bone loss beyond the transverse openings in hollow implants;
- Implant mobility;
- Implants at which no position could be identified where proper probing measurements could be performed;
- Previous surgical treatment of the peri-implantitis lesions.

Interventions

The study protocol was based on the study protocols of two previous studies evaluating the decontaminating effect of chlorhexidine during surgical peri-implantitis treatment [10, 32] and is briefly described below.

Within 1 month before surgical treatment, all patients received extensive oral hygiene instructions and mechanical non-surgical debridement of implants and remaining dentition using hand instrumentation and/or an ultrasonic device. Immediately before surgical treatment screw-retained suprastructures were removed. In order to obtain an optimal overview of the peri-implant area during surgery, prior to the procedure, only screw-retained suprastructures were removed. Cemented single crowns or bridges on mesostructures were left in place to prevent any damage to these structures. Directly after surgery, the screw-retained suprastructures were placed back. Cemented single crowns or bridges on mesostructures were left in place to prevent any damage to these structures. Vertical releasing incisions extending into the alveolar mucosa were placed using a surgical blade (no. 15), and full thickness mucoperiosteal flaps were raised buccally and lingually. Flaps were designed to allow optimal access to the peri-implant bone defect. Granulation tissue was removed using titanium curettes (Gracey; Hu-Friedy®, Chicago, IL, USA). The implant surfaces were mechanically cleaned using titanium curettes and gauzes and cotton pellets soaked in saline. Next, the patients were randomly allocated to either the test or control group. Subsequently, implants were cleaned with either local application of 35% phosphoric acid gel (pH 1) for 1 min (Temrex gel, Temrex, Freeport, NY, USA) (test group) or by rinsing with an abundant amount of sterile saline for 1 min (control group). Care was taken to apply the phosphoric etching gel precisely on the implant surface using a syringe with a small tip. During 1 min, the etching gel was continuously rubbed on to the implant surface with a small brush. In both groups, the intervention continued with rinsing of the implant surface with an abundant amount of sterile saline for 1 min.

Angular bony defects were eliminated, and bone was recontoured using a rotating round bur under saline irrigation. Mucosal flaps were apically positioned and firmly sutured (Vicryl Plus® 3-0; Ethicon Inc., Somerville, NJ, USA), and suprastructures were re-positioned. For both control and test group, surgery was followed by 2 weeks of mouth rinsing with 0.12% CHX + 0.05% CPC without alcohol two times daily for 30 s. Sutures were removed after 2 weeks. Follow-up visits were scheduled after 3 (T_3) months. Patients were all surgically treated by one experienced oral and maxillofacial surgeon (GR).

Outcomes

Primary outcome variable

The primary outcome variable was the difference in anaerobic bacterial load of the implant surface before and after mechanical and chemical debridement and decontamination. After flap deflection and granulation tissue removal, a sample was obtained from the implant surface by rubbing a sterilized brush (Microbrush® International, Grafton, WI, USA) across the implant surface (T_{pre}). A second sample was obtained after mechanical debridement, decontamination of the implant surface with the test or control substance, and subsequent rinsing with sterile saline (Tpost). After sampling, the top part of the brush was cut off and collected in a vial containing reduced transport fluid [33]. From every implant presenting peri-implantitis, separate samples were obtained. All microbiological samples were processed within 24 h [34]. The total anaerobic bacterial load and the presence and numbers of the periodontal pathogens [35] *Aggregatibacter actinomycetemcomitans, Porphyromonas gingivalis, Prevotella intermedia, Tannerella forsythia, Fusobacterium nucleatum, Parvimonas micra,* and *Campylobacter rectus* were determined by laboratory technicians who were blind to treatment allocation.

Secondary outcome variables

Secondary outcome variables were percentage of sites with bleeding on probing (% sites BoP), percentage of sites with suppuration on probing (% sites SoP), mean probing pocket depth (mean PPD), and microbial composition of the peri-implant sulcus. Measurements were performed before (pre) treatment (baseline, T_0) and at 3 months (T_3) after surgery by one and the same examiner (DH) who was blind to treatment allocation. Peri-implant pocket depth was measured at four sites per implant (mesial, buccal, distal, and lingual) using a pressure sensitive probe (KerrHawe Click Probe®, Bioggo, Switzerland) (probe force of 0.25 N). Bleeding and suppuration were scored up to 30s after pocket probing. Microbiological peri-implant sulcus samples were collected from each implant with peri-implantitis using four sterile paperpoints per implant. Paperpoints were collected in a vial containing RTF and were analyzed in the same manner as the intra-operative samples. Outcome variables were total anaerobic bacterial load and the presence and numbers of the periodontal pathogens *A. actinomycetemcomitans*, *P. gingivalis*, *P. intermedia*, *T. forsythia*, *F. nucleatum*, *P. micra*, and *C. rectus*.

Randomization

Fourteen notes with the word "phosphoric acid" and 14 notes with the word "saline" were put into 28 identical, sequentially numbered, non-transparent envelopes according to a randomization list generated by a computer program. The envelopes were irreversibly sealed. During the surgical procedure, after flap deflection and mechanical cleansing, the surgeon temporarily left the operating room. The surgical assistant opened an envelope and prepared the materials as needed according to the information on the note. A third person (YDW) performed the decontamination procedure according to group allocation. The materials were removed, and the surgeon continued the surgical procedure. The researcher (performing the clinical measurements, DH) was blind to treatment allocation and did not have access to the randomization code until the end of the research period.

Statistical methods
Sample size

Sample size was based on the microbiological data from a previous study evaluating the effect of implant surface decontamination with a chlorhexidine solution versus a placebo solution [10]. The decontaminating effect of phosphoric acid was expected to be similar to the decontaminating effect of chlorhexidine (reduction in log-transformed mean anaerobic bacterial load = 4.21 (chlorhexidine group) versus 2.77 (placebo group), SD = 2.12). Assuming a two-sided two sample t test with a significance level (α) of 0.05 and a power (β) of 80% required a sample size of 34 implants. A 20% compensation for dropouts was taken into account (34/0.8 = 42.5 implants). Based on a previous study [10], it was expected that not all baseline microbiological samples would yield a detectable number of cultivable bacteria ([10], 19 out of 79 = 24% of samples showed no bacterial growth). Because "negative" samples cannot be used to determine a decontaminating effect, the sample size was compensated for these potential unusable samples (24%), yielding a sample size of 56 implants (42.5/0.76). According to the assumption that each patient has on average more than two implants with peri-implantitis [10], a sample size of 28 patients was chosen (56/2, 14 patients per group).

Statistical analysis

For the analysis of the primary outcome variable and the secondary *microbiological* outcome variable linear regression analysis was performed. The implant was taken as the statistical unit. Total anaerobic bacterial loads at baseline (T_{pre} and T_0) were distributed normally after logarithmic

transformation. Baseline values were included in the regression model. For the comparison of the number of culture-positive implants after the decontamination period, the chi-square test was used. The secondary *clinical* outcome variables were analyzed using a two-level hierarchical random intercepts model. The two levels of analysis were implant level and patient level. With the crude analysis, the effect of the intervention was determined, while controlling for baseline value. Because a previous study [9] has shown that mean bone loss at baseline and smoking are prognostic indicators for the outcome of resective peri-implantitis treatment, these factors were additionally included in the model (adjusted analysis).

Descriptive data and data regarding the microbiological outcome variables were analyzed using IBM SPSS Statistics 22 Version 22.0 (IBM Corp. Armonk, NY: IBM Corp.). Multilevel models were analyzed using MLwiN version 2.12 (Centre for Multilevel Modeling, University of Bristol, Bristol, UK).

Results

The progress of patients throughout the different phases of the study is illustrated in Fig. 1. Table 1 depicts the baseline demographic patient and implant characteristics. The included patients had a total of 128 implants of which 53 implants showed signs of peri-implantitis. Different implant brands and types with different implant surfaces were present, including Straumann (Straumann AG, Basel, Switserland; SLA® and SLActive® surface), Nobel Biocare (Nobel Biocare AB, Göteborg, Sweden; TiUnite® surface), Biomet 3i (Biomet Inc., Warsaw, Indiana, USA; OSSEOTITE® surface), Frialit-2, (Dentsply Friadent, Mannheim, Germany; FRIADENT® plus surface), and Pitt-Easy (Sybron Implant Solutions GmbH, Bremen, Germany; Puretex® surface). Three patients with each one implant with peri-implantitis were lost to follow-up (2 patients from the control group, 1 from the test group).

Microbiological outcomes

[10]Log-transformed mean bacterial anaerobic counts of the culture-positive implants for the control and test group before and after debridement and decontamination of the implant surface during the surgical procedure are depicted in Table 2. In both groups, the debridement and decontamination procedure resulted in a significant immediate reduction in counts of anaerobic bacteria on the implant surface. Although the reduction in total anaerobic load was greater in the test group, the difference did not reach the level of statistical significance ($p = 0.108$). However, in the test group, the total anaerobic load was significantly more often reduced below detection level than in the control group (20 out of 23 in the test group, 10 out of 17 in the control

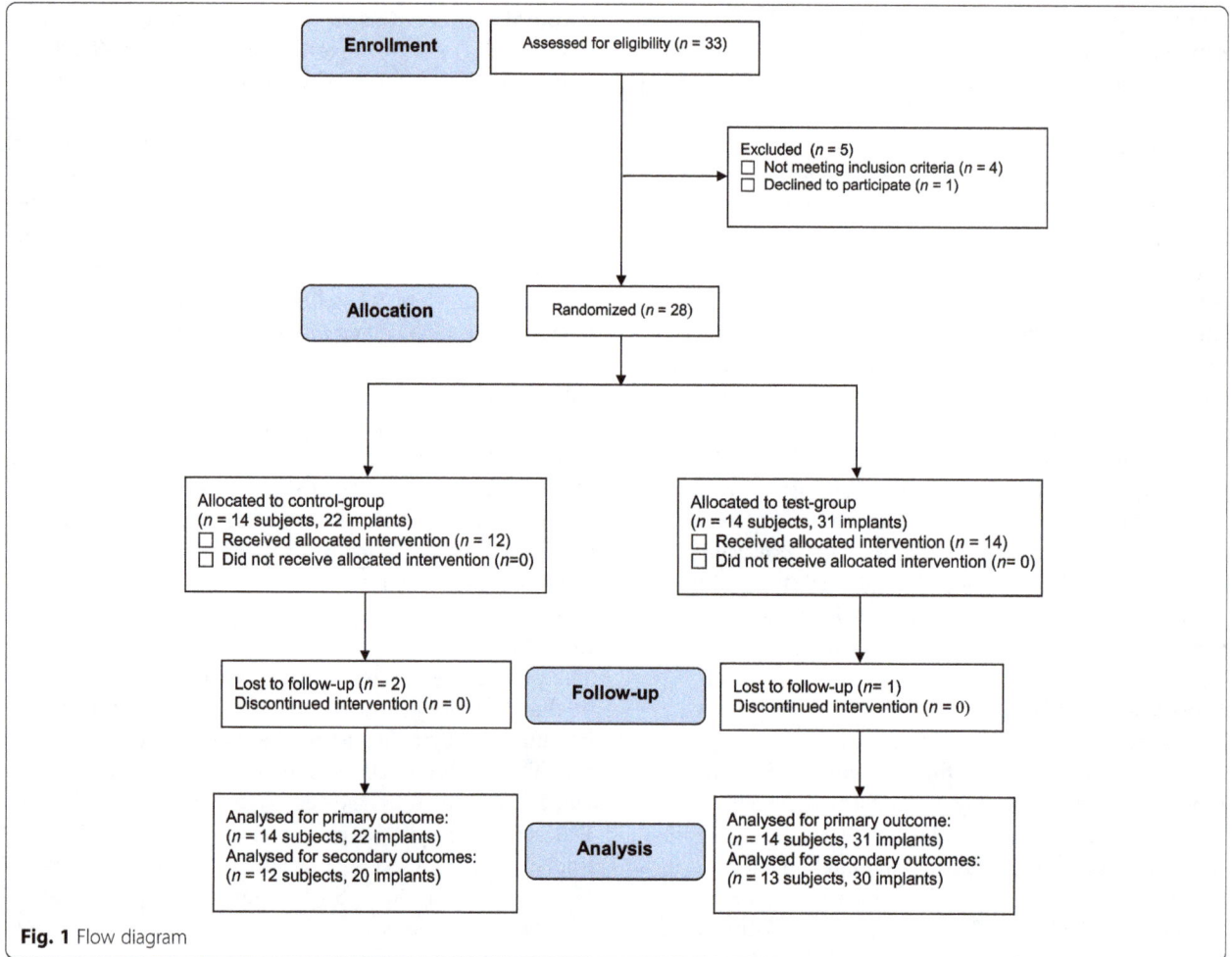

Fig. 1 Flow diagram

group, $p = 0.042$). No significant differences were observed in the ^{10}Log-transformed mean bacterial anaerobic counts of the peri-implant sulcus, neither between control and test group nor between baseline and 3 months after surgery (Table 3).

Table 1 Characteristics of included patients/implants

Characteristics	Control	Test
Number of patients	14	14
Age (years; mean [SD])	57.0 (13.7)	60.9 (7.2)
Gender; M (male), F (female)	M5, F9	M7, F7
Smoking; n subjects (%)	1 (7%)	3 (21%)
History of periodontitis; n subjects (%)	4 (29%)	5 (36%)
Dental status; n subjects (%)		
- Partially edentulous	13 (93%)	12 (86%)
- Fully edentulous	1 (7%)	2 (14%)
Total number of implants (range)	68 (1–9)	60 (1–10)
Number of implants with peri-implantitis (range)	22 (1–4)	31 (1–5)
Mean bone loss at baseline in mm (SD)	2.73 (1.49)	3.58 (1.57)

Clinical outcomes

Descriptive statistics of the clinical outcomes at baseline and follow-up are depicted in Table 4. At 3-month follow-up, 75% of the implants (66.7% of the patients) in the control group and 63.3% of the implants (53.8% of the patients) in the test group showed no clinical signs of inflammation (PPD ≤4 mm without bleeding and/or suppuration on probing) (Table 4). The results from the multilevel analyses regarding the effects of the intervention on BoP, SoP, and PPD are shown in Table 5. No significant differences in BoP, SoP, and mean PPD were detected between control and test group at 3 months after surgery, neither in the "crude" nor in the "adjusted" analysis.

Discussion

This randomized controlled trial aimed to determine the effect of 35% phosphoric etching gel on decontamination of the implant surface during resective surgical treatment of peri-implantitis. Both decontamination procedures (mechanical debridement with curettes and gauzes combined with phosphoric acid 35% and mechanical

Table 2 Log-transformed mean bacterial anaerobic counts (SD) of culture-positive implants for the control and test group before (T_{pre}) and after (T_{post}) debridement and decontamination of the implant surface (intra-operative microbrush samples)

$N = 40$[a]	Total anaerobic bacterial load Log-transformed mean (SD)				
	T_{pre}	T_{post}	Difference	β (95% CI)[b]	p value
Control	5.57 (0.93) [17]	2.25 (2.98)[c] [7][d]	2.68 (3.25)	−1.39 (−3.09–0.32)	0.108
Test	5.35 (0.98) [23]	0.81 (2.25)[c] [3][d]	4.19 (3.31)		

SD standard deviation, [n] number of culture-positive implants
[a] Implants with baseline values of 0 excluded from analysis
[b] Linear regression analysis, adjusted for baseline values
[c] Significant difference from baseline
[d] Significant difference in number of culture-positive implants after decontamination between test and control group ($p = 0.042$)

debridement combined with sterile saline) resulted in a significant immediate reduction in counts of anaerobic bacteria on the implant surface. This immediate reduction was greater when phosphoric acid was used. Although the difference in log-transformed mean anaerobic counts between both decontaminating procedures did not reach the level of statistical significance ($p = 0.108$), there were significantly less culture-positive implants after the decontamination procedure in the phosphoric acid group ($p = 0.042$). As our study focused on the decontaminating effect of phosphoric acid on implant surfaces, we used the microbiological parameter as primary outcome variable. To evaluate the effect of the intervention on this microbiological parameter, an in vivo situation was chosen to benefit the influence of a clinical situation. In addition, we evaluated secondary outcome parameters indicating the clinical effect of the treatment procedure, i.e., disease resolution 3 months after active treatment.

At 3 months post-surgery, disease resolution was more frequently observed in the control group (75% of implants) than in the test group (63.3% of implants). However, no significant differences in clinical and microbiological outcomes between control and test group were found. Although the study was "a priori" not powered to detect clinical differences, no trend was observed for superior results of one decontamination procedure over the other.

To our knowledge, this is the first randomized controlled clinical trial reporting on the effect of phosphoric

Table 3 Log-transformed mean bacterial anaerobic counts (SD) for the control and test group before (T_0) and 3 months after (T_3) the surgical treatment (paperpoint samples)

$N = 47$[a]	Total anaerobic bacterial load Log-transformed mean (SD)				
	T_0	T_3	Difference	β (95% CI)[b]	p value
Control	6.69 (1.32)	6.31 (1.30)	0.38 (1.36)	−0.26 (−0.84–0.33)	0.377
Test	6.53 (1.06)	5.98 (0.94)	0.55 (0.99)		

SD standard deviation
[a] Three samples without bacterial growth and three samples without follow-up excluded from analysis
[b] Linear regression analysis, adjusted for baseline values

acid in relation to peri-implantitis treatment. The reason for choosing phosphoric acid as decontaminating agent was that acids with low pH exert a strong bactericidal effect [22, 36], and phosphoric acid does not seem to chemically damage titanium implant surface [37]. A gel as application mode has the great advantage of being precisely applicable with minimal touching of the surrounding bone or connective tissue. A disadvantage of a gel might be the limited flow in deeper areas of the rough implant surface. To overcome this problem, it was decided to continuously rub the etching gel onto the implant surface with a small brush during the decontamination period.

Phosphoric acid gel as agent for implant surface decontamination has only been investigated in two other clinical studies [26, 27]. Strooker et al. [26] used phosphoric acid 35% for peri-implant supportive therapy and found greater reductions in bacterial load, but no significant clinical differences compared to conventional mechanical supportive therapy. They concluded that local application of 35% phosphoric acid gel can be as effective as conventional mechanical therapy in the professional supportive care of oral implants. In the study of Wiltfang et al. [27], 20% etching gel was used for implant surface decontamination in a combined surgical protocol for treatment of peri-implantitis. Thirty-six implants with peri-implantitis in 22 patients were followed for 1 year. The implants were decontaminated with etching gel, and the defects were filled with autologous bone mixed with an osteoinductive material for regenerative treatment of bone defects. In their study, previous microbiological tests (not published) of implants in situ had revealed complete elimination of the bacterial microflora after decontamination with etching gel, which is close to our results of "complete" elimination (reduction below detection level) in 20 out of 23 implants. They concluded that their surgical protocol in combination with phosphoric etching gel provides a reliable method to treat peri-implant bone defects.

Phosphoric acid used in an in vitro setting has only been described in a study by Tastepe et al. [37]. The use

Table 4 Descriptive statistics of clinical parameters

		Control		Test	
		T_0 ($n = 22$)	T_3 ($n = 20$)	T_0 ($n = 31$)	T_3 ($n = 30$)
Plaque	% of sites (SD)	4.5 (12.5)	10.0 (18.8)	4.0 (9.3)	2.5 (7.6)
	% of implants (n)	13.6 (3)	25.0 (5)	16.1 (5)	9.7 (3)
BoP	% of sites (SD)	86.4 (18.5)	28.8 (35.6)	66.1 (29.3)	39.2 (31.3)
	% of implants (n)	100 (22)	50 (10)	96.8 (30)	76.7 (23)
SoP	% of sites (SD)	22.7 (24.3)	5.0 (15.4)	30.7 (20.1)	8.3 (20.1)
	% of implants (n)	54.5 (12)	10.0 (2)	80.6 (25)	20.0 (6)
Mean PPD	Mean (SD)	5.3 (1.1)	3.5 (1.5)	5.2 (1.1)	4.1 (1.6)
PPD ≥5 mm	% of sites (SD)	67.1 (26.0)	18.8 (30.2)	61.3 (22.2)	28.3 (33.9)
	% of implants (n)	100 (22)	35.0 (7)	100 (31)	46.7 (14)
PPD ≥6 mm	% of sites (SD)	50.0 (27.8)	12.5 (26.3)	46.8 (26.4)	24.2 (33.1)
	% of implants (n)	100 (22)	25.0 (5)	90.3 (28)	40.0 (12)
PPD ≥5 mm + BoP/SoP (same site)	% of sites (SD)	65.9 (26.2)	12.5 (25.0)	54.8 (22.7)	20.0 (29.7)
	% of implants (n)	100 (22)	25.0 (5)	100 (31)	36.7 (11)
	% of patients (n)	100 (14/14)	33.3 (4/12)	100 (14/14)	46.2 (6/13)
PPD ≥6 mm + BoP/SoP (same site)	% of sites (SD)	50.0 (27.8)	8.8 (20.3)	41.1 (24.6)	17.5 (28.7)
	% of implants (n)	100 (22)	20.0 (4)	90.3 (28)	33.3 (10)
	% of patients (n)	100 (14/14)	33.3 (4/12)	100 (14/14)	46.2 (6/13)

of an air abrasive device with four different powders was compared to phosphoric acid. In contrast to our study and the previous described clinical studies, the use of phosphoric acid was not efficient in removing biofilm. The residual biofilm area was significantly greater after treatment with phosphoric acid compared to air abrasive treatment with powder or even control treatment without powder. Apparently, only water and air might be effective in reducing the biofilm. Nonetheless, when the titanium surface was viewed under a scanning electron microscopy (SEM), no visible titanium surface change was seen after phosphoric acid application while some minor changes (dependent on the character and size of the particles) were observed after air powder abrasive treatment.

Recent studies that zoom in on titanium surface physico-chemistry reveal interesting results [38, 39]. Kotsakis et al. [38] hypothesized that chemical residues alter the titanium surface physicochemistry and subsequently compromise cellular response to these decontaminated surfaces. However, they report on effective restoring of biocompatibility when sterile saline, citric acid, and EDTA/sodium hypochlorite (NaOCl-EDTA) were used, in contrast to chlorhexidine. Therefore, they propose the use of sterile saline, citric acid, and NaOCl-EDTA in the treatment of peri-implantitis not only for their antimicrobial properties but also for the preservation of the titanium material properties. In contrast, a study by [39] found noticeable morphological changes and corrosion on the titanium surface when the synergistic effect of acidic environments (i.e., citric acid, 15% hydrogen peroxide, tetracycline, peroxyacetic acid) and mechanical forces (rubbing with cotton swabs) was investigated. Dissolution of the oxide layer (which can result in corrosion) was observed when using peroxyacetic and citric acid. It is therefore hypothesized that surface damage of dental alloys may potentially be induced after detoxification and maintenance treatments with acidic solutions and subsequently might hinder re-osseointegration. No visibly evident damage of the surfaces was shown by [39] when neutral or basic treatments such as sodium fluoride 0.12, 0.20, and 1.10% were used, which might be explained by the neutral electrochemical environment [40].

Table 5 Average differences in BoP, SoP, and PPD between the control and test group at 3-month follow-up

Outcome variable	Crude model[a] β (95% CI)	p value	Adjusted model[b] β (95% CI)	p-value
% Sites BoP	16.2 (−7.9 to 40.3)	0.743	7.9 (−16.4 to 32.3)	0.821
% Sites SoP	0.0 (−10.9 to 10.9)	1.000	0.7 (−10.1 to 11.4)	0.882
Mean PPD	0.6 (−0.6 to 1.8)	0.205	0.2 (−1.0 to 1.3)	0.470

The reference category for intervention effect is the control group. The regression coefficients (β) indicate the average differences in clinical outcomes between the control and test group at 3-month follow-up

BoP bleeding on probing, SoP suppuration on probing, PPD probing pocket depth, 95% CI 95% confidence interval

[a]Adjusted for baseline values

[b]Adjusted for baseline values, smoking, and mean bone loss at baseline

Interpreting the results of these in vitro studies has to be done cautiously since the results among the studies are not homogenous and the effects of the chemical environment coupled with mechanical force in the oral environment has to be further evaluated. In our study, however, phosphoric acid neither seemed to have a positive nor a negative effect on clinical outcomes.

The current study is based on a follow-up time of 3 months and therefore the long-term results on the use of phosphoric acid remain unclear.

Conclusions

Implant surface decontamination is considered a highly susceptible step in the treatment of peri-implantitis. The application of 35% phosphoric acid after mechanical debridement is superior to mechanical debridement combined with sterile saline rinsing for decontamination of the implant surface during surgical peri-implantitis treatment. However, phosphoric acid as implant surface decontaminant does not seem to enhance clinical outcomes on a 3-month follow-up. Larger studies with a longer follow-up period are needed to validate these findings.

Abbreviations

GR: Gerry Raghoebar; DH: Diederik Hentenaar; YDW: Yvonne de Waal

Funding

The study was self-funded by the authors and their institution.

Authors' contributions

DH and YdW drafted the manuscript. DH collected the data. YdW performed the statistical analysis. AJvW analyzed the microbiological samples. GM surgically treated the participants. HS participated in the design of the study. HM conceived the study and participated in its design and coordination. All authors read and approved the final manuscript.

Competing interests

Diederik F. M. Hentenaar, Yvonne C. M. de Waal, Hans Strooker, Henny J. A. Meijer, Arie-Jan van Winkelhoff, and Gerry M. Raghoe declare that they have no competing interests.

Author details

[1]Department of Oral and Maxillofacial Surgery, University of Groningen, University Medical Center Groningen, PO Box 30.001, 9700 RB Groningen, The Netherlands. [2]Center for Dentistry and Oral Hygiene, University of Groningen, University Medical Center Groningen, Groningen, The Netherlands. [3]Department of Medical Microbiology, University of Groningen, University Medical Center Groningen, Groningen, The Netherlands.

References

1. Lang NP, Berglundh T, Working Group 4 of Seventh European Workshop on Periodontology. Periimplant diseases: where are we now?—Consensus of the Seventh European Workshop on Periodontology. J Clin Periodontol. 2011;38(Suppl):11,178–181.

2. Derks J, Tomasi C. Peri-implant health and disease. A systematic review of current epidemiology. J Clin Periodontol. 2015;42:158–71.

3. Derks J, Schaller D, Håkansson J, Wennström JL, Tomasi C, Berglundh T. Peri-implantitis—onset and pattern of progression. J Clin Periodontol. 2016;43:383–8.

4. Lindhe J, Meyle J, Group D of European Workshop on Periodontology. Peri-implant diseases: Consensus Report of the Sixth European Workshop on Periodontology. J Clin Periodontol. 2008;35:282–5.

5. Leonhardt A, Dahlén G, Renvert S. Five-year clinical, microbiological, and radiological outcome following treatment of peri-implantitis in man. J Periodontol. 2003;74:1415–22.

6. Máximo MB, de Mendonça AC, Renata Santos V, Figueiredo LC, Feres M, Duarte PM. Short-term clinical and microbiological evaluations of peri-implant diseases before and after mechanical anti-infective therapies. Clin Oral Implants Res. 2009;20:99–108.

7. Serino G, Turri A. Outcome of surgical treatment of peri-implantitis: results from a 2-year prospective clinical study in humans. Clin Oral Implants Res. 2011;22:1214–20.

8. Bassetti M, Schär D, Wicki B, Eick S, Ramseier SA, Arweiler NB, Sculean A, Salvi GE. Anti-infective therapy of peri-implantitis with adjunctive local drug delivery or photodynamic therapy: 12-month outcomes of a randomized controlled clinical trial. Clin Oral Implants Res. 2014;25:279–87.

9. De Waal YC, Raghoebar GM, Meijer HJ, Winkel EG, van Winkelhoff AJ. Prognostic indicators for surgical peri-implantitis treatment. Clin Oral Implants Res. 2016;27:1485–91.

10. De Waal YC, Raghoebar GM, Huddleston Slater JJ, Meijer HJ, Winkel EG, van Winkelhoff AJ. Implant decontamination during surgical peri-implantitis treatment: a randomized, double-blind, placebo-controlled trial. J Clin Periodontol. 2013;40:186–95.

11. Riben-Grundstrom C, Norderyd O, André U, Renvert S. Treatment of peri-implant mucositis using a glycine powder air-polishing or ultrasonic device: a randomized clinical trial. J Clin Periodontol. 2015;42:462–9.

12. Heitz-Mayfield LJA, Salvi GE, Mombelli A, Faddy M, Lang NP. Anti-infective surgical therapy of peri-implantitis. A 12-month prospective clinical study. Clin Oral Implants Res. 2012;23(2):205–10.

13. Esposito M, Grusovin MG, Worthington HV. Treatment of peri-implantitis: what interventions are effective? A Cochrane systematic review. Eur J Oral Implantol. 2012;5:21–41.

14. Louropoulou A, Slot DE, Van der Weijden F. The effects of mechanical instruments on contaminated titanium dental implant surfaces: a systematic review. Clin Oral Implants Res. 2014;25:1149–60.

15. Ramanauskaite A, Daugela P, Faria de Almeida R, Saulacic N. Surgical non-regenerative treatments for peri-implantitis: a systematic review. J Oral Maxillofacial Res. 2016;7:e14.

16. Schwarz F, Becker K, Bastendorf KD, Cardaropoli D, Chatfield D, Dunn I, Fletcher P, Einwag J, Louropoulou A, Mombelli A, Ower P, Pavlovic P, Sahrmann P, Salvi GE, Schmage P, Takeuchi Y, Van Der Weijden F, Renvert S. Recommendations on the clinical application of air polishing for the management of peri-implant mucositis and peri-implantitis. Quintessence Int J Pract Dent. 2015;47:293–6.

17. Subramani KK. Decontamination of titanium implant surface and re-osseointegration to treat peri-implantitis: a literature review. Int J Oral Maxillofac Implants. 2012;27:1043–54.

18. Gosau M, Hahnel S, Schwarz F, Gerlach T, Reichert TE, Bürgers R. Effect of six different peri-implantitis disinfection methods on in vivo human oral biofilm. Clin Oral Implants Res. 2010;21:866–72.

19. Heitz-Mayfield LJ, Salvi GE, Mombelli A, Faddy M, Lang NP. Implant Complication Research Group. Anti-infective surgical therapy of peri-implantitis. A 12-month prospective clinical study. Clin Oral Implants Res. 2012;23:205–10.

20. Meyle J. Mechanical, chemical and laser treatments of the implant surface in the presence of marginal bone loss around implants. Eur J Oral Implantol. 2012;5:71–81.

21. Ntrouka VI, Slot DE, Louropoulou A, Van der Weijden F. The effect of chemotherapeutic agents on contaminated titanium surfaces: a systematic review. Clin Oral Implants Res. 2011;22:681–90.

22. Chen CJ, Chen CC, Ding SJ. Effectiveness of hypochlorous acid to reduce the biofilms on titanium alloy surfaces in vitro. Int J Mol Sci. 2016;17:1161.

23. Dennison DK, Huerzeler MB, Quinones C, Caffesse RG. Contaminated implant surfaces: an in vitro comparison of implant surface coating and treatment modalities for decontamination. J Periodontol. 1994;65:942–8.

24. Htet M, Madi M, Zakaria O, Miyahara T, Xin W, Lin Z, Aoki K, Kasugai S. Decontamination of anodized implant surface with different modalities for

peri-implantitis treatment: lasers and mechanical debridement with citric acid. J Periodontol. 2016;87:953–61.

25. Mouhyi J, Sennerby L, Van Reck J. The soft tissue response to contaminated and cleaned titanium surfaces using CO2 laser, citric acid and hydrogen peroxide. An experimental study in the rat abdominal wall. Clin Oral Implants Res. 2000;11:93–8.

26. Strooker H, Rohn S, Van Winkelhoff AJ. Clinical and microbiologic effects of chemical versus mechanical cleansing in professional supportive implant therapy. Int J Oral Maxillofac Implants. 1998;13:845–50.

27. Wiltfang J, Zernial O, Behrens E, Schlegel A, Wamke PH, Becker ST. Regenerative treatment of peri-implantitis bone defects with a combination of autologous bone and a demineralized xenogenic bone graft: a series of 36 defects. Clin Implant Dent Relat Res. 2012;14:421–7.

28. Wohlfahrt JC, Lyngstadaas SP, Rønold HJ, Saxegaard E, Ellingsen JE, Karlsson S, Aass AM. Porous titanium granules in the surgical treatment of peri-implant osseous defects: a randomized clinical trial. Int J Oral Maxillofac Implants. 2012;27:401–10.

29. Zablotsky MH, Diedrich DL, Meffert RM. Detoxification of endotoxin-contaminated titanium and hydroxyapatite-coated surfaces utilizing various chemotherapeutic and mechanical modalities. Implant Dent. 1992;1:154–8.

30. Alhag M, Renvert S, Polyzois I, Claffey N. Re-osseointegration on rough implant surfaces previously coated with bacterial biofilm: an experimental study in the dog. Clin Oral Implants Res. 2008;19:182–7.

31. Kolonidis SG, Renvert S, Hämmerle CH, Lang NP, Harris D, Claffey N. Osseointegration on implant surfaces previously contaminated with plaque. An experimental study in the dog. Clin Oral Implants Res. 2003;14:373–80.

32. De Waal YC, Raghoebar GM, Meijer HJ, Winkel EG, van Winkelhoff AJ. Implant decontamination with 2% chlorhexidine during surgical peri-implantitis treatment: a randomized, double-blind, controlled trial. Clin Oral Implants Res. 2015;26:1015–23.

33. Syed SA, Loesche WJ. Survival of human dental plaque flora in various transport media. Appl Microbiol. 1972;24:638–44.

34. Van Winkelhoff AJ, van Steenbergen TJ, Kippuw N, De Graaff J. Further characterization of Bacteroides endodontalis, an asaccharolytic black-pigmented Bacteroides species from the oral cavity. J Clin Microbiol. 1985;22:75–9.

35. Zambon JJ. Periodontal diseases: microbial factors. Ann Periodontol. 1996;1:879–925.

36. Héritier M. Effects of phosphoric acid on root dentin surface. A scanning and transmission electron microscopic study. J Periodontal Res. 1984;19:168–76.

37. Tastepe CS, Lui Y, Visscher CM, Wismeijer D. Cleaning and modification of intraorally contaminated titanium discs with calcium phosphate powder abrasive treatment. Clin Oral Implants Res. 2013;24:1238–46.

38. Kotsakis GA, Lan C, Barbosa J, Lill K, Chen R, Rudney J, Aparicio C. Antimicrobial agents used in the treatment of peri-implantitis alter the physicochemistry and cytocompatibility of titanium surfaces. J Periodontol. 2016;87:809–19.

39. Wheelis SE, Gindri IM, Valderrama P, Wilson Jr TG, Huang J, Rodrigues DC. Effects of decontamination solutions on the surface of titanium: investigation of surface morphology, composition, and roughness. Clin Oral Implants Res. 2016;27:329–40.

40. Suito H, Iwawaki Y, Goto T, Tomotake Y, Ichikawa T. Oral factors affecting titanium elution and corrosion: an in vitro study using simulated body fluid. PLoS One. 2013;8:e66052.

19

Evaluation of dimensional behavior of peri-implant tissues in implants immediately exposed or submerged in fresh extraction and healed sites: a histological study in dogs

Sergio Alexandre Gehrke[1,2]* (iD), Leana Kathleen Bragança[3], Eugenio Velasco-Ortega[4,5] and José Luis Calvo-Guirado[6]

Abstract

Background: The aim of this study was to compare histologically the dimensional behavior of peri-implant tissues during osseointegration of immediately exposed or submerged implant placement in fresh extraction and healed sites.

Methods: Four fresh extraction and four delayed implant sites were placed in each hemimandible of five dogs at the bone crest level. In 2 implants of each side were installed a healing abutment (exposed) and two cover screw (submerged) and formed four groups: implant installed in fresh extraction submerged (group 1), implants in fresh extraction immediately exposed (group 2), implants installed in healed site submerged (group 3), and implants in healed site immediately exposed (group 4). After 12 weeks of healing period, histomorphometric analyses of the specimens were carried out to measure the crestal bone level values and the tissue thickness in the implant shoulder portion.

Results: The measure of crestal bone level showed some higher values for implants installed in fresh extraction sites in the buccal aspect: 1.88 ± 0.42 mm for group 1 and 2.33 ± 0.33 mm for group 2, with statistical significance among all four groups tested ($P < 0.001$). For peri-implant tissue thickness, a significative higher statistical difference ($P < 0.001$) for implants installed in healed sites (groups 3 and 4) was found.

Conclusions: Within the limitations of the present animal study, our findings suggest that the implants placed in fresh extraction or healed site and with regards to the moment of exposition (immediately or no) are important factors to the amount of peri-implant tissues after remodeling over a period of 12 weeks. The null hypothesis was rejected.

Keywords: Crestal bone behavior, Fresh extraction sites, Exposed implants, Submerged implants

Background

After the tooth loss, there is a progressive involution of the alveolar bone both in the horizontal and the vertical dimensions [1, 2]. Moreover, the most rapid reduction in the alveolar bone after tooth extraction occurs during the first 3 months [3, 4]. Implants immediately positioned in alveolus after the surgical extraction of the tooth exhibit a success ranging from 92.7 to 98.0% [5]. Some authors suggested that immediate implant placement may counteract the bone remodeling process and preserve the dimension of the alveolar ridge [6–8]. However, multiple animal investigations have failed to support this hypothesis [3, 9]. In this sense, studies by Araújo et al. [3, 10] found a pronounced resorption of the buccal and lingual bony walls after immediate placement in fresh extraction sockets. In long-term observations, no significant differences in the success and esthetic outcomes have been reported between immediate and delayed implants [11–13].

* Correspondence: sergio.gehrke@hotmail.com
[1]Biotecnos Research Center, Calle Cuareim, 1483, CP: 11.100, Montevideo, Uruguay
[2]University Catholica San Antonio de Murcia (UCAM), Murcia, Spain

The surgical requirements for ideal immediate implants in fresh alveolus include atraumatic tooth extraction, preservation of the extraction socket walls, and thorough alveolar curettage to eliminate any possible pathological material [14, 15]. Also, primary implant stability is also an essential requirement and is achieved through the use of implants that exceed the alveolar apex by 3–5 mm or by placing a dental implant with a greater diameter than the alveolar socket [16, 17]. Gehrke et al. [18] demonstrate that the stabilities of the implants placed into fresh extraction sockets or at healed alveolar sites exhibited similar ISQ value evolutions across the three investigated time points (0, 90, and 150 days).

Non-submerged implants showed comparable clinical results to submerged implants and resulted in higher patient satisfaction due to decreased surgical intervention [19]. In this regard, Abrahamsson et al. [20] compared the mucosa and the bone tissue surrounding implants non-submerged or submerged and observed that parameters such as the length of the barrier epithelium of the peri-implant mucosa, the height of the zone of connective tissue integration, the level of the marginal bone, and the density of bone between threads were almost identical in the two experimental groups at the end of the healing period.

Then, the good results were obtained with both techniques (implants placed into fresh alveolus and implants non-submerged); these have been joined together with the objective to reduce the time of the treatment. However, the esthetic results can directly influence by the peri-implant tissue dimension (vertical or horizontal) and position in relationship of the cervical implant portion. In this way, the objective of the present study was to compare the dimensional changes of crestal bone level and peri-implant soft tissue during osseointegration of immediately exposed and submerged implants placement in fresh extraction or healed sites using a mandible dog model. The null hypothesis was the moment of implant placement after tooth extraction (immediate or after healing) or leaving the implant exposed or submerged not affecting the behavior of the peri-implant tissues.

Methods

Implants and abutments

A total of 40 implants were installed (ICI implant, Galimplant, Sarria, Spain), with 3.5 mm in diameter by 10 mm in length. Eight implants in each dog, half per hemimandible. The surface treatment of this implant model is developed by blasting with three different granulometries of Al_2O_3 and pickling using a hydrofluoric solution (HF) at low temperature and short time, which aims to remove any traces of Al_2O_3. Plus, the conditioning of the surface was performed using hydrochloric acid solution (HCl) and sulfuric acid (H_2SO_4) at high temperature and short time (Fig. 1). Twenty titanium healing abutments with 3.5 mm in diameter and 6 mm in length were used.

Surgical procedure and animals care

Five American foxhound dogs of approximately 1 year of age were used in this study. The Ethics Committee for Animal Research at The University of Murcia (Spain) approved the study protocol, which followed the guidelines established by the European Union Council Directive of February 2013 (R.D.53/2013). Clinical examination determined that all animals were in good general health; moreover, all animals presented intact maxillae, without occlusal trauma or mucosal lesions.

The animals were pre-anesthetized with acepromazine 0.12–0.25 mg/kg, buprenorphine 0.01 mg/kg, and medetomidine 35 mg/kg. This mixture was injected

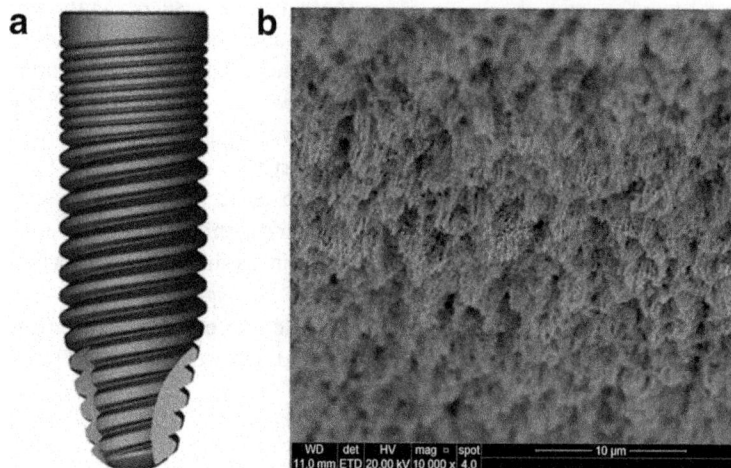

Fig. 1 Image of the implant (**a**) and surface (**b**) used in the present study

intramuscularly in the femoral quadriceps. Animals were then taken to the operating theater, where an intravenous catheter was inserted into the cephalic vein, and propofol (0.4 mg/kg/ min) was continuously infused to maintain the general anesthesia. Conventional dental infiltration anesthesia (articaine 40 mg, 1% epinephrine) was injected at the surgical intraoral sites. All procedures were carried out under the supervision of a veterinary surgeon.

Initially, an impression of each hemimandible was performed to make a surgical guide indicate the implant position, which was predetermined to correspond with the distal root and the center of the crown teeth. Sixty days previous to the surgery, the left mandibular premolars (P2, P3, P4) and molar (M1) were extracted to heal the alveolus sites [21]. In the surgery to place the implants, equally to previous surgery, the teeth of the right hemimandibles were sectioned in a bucco-lingual direction using a tungsten carbide bur so that the roots could be extracted individually without damaging the remaining bony walls. After that, full-thickness mucoperiosteal flaps were increased. The socket of the distal root of each premolar was used as experimental site. For the left sides, a full-thickness mucoperiostal flap was used. All implants were positioned in the crestal bone level. After implant placement, a randomization (randomization.com) was performed to determine which implants received healing abutment and the submerged implants, forming four groups: implant installed in fresh extraction and submerged (group 1), implants in fresh extraction and immediately exposed (group 2), implants installed in healed site and submerged (group 3), and implants in healed site and immediately exposed (group 4). The height of the healing abutments was determined to stay 0.5 mm less of the contact with the corresponding antagonist teeth. No grafting materials were used between the implants and the bony plates. The flaps were closed using single nonabsorbable sutures (Silk® 4-0, Sweden & Martina, Due Carrare). After the surgical procedures, animals received antibiotic treatment (amoxicillin 500 mg, twice a day) and analgesics (ibuprofen 600 mg, three times a day) via the systemic route. Moreover, dogs were fed a soft diet for 7 days, and plaque control was maintained by the application of Sea 4 (Sea 4 teeth, Blue Sea Laboratories, Alicante, Spain). Wounds were inspected daily for clinical postsurgical complications. Two weeks after surgery, sutures were removed. All animals were sacrificed at 12 weeks after the implant insertion by means of an overdose of Pentothal Natrium® (Abbott Laboratories, Madrid, Spain).

Histological preparation and histomorphometric analysis

The hemimandibles were removed with care to preserve the integrity of both peri-implant hard and soft tissues, washed in saline solution and fixed in 10% buffered formalin, and sent for processing at the Laboratory of Ucam-Biotecnos (Murcia, Spain). Specimens were dehydrated in ascending series of alcohol rinses and embedded in a glycol methacrylate resin (Technovit 7200 VLC; Kulzer, Wehrheim, Germany). After polymerization, the specimens were sectioned along its longitudinal axis with a high-precision diamond disk in the IsoMet® 1000 (Buehler, Lake Bluff, IL, USA), at about 150 μm down to 30 μm. A total of two slides were obtained for each implant. The slides were stained with Picrosirius Red Stain (Polysciences, Inc., Warrington, USA) and observed in a normal transmitted light microscope and a polarized light microscope (Nikon, Tokyo, Japan). Buccal bone wall level in comparison with lingual bone wall height after remodeling was expressed as a linear measurement from the implant shoulder to the first bone-implant contact, showed in the Fig. 2 corresponding with the A-B distance. The buccal and lingual tissue thickness was measured in the level corresponding with the implant

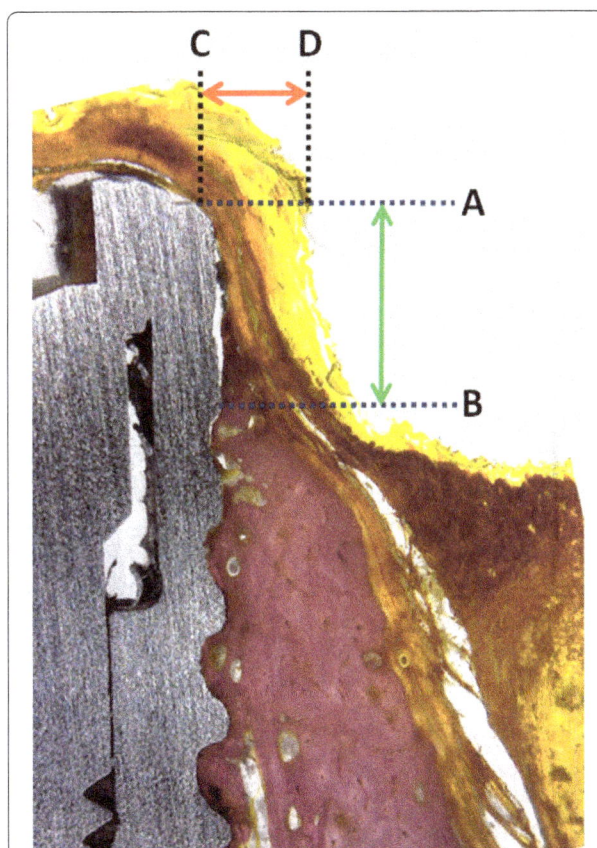

Fig. 2 Parameters measured in each group. Crestal bone loss is the distance between the implant collar (A) and the first bone contact of the crestal bone (B) = A-B bone height; and, the tissue thickness that is the distance from the implant collar (C) to the more external portion of the tissues (D) = C-D tissue thickness. Picrosirius red staining. Original magnification × 16

shoulder (A line) from the implant to the external epithelium portion of the mucosa, showed in the Fig. 2 corresponding with the C-D distance. The measurements were performed by an expert examiner in histology (SG).

Metric evaluation of the predetermined parameters was carried out using a light microscope (Nikon, Tokyo, Japan) connected to a high-resolution video camera (3CCD, JVC KY-F55B, JVC®; JVC, Yokohama, Japan). After digitizing the phase of each specimen under the light microscope, all proposed details were measured in the images using the program Image Tool version 5.02 for *Microsoft Windows*™ (UT Health Science Center School of Dentistry, San Antonio, TX, USA).

Statistical analysis

Means, medians, and standard deviations of crestal bone height and tissue thickness were calculated for all groups. All data sets ($n = 10$) were tested for normality using the Shapiro–Wilk test, and the data did not show normal distribution. The Friedman test was performed for intergroup comparisons in buccal or lingual recorded measures for A-B and C-D parameters followed by the Dunn's multiple comparison test for further comparison of different groups. Furthermore, Wilcoxon matched-pairs signed-rank test was used for the comparison of two groups. The significance level was set at $P < 0.05$.

A power analysis was conducted to determine appropriate sample size; although it was determined that 6 samples from each group would generate a 95% confidence limit (G3Power), 10 samples were proposed for each situation to increase the level of significance.

Results

The surgical sites healed uneventfully. All animals presented appropriate healing during the first week following the surgical procedure. Post-surgical inspections for 2 weeks post-operatively indicated the absence of infection or inflammation. All implants presented osseointegration after the proposed period and were available for histological analysis.

Histological observations

Direct contact was observed between living bone, and all implants without the presence of soft tissues were observed in all groups. However, during the healing, the crestal areas were accompanied by decreases in the dimensions of the buccal as well as the lingual bone walls in different proportions for each group (Figs. 3 and 4). For all implants, keratinized oral epithelium was continuous with junctional epithelium facing the implants and the

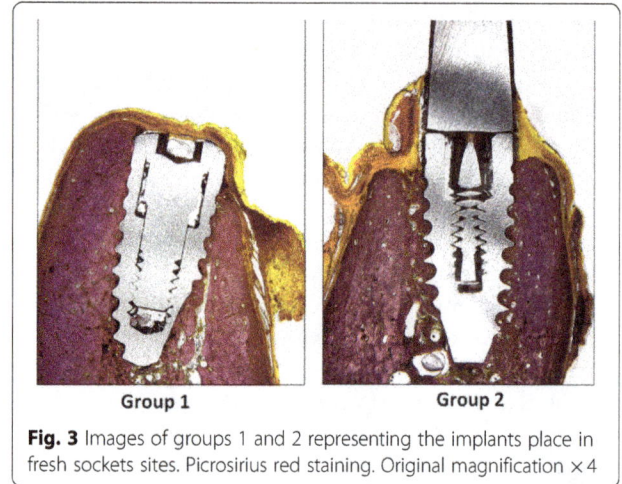

Fig. 3 Images of groups 1 and 2 representing the implants place in fresh sockets sites. Picrosirius red staining. Original magnification × 4

healing abutments. Subjacent connective tissue with a dense network of collagen fibers was observed.

Bone-to-shoulder height measurements

After evaluating all measurements, the distance from the top of the implant collar (line A) to the first contact of the implant with the bone (line B) was measured for buccal and lingual aspect. Mean, median, standard deviation, and standard error for each group evaluated for lingual as well as buccal sites are summarized in Table 1 and showed in the Fig. 5. The buccal and lingual dimensions showed statistically significant differences at 12 weeks among the groups, which are showed in the Table 3 and the distribution data represented in the Fig. 7a. A-B distance evaluated in the group 3 was significantly lower in both buccal and lingual measured groups, whereas for group 2, A-B distance resulted higher than the other groups.

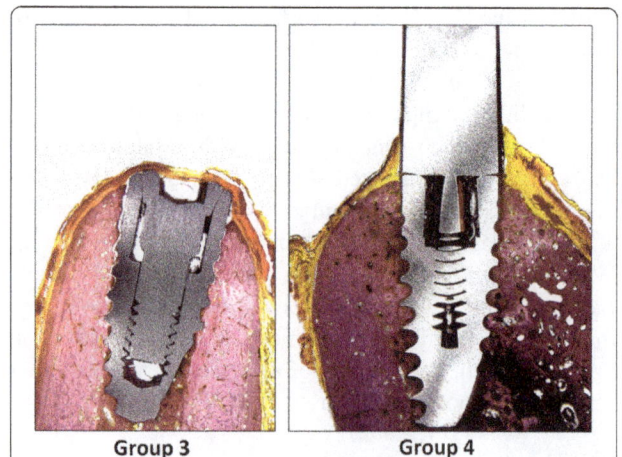

Fig. 4 Images of groups 3 and 4 representing the implants place in healed alveolar sites. Picrosirius red staining. Original magnification × 4

Table 1 Mean, median, standard deviation, and standard error for each group evaluated for lingual as well as buccal sites of the crestal bone height (in mm) for all groups

| | Crestal bone loss (A-B distance in mm) | | | | | | | |
| | Buccal | | | | Lingual | | | |
	Group 1	Group 2	Group 3	Group 4	Group 1	Group 2	Group 3	Group 4
Median	1.95	2.25	0.40	0.65	1.00	1.40	0.30	0.55
Mean	1.88	2.23	0.34	0.69	0.93	1.41	0.31	0.57
Std. deviation	0.42	0.33	0.30	0.21	0.41	0.38	0.27	0.32
Std. error	0.13	0.11	0.10	0.07	0.13	0.12	0.09	0.10
Lower 95% CI of mean	1.58	1.99	0.12	0.54	0.63	1.14	0.12	0.34
Upper 95% CI of mean	2.18	2.47	0.56	0.84	1.23	1.69	0.51	0.80

Buccal and lingual tissue thickness measurements

The overall mean of the tissue thickness from the top of the implant collar (line C) to the more external portion of the tissues (line D) was also calculated. Parameters such as mean, median, standard deviation, and standard error for each group evaluated for lingual as well as buccal sites are summarized in Table 2 and showed in the Fig. 6. Crestal bone height was higher for group 2 both at buccal and lingual sites. The statistical analysis also revealed differences among groups of the measured parameters, which are presented in the Table 3 and the distribution data represented in the Fig. 7b.

Discussion

The immediate implants in fresh sockets have demonstrated a great success rate [18, 22–24]. However, the removal of a single tooth followed by immediate placement of an implant results in marked alterations of the ridge in the horizontal as well as in the vertical dimension. The early phases of tissue integration in immediate post-extraction implants have been well documented [1, 25, 26]. The implants non-submerged are used with the intention of reducing the treatment time and decrease the quantity of surgical interventions, fleeing the protocol initially proposed by Branemark. Also, several studies have demonstrated a high rate of success when compared with the traditional technique [27–29]. However, it is a consensus that the implantation technique in alveolus immediately after tooth extraction and the use of immediate load is predictable in terms of osseointegration, standing as the main point of the behavior of the peri-implant tissue around of these implants. In this sense, the present investigation showed the tissues' behavior after 12-week healing period which affected both buccal and lingual crestal bone and the tissue thickness in the portion corresponding to the implant collar and so the null hypothesis was rejected.

The conservation of bone around the implant especially in the buccal plate plays a crucial role on esthetics. Resorption of buccal plate may lead to exposed threads thus affecting the esthetic of the treatment, even if prostheses are not still connected [30]. In this sense,

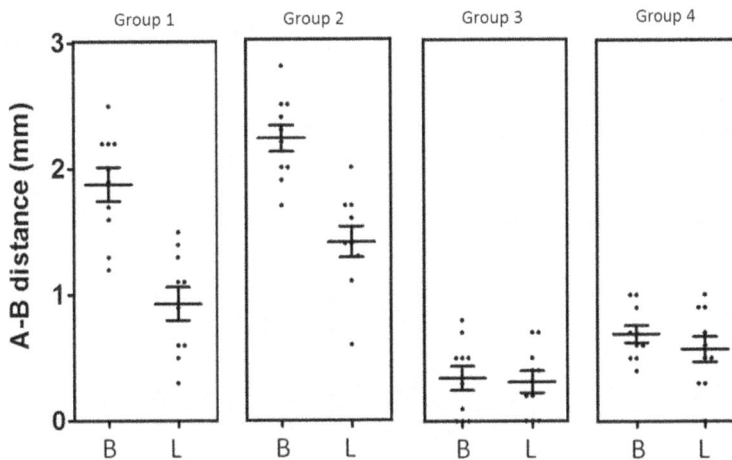

Fig. 5 Graph comparing the data of buccal (B) and lingual (L) measured the A-B distance (bone height). Group 1 = implant installed in fresh extraction and submerged; group 2 = implants in fresh extraction and immediately exposed; group 3 = implants installed in healed site and submerged; and group 4 = implants in healed site and immediately exposed

Table 2 Mean, median, standard deviation, and standard error for each group evaluated for lingual as well as buccal sites of the tissue thickness (in mm) for all groups

| | Tissue thickness (C-D distance in mm) | | | | | | | |
| | Buccal | | | | Lingual | | | |
	Group 1	Group 2	Group 3	Group 4	Group 1	Group 2	Group 3	Group 4
Median	0.60	0.70	1.35	1.45	0.90	0.90	1.80	1.75
Mean	0.70	0.75	1.34	1.36	0.95	1.01	1.82	1.68
Std. deviation	0.25	0.25	0.35	0.46	0.30	0.33	0.41	0.39
Std. error	0.08	0.08	0.11	0.14	0.10	0.10	0.13	0.12
Lower 95% CI of mean	0.52	0.57	1.09	1.03	0.73	0.77	1.53	1.40
Upper 95% CI of mean	0.88	0.93	1.59	1.69	1.17	1.25	2.11	1.96

Calvo-Guirado et al. [31] showed that the resorption of the buccal plate was more pronounced in implants installed in fresh sockets, corroborated by the results of the present study, which revealed greater depth of crestal bone resorption at the buccal crest than at the lingual crest. Moreover, this bone dehiscence following implant placement corroborates findings reported previously [2, 3, 31–33]. In the present study, the crestal buccal and lingual bone height after the remodelation decreased in the implants without immediate load and, mainly, in implants placed in healed alveolar sites from the 12-week healing period. The study of Araújo et al. [10] corroborated this fact; the authors concluded that the implant placement failed to preserve the hard tissue dimension of the ridge following tooth extraction, both in the buccal and the lingual bone walls that were resorbed.

In the present study, the implants were positioned in the crestal bone level, by following Bornstein et al. [34, 35] which reported that the implants are often inserted within the bone crest. Tomasi et al. [36] in a clinical trial observed that the implant position conditioned the amount of buccal crest resorption. Moreover, the thickness of the buccal bone plate and the tridimensional positioning of the implant must be considered because these are important factors that influence the response of hard tissues during healing. In this sense, each animal was performed a surgical guide, based in the previous natural teeth, to position the implants in all groups and conditions in the same place because mainly in the site with the presence of alveolus post-extraction, this condition induces the error of the ideal position during the implant osteotomy.

In relation to the non-submerged implants, it has become a widely reported practice with success rates ranging from 82.9 to 95.7% [37–39]. Theoretically, submerged implant during the osseointegration period are less susceptible to complications; however, some studies comparing submerged implants and non-submerged showed no difference in the implant failure rate, postoperative infection, and marginal bone loss [40]. In the present study, the two groups with non-submerged implants compared between them (groups 1

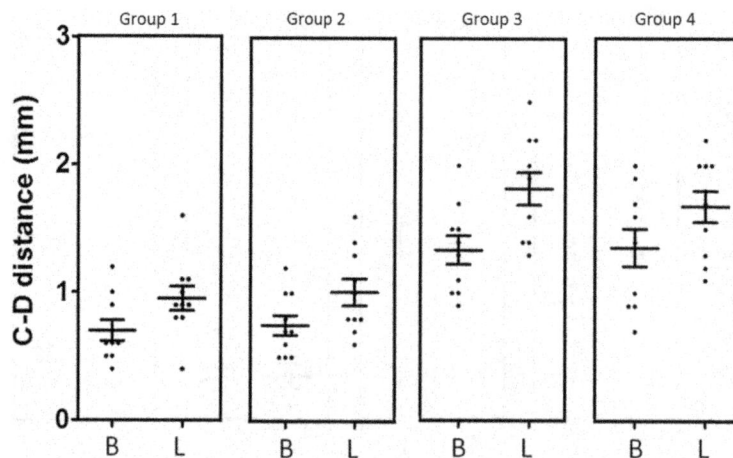

Fig. 6 Graph comparing the data of buccal (B) and lingual (L) measured the C-D distance (tissue thickness). Group 1 = implant installed in fresh extraction and submerged; group 2 = implants in fresh extraction and immediately exposed; group 3 = implants installed in healed site and submerged; and group 4 = implants in healed site and immediately exposed

---

Table 3 Statistical analysis comparing measured distances (A-B and C-D) among different groups in buccal and lingual sites

		Group 1 Mean ± SD	Group 2 Mean ± SD	Group 3 Mean ± SD	Group 4 Mean ± SD	Friedman test	Friedman statistic
Crestal bone loss (A-B distance)	Buccal	1.88 ± 0.42[a]	2.23 ± 0.33[bc]	0.34 ± 0.30[ab]	0.69 ± 0.21[c]	$P < 0.0001$	26.45
	Lingual	0.93 ± 0.41[d]	1.41 ± 0.38[ef]	031 ± 0.27[de]	0.57 ± 0.32[f]	$P < 0.0001$	21.43
Tissue thickness (C-D distance)	Buccal	0.70 ± 0,.25[gh]	0.75 ± 0.25	1.34 ± 0.35[g]	1.36 ± 0.46[h]	$P = 0.0005$	17.79
	Lingual	0.95 ± 0.30[i]	1.01 ± 0.33[j]	1.82 ± 0.41[ij]	1.68 ± 0.39	$P = 0.0003$	18.68

Different superscript letters in the same row indicate significant differences between groups assessed by Dunn's multiple comparison test ($P < 0.05$) and Wilcoxon signed rank test for comparison of different groups

[a] $P = 0.0059$
[b] $P = 0.0055$
[c] $P = 0.0053$
[d] $P = 0.0125$
[e] $P = 0.0056$
[f] $P = 0.0058$
[g] $P = 0.0039$
[h] $P = 0.0080$
[i] $P = 0.0058$
[j] $P = 0.0039$

vs 2 and, groups 3 vs 4), the bone height was smaller, which is likely related to the presence of micromovements generated during mastication during the initial period of osseointegration [41].

Today, implants with expanded platform have demonstrated better crestal bone preservation. Then, in this study, it was carried out by the insertion of implants with an expanded platform and a surface characterized for presenting light roughness in the upper part of the neck, different parts of the body, and apical portion where showed a highly roughness. Previous studies had established that the use of implants with a rough surface

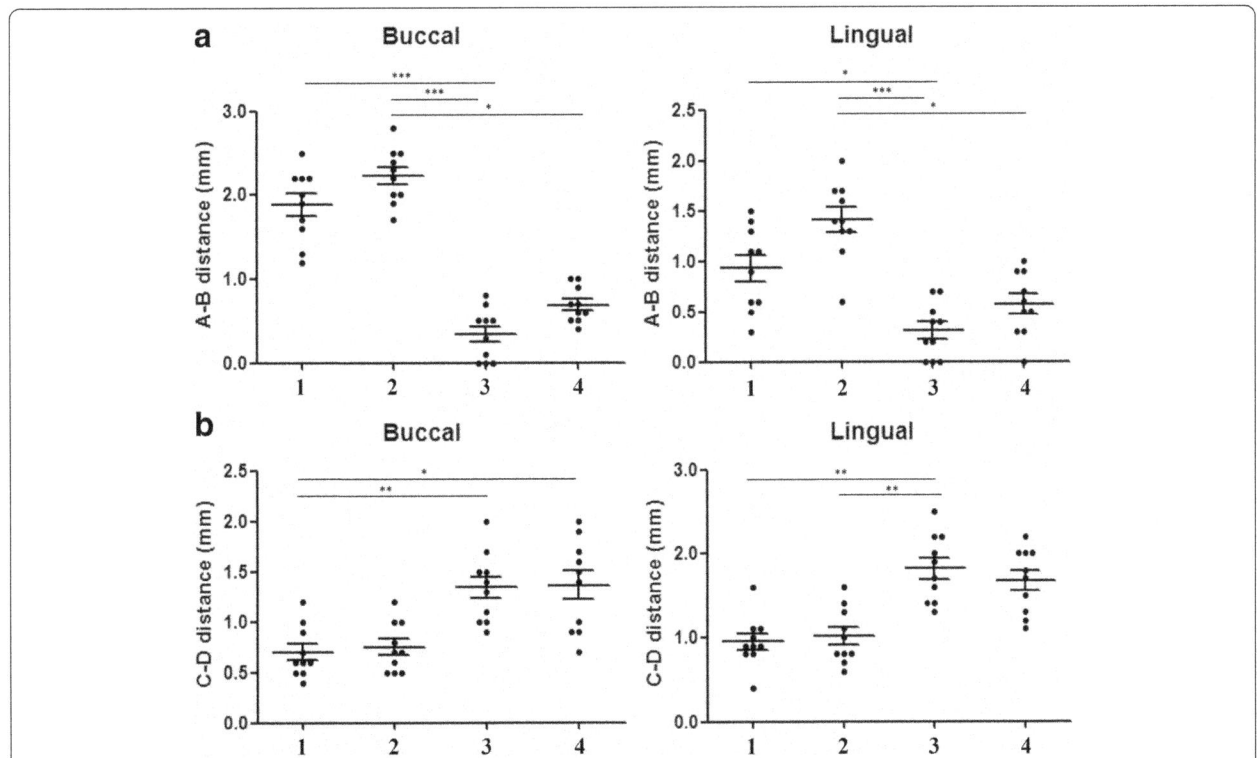

Fig. 7 Multiple graphs comparing A-B distance (height bone) (**a**) and the C-D distance (tissue thickness) (**b**) among different groups. Differences between groups were assessed by Dunn's multiple comparison test (*$P < 0.05$; **$P < 0.01$; ***$P < 0.001$). 1 = (group 1) implant installed in fresh extraction and submerged; 2 = (group 2) implants in fresh extraction and immediately exposed; 3 = (group 3) implants installed in healed site and submerged; and 4 = (group 4) implants in healed site and immediately exposed

may influence the amount of bone regeneration and the values of BIC during healing [9, 20, 42]. Different studies have assessed that implants presenting a rough surface may influence the degree of bone regeneration and the percentages of BIC during healing [9, 43, 44]. Calvo-Guirado et al. [31, 45] concluded that the surface treatment can reduce the crestal bone resorption. Cooper [46] found that an increased surface roughness improves bone integration of the implant, increases osteoconduction, and increases osteogenesis.

New studies are needed to define the influence of other surface compositions and neck configurations for implants placed in fresh extraction sockets with/or without submerged and the influence of abutment change on crestal bone stabilization during the remodeling process. These would appear to be important factors for improving peri-implant bone and soft tissue stability and clinical outcomes, including esthetics, which are of particular importance in the anterior zone.

Conclusions
Within the limitations of this study, our findings suggest that the crestal bone height is larger when implants are inserted in healed areas in comparison with implants installed in fresh extraction sites. Moreover, significant differences were found between non-exposed and immediately exposed implants with regards to crestal bone height position, and higher thickness tissue values in the groups of healed sites implants were found.

Authors' contributions
SAG and JLCG initiated and designed the retrospective study and drafted the manuscript including the preparation of figures and tables. SAG, LKB, EVO, and JLCG reviewed the medical records and collected the data. All authors revised the manuscript and approved the final manuscript.

Competing interests
Sergio Alexandre Gehrke, Leana Kathleen Bragança, Eugenio Velasco-Ortega, and Jose Luis Calvo-Guirado declare that they have no competing interests.

Author details
[1]Biotecnos Research Center, Calle Cuareim, 1483, CP: 11.100, Montevideo, Uruguay. [2]University Catholica San Antonio de Murcia (UCAM), Murcia, Spain. [3]Implant Dentistry, Seville University, Seville, Spain. [4]General Dentistry, Seville University, Seville, Spain. [5]Implant Dentistry Master, Seville University, Seville, Spain. [6]International Dentistry Research Cathedra, Faculty of Medicine and Dentistry, San Antonio Catholic University of Murcia (UCAM), Murcia, Spain.

References
1. Botticelli D, Berglundh T, Lindhe J. Hard-tissue alterations following immediate implant placement in extraction sites. J Clin Periodontol. 2004; 31(10):820–8.
2. Araújo MG, Lindhe J. Dimensional ridge alterations following tooth extraction. An experimental study in the dog. J Clin Periodontol. 2005;32(2):212–8.
3. Araújo MG, Sukekava F, Wennström JL, Lindhe J. Ridge alterations following implant placement in fresh extraction sockets. J Clin Periodontol. 2005;32(6):645–52.
4. Schropp L, Wenzel A, Kostopoulos L, Karring T. Bone healing and soft tissue contour changes following single-tooth extraction: a clinical and radiographic 12-month prospective study. Int J Periodontics Restorative Dent. 2009;23(4): 313–23.
5. Peñarrocha M, Uribe R, Balaguer J. Immediate implants after extraction. A review of the current situation. Med Oral. 2004;9(3):234–42.
6. Paolantonio M, Dolci M, Scarano A, d'Archivio D, di Placido G, Tumini V, Piattelli A. Immediate implantation in fresh extaction sockets. A controlled clinical and histological study in man. J Periodontol. 2001;72(11):1560–71.
7. Hermann F, Lerner H, Palti A. Factors influencing the preservation of the periimplant marginal bone. Implant Dent. 2007;16(2):165–75.
8. Barone A, Orlando B, Cingano L, Marconcini S, Derchi G, Covani U. A randomized clinical trial to evaluate and compare implants placed in augmented versus non-augmented extraction sockets: 3-year results. J Periodontol. 2012;83(7):836–46.
9. Botticelli D, Berglundh T, Persson LG, Lindhe J. Bone regeneration at implants with turned or rough surfaces in self-contained defects. An experimental study in the dog. J Clin Periodontol. 2005;32(10):448–55.
10. Araújo MG, Wennström JL, Lindhe J. Modeling of the buccal and lingual bone walls of fresh extraction sites following implant installation. Clin Oral Implants Res. 2006;7(6):606–14.
11. Grunder U, Polizzi G, Goené R, Hatano N, Henry P, Jackson WJ, Kawamura K, Köhler S, Renouard F, Rosenberg R, Triplett G, Werbitt M, Lithne B. A 3-year prospective multicenter follow-up report on the immediate and delayed-immediate placement of implants. Int J Oral Maxillofac Implants. 1999;14(2):210–6.
12. Mangano F, Mangano C, Ricci M, Sammons RL, Shibli JÁ, Piattelli A. Single-tooth Morse taper connection implants placed in fresh extraction sockets of the anterior maxilla: an aesthetic evaluation. Clin Oral Implants Res. 2012; 23(11):1302–7.
13. Chen ST, Buser D. Esthetic outcomes following immediate and early implant placement in the anterior maxilla—a systematic review. Int J Oral Maxillofac Implants. 2014;29(Suppl):186–215.
14. Berberi AN, Tehini GE, Noujeim ZF, Khairallah AA, Abousehlib MN, Salameh ZA. Influence of surgical and prosthetic techniques on marginal bone loss around titanium implants. Part I: immediate loading in fresh extraction sockets. J Prosthodont. 2014;23(7):521–7.
15. Al-Sabbagh M. Implants in the esthetic zone. Dent Clin N Am. 2006; 50(3):391–407.
16. Becker W, Becker BE. Flap designs for minimization of recession adjacent to maxillary anterior implant sites: a clinical study. Int J Oral Maxillofac Implants. 1996;11(1):46–54.
17. Barone A, Rispoli L, Vozza I, Quaranta A, Covani U. Immediate restoration of single implants placed immediately after tooth extraction. J Periodontol. 2006;77(11):1914–20.
18. Gehrke SA, da Silva Neto UT, Rossetti PH, Watinaga SE, Giro G, Shibli JA. Stability of implants placed in fresh sockets versus healed alveolar sites: early findings. Clin Oral Implants Res. 2016;27(5):577–82.
19. Nemli SK, Güngör MB, Aydın C, Yılmaz H, Türkcan I, Demirköprülü H. Clinical evaluation of submerged and non-submerged implants for posterior single-tooth replacements: a randomized split-mouth clinical trial. Int J Oral Maxillofac Surg. 2014;43(12):1484–92.
20. Abrahamsson I, Berglundh T, Linder E, Lang NP, Lindhe J. Early bone formation adjacent to rough and turned endosseous implant surfaces. An experimental study in the dog. Clin Oral Implants Res. 2004;15(4):381–92.
21. Discepoli N, Vignoletti F, Laino L, de Sanctis M, Muñoz F, Sanz M. Early healing of the alveolar process after tooth extraction: an experimental study in the beagle dog. J Clin Periodontol. 2013;40(6):638–44.
22. Polizzi G, Grunder U, Goené R, Hatano N, Henry P, Jackson WJ, Kawamura K, Renouard F, Rosenberg R, Triplett G, Werbitt M, Lithner B. Immediate and delayed implant placement into extraction sockets: a 5-year report. Clin Implant Dent Relat Res. 2000;2(2):93–9.
23. Alves CC, Correia AR, Neves M. Immediate implants and immediate loading in periodontally compromised patients—a 3-year prospective clinical study. Int J Periodontics Restorative Dent. 2010;30(5):447–55.
24. Lang NP, Pun L, Lau KY, Li KY, Wong MC. A systematic review on survival and success rates of implants placed immediately into fresh extraction sockets after at least 1 year. Clin Oral Implants Res. 2012;23(Suppl 5):39–66.
25. Bornstein MM, Valderrama P, Jones AA, Wilson TG, Seibl R, Cochran DL. Bone apposition around two different sandblasted and acid-etched

titanium implant surfaces: a histomorphometric study in canine mandibles. Clin Oral Implants Res. 2008;19(3):233–41.

26. Negri B, Calvo-Guirado JL, Ramírez-Fernández MP, Maté Sánchez-de Val J, Guardia J, Muñoz-Guzón F. Peri-implant bone reactions to immediate implants placed at different levels in relation to crestal bone. Part II: a pilot study in dogs. Clin Oral Implants Res. 2012;23(2):236–44.

27. Degidi M, Piattelli A. Immediate functional and non-functional loading of dental implants: a 2- to 60-month follow-up study of 646 titanium implants. J Periodontol. 2003;74(2):225–41.

28. Degidi M, Piattelli A. Comparative analysis study of 702 dental implants subjected to immediate functional loading and immediate nonfunctional loading to traditional healing periods with a follow-up of up to 24 months. Int J Oral Maxillofac Implants. 2005;20(1):99–107.

29. Nkenke E, Lehner B, Fenne M, Roman FS, Thams U, Neukam FW, Radespiel-Tröger M. Immediate versus delayed loading of dental implants in the maxillae of minipigs: follow-up of implant stability and implant failures. Int J Oral Maxillofac Implants. 2005;20(1):39–47.

30. Boquete-Castro A, Gómez-Moreno G, Aguilar-Salvatierra A, Delgado-Ruiz RA, Romanos GE, Calvo-Guirado JL. Influence of the implant design on osseointegration and crestal bone resorption of immediate implants: a histomorphometric study in dogs. Clin Oral Implants Res. 2015;26(8):876–81.

31. Calvo-Guirado JL, Gómez-Moreno G, Aguilar-Salvatierra A, Guardia J, Delgado-Ruiz RA, Romanos GE. Marginal bone loss evaluation around immediate non-occlusal microthreaded implants placed in fresh extraction sockets in the maxilla: a 3-year study. Clin Oral Implants Res. 2015;26(7):761–7.

32. Cardaropoli G, Lekholm U, Jl W. Tissue alterations at implant supported single-tooth replacements: a 1-year prospective clinical study. Clin Oral Implants Res. 2006;17(2):165–71.

33. Spray JR, Black CG, Morris HF, Ochi S. The influence of bone thickness on facial marginal bone response: stage 1 placement through stage 2 uncovering. Ann Periodontol. 2000;5(1):119–28.

34. Bornstein MM, Lussi A, Schmid B, Belser UC, Buser D. Early loading of nonsubmerged titanium implants with a sandblasted and acid-etched (SLA) surface: 3-year results of a prospective study in partially edentulous patients. Int J Oral Maxillofac Implants. 2003;18(5):659–66.

35. Bornstein MM, Schmid B, Belser UC, Lussi A, Buser D. Early loading of non-submerged titanium implants with a sandblasted and acid-etched surface. 5-year results of a prospective study in partially edentulous patients. Clin Oral Implants Res. 2005;16(6):631–8.

36. Tomasi C, Sanz M, Cecchinato D, Pjetursson B, Ferrus J, Lang NP, Lindhe J. Bone dimensional variations at implants placed in fresh extraction sockets: a multilevel multivariate analysis. Clin Oral Implants Res. 2010;21(1):30–6.

37. Buser D, Mericske-Stern R, Dula K, Lang NP. Clinical experience with one-stage, non-submerged dental implants. Adv Dent Res. 1999;13:153–61.

38. Hellem S, Karlsson U, Almfeldt I, Brunell G, Hamp SE, Astrand P. Nonsubmerged implants in the treatment of the edentulous lower jaw: a 5-year prospective longitudinal study of ITI hollow screws. Clin Implant Dent Relat Res. 2001;3(1):20–9.

39. Simonis P, Dufour T, Tenenbaum H. Long-term implant survival and success: a 10-16-year follow-up of non-submerged dental implants. Clin Oral Implants Res. 2010;21(7):772–7.

40. Chrcanovic BR, Albrektsson T, Wennerberg A. Immediately loaded non-submerged versus delayed loaded submerged dental implants: a meta-analysis. Int J Oral Maxillofac Surg. 2015;44(4):493–506.

41. Duyck J, Vandamme K. The effect of loading on peri-implant bone: a critical review of the literature. J Oral Rehabil. 2014;41(10):783–94.

42. Abrahamsson I, Cardaropoli G. Peri-implant hard and soft tissue integration to dental implants made of titanium and gold. Clin Oral Implants Res. 2007; 18(3):269–74.

43. Wennerberg A, Albrektsson T, Johansson C, Andersson B. Experimental study of turned and grit-blasted screw-shaped implants with special emphasis on effects of blasting material and surface topography. Biomaterials. 1996;17(1):15–22.

44. Trisi P, Lazzara R, Rao W, Rebaudi A. Bone-implant contact and bone quality: evaluation of expected and actual bone contact on machined and osseotite implant surfaces. Int J Periodontics Restorative Dent. 2002;22(6):535–45.

45. Calvo-Guirado JL, Ortiz-Ruiz AJ, Negri B, López-Marí L, Rodriguez-Barba C, Schlottig F. Histological and histomorphometric evaluation of immediate implant placement on a dog model with a new implant surface treatment. Clin Oral Implants Res. 2010;21(3):308–15.

46. Cooper LF. Systemic effectors of alveolar bone mass and implications in dental therapy. Periodontol. 2000;23:103–9.

20

Dental implants and grafting success remain high despite large variations in maxillary sinus mucosal thickening

Bartosz Maska[1†], Guo-Hao Lin[1,2†], Abdullah Othman[1,3], Shabnam Behdin[1,4], Suncica Travan[1], Erika Benavides[1] and Yvonne Kapila[1,5*]

Abstract

Background: Although mucosal thickening is the most common radiographic finding observed regarding sinus pathology, the knowledge regarding its clinical significance on the outcomes of dental implants and grafting in the maxillary sinuses is still limited. We hypothesized that mucosal thickening would not alter the predictability for sinus floor augmentation and dental implant placement. The purpose of this retrospective study was to evaluate the outcomes of dental implant placement in sinus-augmented areas with preexisting sinus mucosal thickening.

Methods: This study involved the review of cone-beam computed tomographic (CBCT) scans taken on patients that underwent both maxillary sinus elevation with grafting and implant placement at the University of Michigan School of Dentistry from 2004 to 2014. Cases with documented radiographic and clinical follow-up were included. The data analyses revealed the following.

Results: A total of 29 CBCT scans met the inclusion criteria for evaluation, and 93.1% of them had maxillary sinus mucosal/tissue thickening. Specifically, 6.9% of cases exhibited no thickening, 6.9% had minimal thickening (1–2 mm), 20.7% of cases had moderate thickening (2–5 mm), and 65.5% had severe thickening (>5 mm). We propose these categorical measurements of tissue thickening as a new "mucosal thickening index." The tissue thickening did not vary based on gender, age, or smoking status, nor did it relate to the underlying alveolar ridge height. However, patients with a history of periodontal diseases demonstrated a significant association with mucosal thickening ($p = 0.0043$). These data indicate that there is high implant and grafting success rate (100%) in the maxillary sinus despite large and varied physiologic sinus mucosal/tissue thickening.

Conclusions: Based on study findings, this research will help guide dental practitioners regarding cases that exhibit mucosal thickening. These data support the concept that physiologic mucosal thickening in varied ranges is not associated with implant or grafting failure in the maxillary sinus.

Keywords: Mucosal thickening, Dental implants, Maxillary sinus, Sinus floor augmentation, Periodontal diseases, Cone-beam computed tomography

* Correspondence: Yvonne.Kapila@ucsf.edu
†Equal contributors
[1]Department of Periodontics and Oral Medicine, School of Dentistry, University of Michigan, 1011 N University Ave, Ann Arbor, MI, USA
[5]Department of Orofacial Sciences, School of Dentistry, University of California San Francisco, 513 Parnassus Ave, S612D, Box 0422, San Francisco 94143, CA, USA
Full list of author information is available at the end of the article

Background

Despite the high survival rate of dental implants inserted in maxillary sinuses that have undergone sinus floor elevation (SFE) with bone grafting, complications still occur [1–3]. Sinus membrane perforation is reported to be the most common complication [4, 5]. Postoperative maxillary sinusitis is less common (0–22%) [6, 7]; nevertheless, it could potentially compromise the outcome of SFE and affect the overall well-being of the patient [8]. Developing postoperative sinusitis is often associated with a reduction in the patency or complete obstruction of the ostium due to inflammatory edema in the sinus or preexisting chronic sinusitis [8–12].

Various cyst-like pathologies can be found in the maxillary sinus, including a pseudocyst and a surgical ciliated cyst [13]. However, a thickened mucous membrane can be physiologic or benign without presentation of symptoms. In contrast, cyst-like entities may need surgical removal due to their pathologic progression [14]. A surgical ciliated cyst is defined as a posterior maxillary cyst found after the surgical treatment of maxillary sinusitis [15]. Pseudocysts are diagnosed as dome-shaped, noncorticated soft tissue opacities with a well-defined border in the maxillary sinus [16].

In the dental literature, sinusitis has most commonly been identified on radiographs as thickening of the sinus membrane [12]. Mucosal thickening >2 mm is considered a threshold for pathological thickness [17]. Although mucosal thickening is the most common radiographic finding observed regarding sinus pathology [18], the knowledge regarding its clinical significance on the outcomes of dental implants and grafting in the maxillary sinuses is still limited [19].

The purpose of this retrospective study was to evaluate the outcomes of dental implant placement in sinus augmented areas with preexisting mucosal thickening of more than 2 mm. The aims of this study were to (1) determine the success rate of dental implant placement in augmented maxillary sinus areas with mucosal thickening, (2) evaluate the effect of gender, age, and smoking on the dimensions of sinus mucosal membranes, and (3) based on the overall findings, develop a written protocol to guide dental practitioners regarding cases that exhibit mucosal thickening (the threshold of safety).

Methods
Study design

Our study hypothesis was that mucosal thickening of more than 2 mm and up to 1/3 of the volume of the sinus would not alter the predictability for SFE and dental implant placement. The primary outcome was to determine the success rate of dental implant placement in augmented maxillary sinus areas with mucosal thickening. A secondary outcome was to evaluate the effect of gender, age, and smoking on the dimensions of sinus mucosal membranes.

This study consisted of performing a retrospective analysis of cone-beam computed tomographic (CBCT) scans taken with a CBCT machine (i-CAT Cone-Beam Computed Tomography machine, Imaging Sciences International, Hatfield, PA) for patients that underwent both maxillary sinus elevation with grafting and implant placement at the University of Michigan School of Dentistry from 2004 to 2014. This study was approved by the University of Michigan Institutional Review Board.

Subject inclusion and exclusion criteria

Subjects that exhibited the following criteria were included in the study: partial edentulism, over 18 years old, received dental implants after sinus grafting, and had clinical and radiographic follow-up. These subjects had at least one CBCT scan prior to a SFE procedure. Subjects that exhibited the following criteria were excluded from the study: under 18 years old, subjects whose CBCT images were not clear enough to read, or had portions of the maxillary sinus not fully captured in the field of view. Subject data that was extracted from the general and medical record included the following: age, gender, and any systemic issues following a review of overall systems for the presence of any pathology (respiratory system, cardiovascular system, diabetes status, smoking history, etc.).

Subject data extracted from the dental records included the following: restorative, endodontic, periodontal, orthodontic, and oral surgery treatment or extractions.

Given these specific inclusion and exclusion criteria and the specific purpose of this study, only 29 cases qualified for inclusion from an original screen of approximately 4000 cases. An initial search of our database resulted in a larger number of cases that would theoretically qualify; however, further investigation revealed the need to exclude a great number of cases. The reasons for exclusion of these cases were as follows: scatter on the CBCT images due to fixed prosthodontics, unclear CBCT images, poor charting that did not allow for proper data gathering, no follow-up radiographs, not enough of the sinus being visible in the image, diagnosed periapical pathosis in the examined areas, implants not being placed in the area of the maxillary sinus, or no grafting completed in the maxillary sinus. Although these factors greatly reduced our sample size, this, in turn, created a stronger data set for analyses.

Subject privacy protection

The study required access to University of Michigan Protected Health Information (PHI). PHI was necessary in order to track and coordinate the CBCT data and dental and medical history for each subject. Corresponding subject charts and electronic records were reviewed for retrieval of relevant implant placement and restorative history, medical history, and demographic information, including gender and age and smoking history. Also, any pertinent dental treatment was received and response to treatment were reviewed and recorded. No other personal information was retrieved. The use of PHI involved no greater than minimal risk because each subject was assigned a coded number that was used for all data analyses, tables, and reports.

Measurement methodology

Using CBCT images, the mucosal thickness/height was measured at the point of maximum height using sagittal views, which were perpendicular to the underlying sinus floor at edentulous sites [12, 20]. Using these sagittal views, measurements were taken at four points: ¼, ½, and ¾ of the widest distance of the maxillary sinus from anterior to posterior. In order to standardize the measurements for each sinus, each scan was carefully oriented in the axial, coronal, and sagittal plane. In the

axial plane, a horizontal line from the right and left zygoma was chosen as the standard. Orienting the hard palate horizontally was the standard in the coronal plane as well as in the sagittal plane. The specific teeth that were to be replaced by implants were then located by reviewing each patient's chart, and the area of implant placement was located in the CBCT. To select the appropriate slice in the sagittal view to measure the mucosal thickening, the vertical line in the axial view was placed in the center of the alveolus where the future implant was to be placed. The appropriate sagittal view was then obtained and measurements of the mucosal thickening were performed. Each measurement was completed with the brightness and contrast set at 50%, and the zoom function was utilized to better visualize the soft tissue.

The sites that were measured are specified in the image below (Fig. 1). The most posterior and anterior aspects of the visible maxillary sinus were measured. The ½ point along with the ¼ and ¾ points were then selected, and the measurements of the mucosal thickening were then

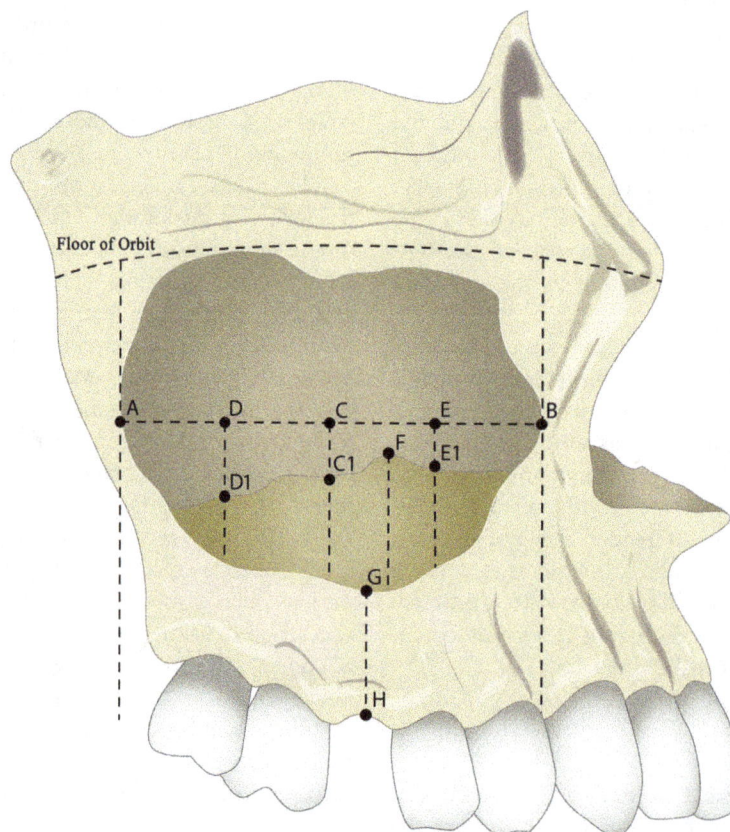

Fig. 1 Figure illustrating the reference points of the CBCT measurements. *A*: most posterior point of the sinus wall; *B*: most anterior point of the sinus wall; *C*: mid-point between *A* and *B*; *C1*: measurement of mucosal thickening perpendicular to *A–B* line at point *C*; *D*: mid-point between *A* and *C*; *D1*: measurement of mucosal thickening perpendicular to *A–B* line at point *D*; *E*: mid-point between *B* and *C*; *E1*: measurement of mucosal thickening perpendicular to *A–B* line at point *E*; *F*: highest extension of thickened sinus membrane; *G–H*: height of residual alveolar bone (measured at the mid-point of the edentulous ridge/implant-planned site)

completed at these three sites. The thickest portion of the mucosa was also measured if it did not coincide with one of the three earlier measurements. Post implant placement radiographs were analyzed to locate the area where the implant was placed, and this area was then estimated on the CBCT and the thickness of the alveolus was measured there.

Statistical analysis

Outcome analyses included the overall implant survival rate and percentage of mucosal thickening at different sites. The associations between the amount of mucosal thickening and the recorded variables, including patients' systemic conditions and dental history, were estimated by linear mixed models. Adjustment for potential inter-variable influence using regression analysis was also performed. A p value of 0.05 was used as the level of significance. All the statistical analyses were calculated using a computer program (SAS Institute Inc. 2011. Base SAS® 9.3 Procedures Guide, Cary, NC).

Results

Twenty-nine CBCT images (11 females and 18 males) were included in this study. All the implants placed in these included cases survived, representing a 100% implant survival rate. With regards to measurements of mucosal thickening, the intra-examiner reproducibility revealed an exact intra-examiner correlation of 99%, with a p value of 0.40 for a t test for independent samples, indicating a high reproducibility and intra-examiner agreement for the radiographic measurements. The study data for the 29 analyzed CBCT scans are presented in Table 1. The mean follow-up time after implant placement was 3.3 ± 2.2 (range 1 to 7) years.

Percentage and amount of mucosal thickening

Among the subjects, 93.1% of patients had maxillary sinus mucosal/tissue thickening. Specifically, 6.9% of cases exhibited no thickening (≤ 1 mm), 6.9% had minimal thickening (>1 mm but ≤ 2 mm), 20.7% of cases had moderate thickening (>2 mm but ≤ 5 mm), and 65.5% had severe thickening (>5 mm). However, only 45.9% of designated implant sites presented sinus mucosal thickening. The average amount of mucosal thickening in the anterior section (point E1 to floor of the sinus) was 4.63 ± 4.95 mm, in the middle section (point C1 to floor of the sinus) it was 4.87 ± 5.10 mm, and in the posterior section (point D1 to floor of the sinus) it was 3.46 ± 3.17 mm. The average mucosal thickening (point F to floor of the sinus) was 8.34 ± 5.70 mm, and it ranged from 1.55 to 22.81 mm.

Table 1 CBCT measurements of sinus mucosal thickening

Patient	Anterior (E1-floor of the sinus)	Middle (C1-floor of the sinus)	Posterior (D1-floor of the sinus)	Thickest (F-floor of the sinus)
1	3.06	0.32	0.76	4.59
2	0.34	0.21	0.20	0.34
3	0.39	0.54	1.38	1.66
4	4.15	3.79	0.61	6.36
5	5.64	1.33	3.73	8.42
6	7.34	0.77	0.86	7.66
7	1.93	9.25	6.17	12.5
8	8.22	7.89	1.62	12.27
9	3.52	10.05	4.76	10.05
10	7.62	0.43	2.03	8.11
11	7.19	2.75	0.77	7.62
12	0.26	9.26	8.38	9.26
13	0.76	19.50	0.46	22.81
14	14.95	11.33	9.67	18.92
15	0.79	0.71	1.36	1.55
16	0.60	3.34	1.52	4.40
17	4.44	1.82	3.60	12.25
18	1.39	0.68	0.52	8.00
19	0.21	0.24	0.24	0.24
20	16.27	11.11	8.07	16.27
21	2.87	5.10	6.40	7.85
22	5.13	0.64	4.12	5.13
23	1.19	1.36	0.25	2.48
24	0.80	2.39	2.08	4.84
25	19.05	16.94	10.14	20.10
26	3.51	4.25	2.63	4.25
27	0.28	1.62	2.85	2.85
28	9.94	7.21	5.29	11.07
29	2.56	6.28	9.98	9.98
Mean (mm)	4.63	4.87	3.46	8.34
Standard deviation (mm)	4.95	5.10	3.17	5.70

Factors associated with mucosal thickening

A significantly higher amount of mucosal thickening was associated with patients with a history of periodontal diseases ($p = 0.004$). Other factors, such as gender ($p = 0.054$), and systemic factors, including respiratory diseases ($p = 0.313$), cardiovascular diseases ($p = 0.438$), diabetes ($p = 0.209$), or smoking ($p = 0.541$), were not significantly associated with mucosal thickening.

In terms of dental history, the presence of tooth restorations ($p = 0.056$), endodontic treatment ($p = 0.379$), orthodontic treatment ($p = 0.125$), edentulism ($p = 0.718$), and underlying alveolar ridge height (point G to H, $p = 0.889$)

were not associated with mucosal thickening. The results of the statistical analyses after inter-variable adjustment are presented in Table 2.

Discussion

CBCT imaging has been recognized as a more sensitive imaging modality for identifying sinus thickening and pathoses in the posterior maxilla compared to panoramic radiography [21, 22]. This could explain why the current study identified a higher prevalence of mucosal thickening compared to earlier studies [23]. However, compared to other similar CBCT studies [21, 24, 25], the prevalence reported in the current study is still much higher than the previously published articles with a similar study design. Ritter et al. [25] in a retrospective CBCT study reported 38.1% of subjects presented with mucosal thickening. Similarly, Pazera et al. [24] reported a prevalence of 23.7% and Janner et al. [20] reported 37% of cases with membrane thickening. In a recent study, Brüllmann et al. [17] found 74% of evaluated sinuses had sinus findings upon CBCT examination. These differences in prevalence might result from the different inclusion criteria among the studies. Another potential explanation for these differences in the reported prevalence of mucosal thickening may be due to the ambiguous definition used in the early studies. Some studies suggested that 2 mm should be considered the threshold for identifying mucosal thickening [20], and thus the prevalence of slight mucosal thickening may have been underestimated. To avoid this situation, the current study analyzed the thickness of sinus membranes based on four different categories: no thickening (≤ 1 mm), minimal (>1 mm but ≤ 2 mm), moderate (>2 mm but ≤ 5 mm), and severe thickening (>5 mm). According to this index (Fig. 2), 93.1% of cases examined had maxillary sinus mucosal/tissue thickening and 65.5% had severe thickening.

The current study demonstrated that sinus mucosal thickening does not correlate with implant survival. This result is consistent with a previously published report by Jungner et al. [26]. In their study, the presence of sinus thickening was not significantly associated with implant failure. Similarly, our study found a 100% implant survival rate for both patients with and without sinus mucosal thickening. It is worth mentioning that none of the CBCT images evaluated in the current study showed

signs of sinusitis or periapical pathoses, despite indications of physiologic mucosal thickening. All the selected images presented clear sinuses without signs of infection. Therefore, it could be postulated that physiologic mucosal thickening does not contribute to implant failure. However, an association between pathologic mucosal thickening and implant survival cannot be drawn. If sinusitis is suspected, it is suggested that clinicians consult the appropriate medical specialists before implant placement.

Based on the findings of the current study, a history of periodontal disease is the only identified parameter significantly associated with sinus mucosal thickening. This finding indicates that clinicians should expect some degree of mucosal thickening when performing sinus augmentation procedures in a previously periodontally involved site. This finding is consistent with several previously published studies [27–29]. Phothikhun et al. [28] reported that sinuses with severe periodontal bone loss were three times more likely to have mucosal thickening. In a more recent study, Ren et al. [29] reported an odds ratio of 4.62 for patients with severe periodontal bone loss with mucosal thickening. A possible explanation for this phenomenon is that increased inflammatory cytokines resulting from periodontal diseases might also reach the maxillary sinus, and thereby trigger an increased membrane thickening. With regards to implant treatment outcomes, while our study found that there is no association between mucosal thickening and future implant survival, a higher chance of sinus membrane perforation during sinus lift procedures has been reported when a thicker membrane is present [3, 30].

Our study did not find a significant association between endodontically treated teeth and mucosal thickening. Though this finding is consistent with some previously published studies [27, 28], other studies [21, 31] did report an association. These discrepant findings could be the result of different inclusion criteria in the study design. Since our study did not include any patients with radiographic signs of pulpal pathoses, these data suggest that successful root canal treatment without signs of apical radiolucency should not be considered as a risk indicator of future mucosal thickening. On the other hand, it has been reported [32, 33] that the presence of apical periodontitis is related to sinus mucosal thickening, which should alert clinicians when planning

Table 2 Statistical results after inter-variable adjustment showing the association between recorded parameters and sinus mucosal thickening; p values that showed statistically significant differences are italicized

	Gender	Respiratory diseases	Cardio-vascular diseases	Diabetes mellitus	Smoking	History of periodontal diseases	Endodontic treatment	History of orthodontic treatment	Alveolar ridge height	Extraction performed
p value	0.054	0.3130	0.4376	0.2090	0.5413	*0.0043*	0.3793	0.1248	0.8896	0.7175

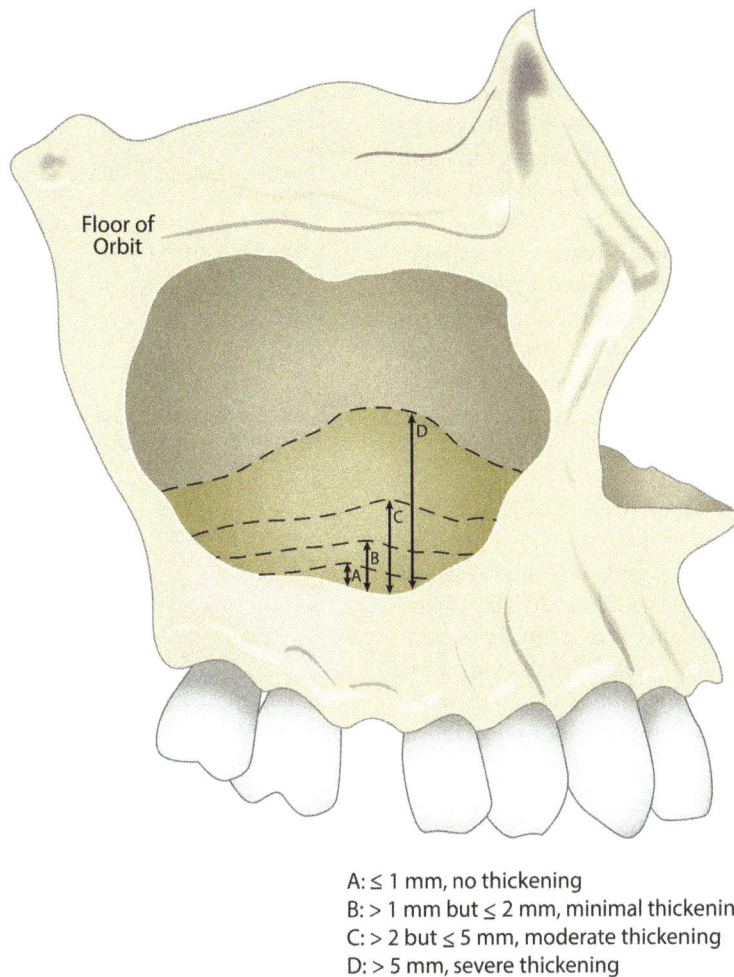

Floor of Orbit

A: ≤ 1 mm, no thickening
B: > 1 mm but ≤ 2 mm, minimal thickening
C: > 2 but ≤ 5 mm, moderate thickening
D: > 5 mm, severe thickening

Fig. 2 Figure illustrating the proposed mucosal thickening index. *A* ≤1 mm, indicating no thickening; *B* >1 mm but ≤2 mm, indicating minimal thickening; *C* >2 mm but ≤5 mm, indicating moderate thickening; *D* >5 mm, indicating severe thickening

future implant-related procedures. Because periapical infections are considered a multifactorial entity, they should be carefully evaluated and treated to ensure a favorable implant treatment outcome [34, 35]. In addition, the influence of a periapical scar of dense collagen tissue, formed after conventional root canal treatment, on implant treatment outcomes has not yet been fully explored. Therefore, additional future investigations are needed to examine these unresolved issues.

Although residual alveolar ridge height has been associated with sinus mucosal thickening [36], our study did not find a significant association between these two parameters. Acharya et al. [36] reported that lower available bone height in the subsinus region was related to thickened sinus membranes within an Asian-Indian and Hong Kong-based Chinese population. Differences in the ethnic composition and geographic location of this population might explain the different findings compared to our study, which was primarily comprised of a

Caucasian cohort in North America. Also, in their study, the majority of patients (80.53%) had some degree of periodontal disease, which might have directly influenced their outcome analysis. Since residual bone height depends highly on the rate of bone remodeling and sinus pneumatization after tooth extraction [37], future prospective clinical trials are needed to investigate the relationship between changes in maxillary sinus dimension and mucosal thickness.

This study presents new data on maxillary sinus mucosal thickening derived from a carefully defined data set; however, there were some limitations in the study. One limitation was the limited sample size. However, as discussed, our stringent case selection criteria yielded a more uniform data set for analyses. Other limitations were related to the actual measurements of the maxillary sinus. In order to normalize the data, specific planes were used as the basis for measurements. However, due to anatomical variations in patients, it was not always possible to orient each plane in the exact position. In those instances, the plane of orientation was set as close to ideal as possible. For example, it was not possible to orient the entire hard palate horizontally in some patients if it had a curvature. In addition, since the maxillary sinus is a three-dimensional structure with many variations among patients, situations arose where mucosal thickening extended from the septa or lateral walls instead of just on the floor of the sinus. In these situations, best judgment was utilized in order to decide if these areas of thickening would have an impact on the implant placement area. Also, variations in the anatomical features made orienting CBCT scans at times challenging, and this may have influenced the study outcomes.

Conclusions

Our study found that the largest tissue thickening was present in the middle section of the maxillary sinus. This tissue thickening did not vary based on gender, age, or smoking status, nor did it relate to the underlying alveolar ridge height. However, patients with a history of periodontal diseases demonstrated a significant association with mucosal thickening. A mucosal thickening index was proposed as a guide for future studies and clinical practice. A high implant and grafting success rate (100%) in the maxillary sinus was noted despite large and varied physiologic sinus mucosal/tissue thickening.

Abbreviations

CBCT: Cone-beam computed tomographic; PHI: Protected Health Information; SFE: Sinus floor elevation

Acknowledgements

The authors thank Ms. Victoria Zakrzewski for her help with the figure generation and preparation.

Authors' contributions

Co-primary author BM contributed to the CBCT measurement and preparation of the manuscript. Co-primary author G-HL contributed to the data analysis and preparation of the manuscript. Second author AO contributed to the protocol preparation, case review, case selection, and preparation of the manuscript. Third author SB contributed to the protocol preparation, case review, case selection, and preparation of the manuscript. Fourth author ST contributed to the preparation of the manuscript. Fifth author EB contributed to the data analysis and CBCT evaluation. Corresponding author YK contributed to the protocol preparation, preparation of the manuscript, and guidance of the study. All authors read and approved the final manuscript.

Competing interests

All authors Bartosz Maska, Guo-Hao Lin, Abdullah Othman, Shabnam Behdin, Suncica Travan, Erika Benavides, and Yvonne Kapila declare that they have no competing interests.

Author details

[1]Department of Periodontics and Oral Medicine, School of Dentistry, University of Michigan, 1011 N University Ave, Ann Arbor, MI, USA. [2]Department of Surgical Sciences, School of Dentistry, Marquette University, 1801 W Wisconsin Ave, Milwaukee, WI, USA. [3]Department of Periodontology & Dental Hygiene, University of Detroit Mercy, 2700 Martin Luther King Jr. Blvd, Detroit, MI, USA. [4]Department of Periodontics, School of Dental Medicine, Case Western Reserve University, 2124 Cornell Rd, Cleveland, OH, USA. [5]Department of Orofacial Sciences, School of Dentistry, University of California San Francisco, 513 Parnassus Ave, S612D, Box 0422, San Francisco 94143, CA, USA.

References

1. Beretta M, Poli PP, Grossi GB, Pieroni S, Maiorana C. Long-term survival rate of implants placed in conjunction with 246 sinus floor elevation procedures: results of a 15-year retrospective study. J Dent. 2015;43:78–86.
2. Del Fabbro M, Corbella S, Weinstein T, Ceresoli V, Taschieri S. Implant survival rates after osteotome-mediated maxillary sinus augmentation: a systematic review. Clin Implant Dent Relat Res. 2012;14 Suppl 1:e159–168.
3. Wen SC, Lin YH, Yang YC, Wang HL. The influence of sinus membrane thickness upon membrane perforation during transcrestal sinus lift procedure. Clin Oral Implants Res. 2015;26:1158–64.
4. Pjetursson BE, Lang NP. Sinus floor elevation utilizing the transalveolar approach. Periodontol 2000 2014;66:59-71.
5. Zijderveld SA, van den Bergh JP, Schulten EA, ten Bruggenkate CM. Anatomical and surgical findings and complications in 100 consecutive maxillary sinus floor elevation procedures. J Oral Maxillofac Surg. 2008;66:1426–38.
6. Bhattacharyya N. Bilateral chronic maxillary sinusitis after the sinus-lift procedure. Am J Otolaryngol. 1999;20:133–5.
7. Tidwell JK, Blijdorp PA, Stoelinga PJ, Brouns JB, Hinderks F. Composite grafting of the maxillary sinus for placement of endosteal implants. A preliminary report of 48 patients. Int J Oral Maxillofac Surg. 1992;21:204–9.
8. Timmenga NM, Raghoebar GM, Boering G, van Weissenbruch R. Maxillary sinus function after sinus lifts for the insertion of dental implants. J Oral Maxillofac Surg. 1997;55:936–9.
9. Carmeli G, Artzi Z, Kozlovsky A, Segev Y, Landsberg R. Antral computerized tomography pre-operative evaluation: relationship between mucosal thickening and maxillary sinus function. Clin Oral Implants Res. 2011;22:78–82.
10. Manor Y, Mardinger O, Bietlitum I, Nashef A, Nissan J, Chaushu G. Late signs and symptoms of maxillary sinusitis after sinus augmentation. Oral Surg Oral Med Oral Pathol Oral Radiol Endod. 2010;110:e1–4.
11. Pignataro L, Mantovani M, Torretta S, Felisati G, Sambataro G. ENT assessment in the integrated management of candidate for (maxillary) sinus lift. Acta Otorhinolaryngol Ital. 2008;28:110–9.
12. Shanbhag S, Karnik P, Shirke P, Shanbhag V. Cone-beam computed tomographic analysis of sinus membrane thickness, ostium patency, and residual ridge heights in the posterior maxilla: implications for sinus floor elevation. Clin Oral Implants Res. 2014;25:755–60.
13. Gardner DG. Pseudocysts and retention cysts of the maxillary sinus. Oral Surg Oral Med Oral Pathol. 1984;58:561–7.
14. Chiapasco M, Palombo D. Sinus grafting and simultaneous removal of large antral pseudocysts of the maxillary sinus with a micro-invasive intraoral access. Int J Oral Maxillofac Surg. 2015;44:1499–505.
15. Cano J, Campo J, Alobera MA, Baca R. Surgical ciliated cyst of the maxilla. Clinical case. Med Oral Patol Oral Cir Bucal. 2009;14:E361–364.
16. Gracco A, Incerti Parenti S, Ioele C, Alessandri Bonetti G, Stellini E. Prevalence of incidental maxillary sinus findings in Italian orthodontic patients: a retrospective cone-beam computed tomography study. Korean J Orthod. 2012;42:329–34.
17. Cagici CA, Yilmazer C, Hurcan C, Ozer C, Ozer F. Appropriate interslice gap for screening coronal paranasal sinus tomography for mucosal thickening. Eur Arch Otorhinolaryngol. 2009;266:519–25.
18. Rege IC, Sousa TO, Leles CR, Mendonca EF. Occurrence of maxillary sinus abnormalities detected by cone beam CT in asymptomatic patients. BMC Oral Health. 2012;12:30.
19. Schneider AC, Bragger U, Sendi P, Caversaccio MD, Buser D, Bornstein MM. Characteristics and dimensions of the sinus membrane in patients referred for single-implant treatment in the posterior maxilla: a cone beam computed tomographic analysis. Int J Oral Maxillofac Implants. 2013;28:587–96.
20. Janner SF, Caversaccio MD, Dubach P, Sendi P, Buser D, Bornstein MM. Characteristics and dimensions of the Schneiderian membrane: a radiographic analysis using cone beam computed tomography in patients referred for dental implant surgery in the posterior maxilla. Clin Oral Implants Res. 2011;22:1446–53.
21. Brullmann DD, Schmidtmann I, Hornstein S, Schulze RK. Correlation of cone beam computed tomography (CBCT) findings in the maxillary sinus with

dental diagnoses: a retrospective cross-sectional study. Clin Oral Investig. 2012;16:1023–9.

22. Shahbazian M, Vandewoude C, Wyatt J, Jacobs R. Comparative assessment of panoramic radiography and CBCT imaging for radiodiagnostics in the posterior maxilla. Clin Oral Investig. 2014;18:293–300.

23. Logan GM, Brocklebank LM. An audit of occipitomental radiographs. Dentomaxillofac Radiol. 1999;28:158–61.

24. Pazera P, Bornstein MM, Pazera A, Sendi P, Katsaros C. Incidental maxillary sinus findings in orthodontic patients: a radiographic analysis using cone-beam computed tomography (CBCT). Orthod Craniofac Res. 2011;14:17–24.

25. Ritter L, Lutz J, Neugebauer J, et al. Prevalence of pathologic findings in the maxillary sinus in cone-beam computerized tomography. Oral Surg Oral Med Oral Pathol Oral Radiol Endod. 2011;111:634–40.

26. Jungner M, Legrell PE, Lundgren S. Follow-up study of implants with turned or oxidized surfaces placed after sinus augmentation. Int J Oral Maxillofac Implants. 2014;29:1380–7.

27. Yoo JY, Pi SH, Kim YS, Jeong SN, You HK. Healing pattern of the mucous membrane after tooth extraction in the maxillary sinus. J Periodontal Implant Sci. 2011;41:23–9.

28. Phothikhun S, Suphanantachat S, Chuenchompoonut V, Nisapakultorn K. Cone-beam computed tomographic evidence of the association between periodontal bone loss and mucosal thickening of the maxillary sinus. J Periodontol. 2012;83:557–64.

29. Ren S, Zhao H, Liu J, Wang Q, Pan Y. Significance of maxillary sinus mucosal thickening in patients with periodontal disease. Int Dent J. 2015;65:303–10.

30. Lin YH, Yang YC, Wen SC, Wang HL. The influence of sinus membrane thickness upon membrane perforation during lateral window sinus augmentation. Clin Oral Implants Res. 2016;27:612–7.

31. Vallo J, Suominen-Taipale L, Huumonen S, Soikkonen K, Norblad A. Prevalence of mucosal abnormalities of the maxillary sinus and their relationship to dental disease in panoramic radiography: results from the Health 2000 Health Examination Survey. Oral Surg Oral Med Oral Pathol Oral Radiol Endod. 2010;109:e80–87.

32. Lu Y, Liu Z, Zhang L, et al. Associations between maxillary sinus mucosal thickening and apical periodontitis using cone-beam computed tomography scanning: a retrospective study. J Endod. 2012;38:1069–74.

33. Shanbhag S, Karnik P, Shirke P, Shanbhag V. Association between periapical lesions and maxillary sinus mucosal thickening: a retrospective cone-beam computed tomographic study. J Endod. 2013;39:853–7.

34. McAllister BS, Masters D, Meffert RM. Treatment of implants demonstrating periapical radiolucencies. Pract Periodontics Aesthet Dent. 1992;4:37–41.

35. Romanos GE, Froum S, Costa-Martins S, Meitner S, Tarnow DP. Implant periapical lesions: etiology and treatment options. J Oral Implantol. 2011;37:53–63.

36. Acharya A, Hao J, Mattheos N, Chau A, Shirke P, Lang NP. Residual ridge dimensions at edentulous maxillary first molar sites and periodontal bone loss among two ethnic cohorts seeking tooth replacement. Clin Oral Implants Res. 2014;25:1386–94.

37. Sharan A, Madjar D. Maxillary sinus pneumatization following extractions: a radiographic study. Int J Oral Maxillofac Implants. 2008;23:48–56.

21

Cellular fluid shear stress on implant surfaces—establishment of a novel experimental set up

P. W. Kämmerer[1†], D. G. E. Thiem[1*†], A. Alshihri[2,3], G. H. Wittstock[4], R. Bader[5], B. Al-Nawas[4] and M. O. Klein[4]

Abstract

Background: Mechanostimuli of different cells can affect a wide array of cellular and inter-cellular biological processes responsible for dental implant healing. The purpose of this in vitro study was to establish a new test model to create a reproducible flow-induced fluid shear stress (FSS) of osteoblast cells on implant surfaces.

Methods: As FSS effects on osteoblasts are detectable at 10 dyn/cm^2, a custom-made flow chamber was created. Computer-aided verification of circulation processes was performed. In order to verify FSS effects, cells were analysed via light and fluorescence microscopy.

Results: Utilising computer-aided simulations, the underside of the upper plate was considered to have optimal conditions for cell culturing. At this site, a flow-induced orientation of osteoblast cell clusters and an altered cell morphology with cellular elongation and alteration of actin fibres in the fluid flow direction was detected.

Conclusions: FSS simulation using this novel flow chamber might mimic the peri-implant situation in the phase of loaded implant healing. With this FSS flow chamber, osteoblast cells' sensitivity to FSS was verified in the form of morphological changes and cell re-clustering towards the direction of the flow. Different shear forces can be created simultaneously in a single experiment.

Keywords: Bioengineering, Biomechanics, Dental implant materials, Implant healing, Cell biology, Osteoblast, Stress analysis

Background

Cells can be influenced by different mechanostimuli, which lead to an activation of cellular and inter-cellular responses. These reactions may be caused by either a direct stimulation of the cell body (mechanoreception) or indirect cellular stimulation (response) [1–3]. Extracellular fluid movement induces fluid shear stress (FSS) that can result in different cellular processes including proliferation, migration and gene expression [4].

There are two different ways of cell stimulation by FSS, where both lead to extracellular signalling. First, fluid-induced cell stimulation occurs when the cell surface is in direct contact with the moving extracellular fluid as seen in the vascular endothelium. Second, it has been hypothesised that indirect stimulation occurs via fluid flow through the lacunar network as seen in bones such as close to loaded dental endosseous implants [1–3]. This extracellular cell stimulation leads to an altered cell morphology as well as altered intracellular signal cascades such as changed gene and protein expression pattern [4–7]. A reorganisation of actin fibres in accordance with the flow direction could be observed as well [8].

To prove the theory of a FSS-triggered effect on different cell lines, several in vitro investigations using different flow chambers were conducted [5, 9–12]. In osteoblasts, biochemical responses on FSS in form of an increased intracellular calcium production [13–15] and an increased release of prostaglandins were reported [15–19]. FSS stimulation of osteoblasts also improved the cell adhesion by enhancing the affinity of intracellular integrins to extracellular matrix ligands as well as to biomaterial surfaces [20, 21]. Shear forces' triggered effects on osteoblasts could be detected at a

---
* Correspondence: daniel.thiem@med.uni-rostock.de
†Equal contributors
[1]Department of Oral and Maxillofacial Surgery, Facial Plastic Surgery, University Medical Centre Rostock, Schillingallee 35, 18057 Rostock, Germany
Full list of author information is available at the end of the article

value of 10 dyn/cm^2, which almost reflects the in vivo situation [4, 22, 23]. Todays' frequently used flow chambers mainly simulate the in vivo formed shear forces. However, it is difficult to ensure the required reproducibility and linear flow conditions. The most distinctive feature of currently used flow chambers is a liquid flow along rigidly fixed cell-bearing surfaces. Some of the above mentioned flow devices are either operating with a constant flow velocity or using pulsating flow profiles, which should be applied in case of analysing blood flow characteristics [9, 24]. Computerised investigations of flow chambers by Anderson et al. [4] have shown that deviating shear forces occur in the same flow chamber after repeating the same experiment twice. Consequently, different results of stimulation and cells response are obtained. Another downside of reported flow chambers is the inability to simultaneously set different shear forces in a single experiment.

Therefore, the aim of the present study was to establish a new cell chamber model for FSS simulation and stimulation. In addition to its ease of use, the reported model in this study should meet the requirements of a simple design, generating reproducible flow characteristics next to laminar flows and clearly defined flow gradients on implant surfaces.

Methods

Experimental setup

A three-dimensional illustration and photography of the plate/plate flow chamber model is shown in Fig. 1. A detailed list of used parts can be found in Appendix 1.

The circulation within the flow chamber was generated by an externally attached electric motor, which rotates up to 500 rounds per minute (rpm). A commercial grade 4 pure medical titanium gear shaft (length = 40 mm, diameter = 4 mm) was connected to the motor by a set screw-fixed gearwheel. For the attachment of the custom-made

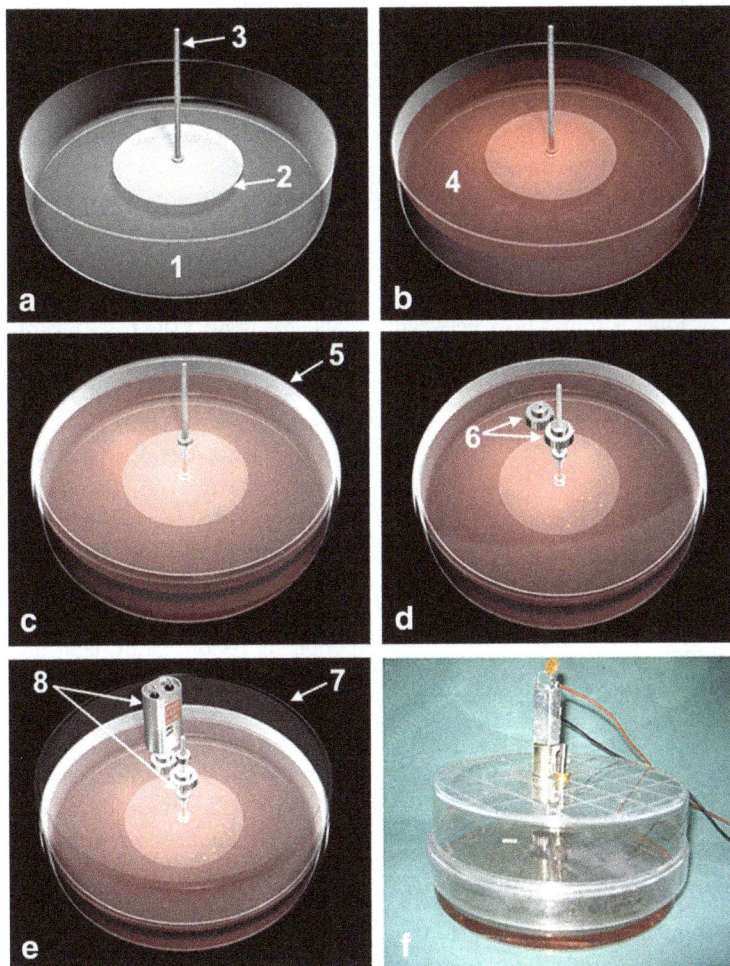

Fig. 1 Three-dimensional illustration (**a–e**) and photography (**f**) of the experimental setup with the components marked numerical. **a** *1* Lower petri dish (s' bottom serving as the lower plate); *2* Rotating glass panel [60 mm diameter (cell bearing)]; *3* Titanium axis. **b** *4* Liquid medium (*red*). **c** *5* Reversed upper petri dish. **d** *6* Gearwheel with set screw. **e** *7* Closing; *8* Electronic motor device and adjusting ring with additional set screw

biocompatible glass panel (diameter = 60 mm, thickness = 2 mm; 4-mm central circular opening), the gear shafts' lower end was disc shaped (diameter = 10 mm). The glass panel was fixed by an adjusting ring with an additional set screw from above. The cover of the lower petri dish contained guiding grooves to stabilise an inverted larger petri dish placed on, which in turn served as a holding device to the electric motor (Fig. 1).

Model assembly

Under sterile conditions, the cell-bearing glass plate was attached to the lower end of the gear shaft with the cells facing the bottom plate. A space of 2 mm between the two plates was determined via computational simulations. After filling the lower petri dish to 70% of its capacity with culture medium, a closing plate with a centred recess for the gear shaft (4 mm) was placed on top to seal the lower compartment. Lastly, a larger petri dish, having a central recess (4 mm), with an externally attached electric motor, was reversely installed above to form the upper compartment. As shown in Fig. 1, the transmission between motor and gear shaft was realised by using two same-sized gear-wheels, one fixed on each of the two components within the non-sterile upper compartment.

Analytical formula for evaluating the flow characteristics

Frequently used flow chambers are characterised by an internal fluid flow along a stationary cell-bearing surface, whereas the osteoblast test cells of this newly developed model are circulating within a resting culture medium.

For constant and fully developed laminar flow between the two parallel plates, the magnitude of the wall shear stress (τ) in between was calculated by formula 1:

$$\tau = \frac{\eta r \omega}{H}$$

in which η is the *dynamic fluid viscosity* (dyn/cm^2), r is the *radius of the plate* (cm), ω stands for *angular velocity* and H for *height* (*vertical distance in between the two plates*).

To get information whether the flow is laminar or turbulent, Reynolds numbers (Re) were calculated for all flow regimes using formula 2 [25]:

$$Re = \frac{\rho v A}{\eta}$$

in which ρ is the liquids' density, η is its dynamic viscosity, v stands for average angular velocity and A is the characteristic area within which liquids flow (vertical distance between the two plates). Re values of >1500 are commonly considered illustrative of turbulent flow as well as values <1500 create laminar flows.

Computational simulation of the flow characteristics

Numerous computerised simulations were performed to verify flow characteristics occurring within the plate/plate flow chamber assisted by the Department of Hydraulic Machines, Faculty of Mechanical Engineering, Technical University of Munich, Germany. For simulation of flow profiles to assess a potential cellular impact by fluid shear stress inside the chamber, graphical illustrations were created by using Ansys CFX° software (Ansys Germany GmbH, Otterfing, Germany).

Test procedure

The experimental process involved three steps. First, a count of $n = 50.000$ commercially available osteoblasts (PromoCell, Heidelberg, Germany) per millilitre of culture medium were cultured on the bottom of the cell-bearing surface (glass panel). Therefore, cells were seeded in a culture medium (cf. Appendix 2 for a detailed composition) at 37 °C. Prior to the test procedure, the cells were manually removed from the culture bottles' bottom by gentle movements while adding 5 ml of Trypsin followed by 10 min of incubation. Finally, Trypsin residues were removed with, first, centrifugation (1600 rpm/5 min) of the cell fluid (culture medium with additives and loose osteoblast cells) and, second, by subsequently adding 10 ml of culture medium. After 24 h of incubation, cells showed adherent to the glass panel. A conventional petri dish was filled to 70% of its capacity with cell fluid (culture medium and additives (Appendix 2). The petri dishs' bottom formed the lower plate and the round glass panel the upper plate placed within the culture medium. Directly after, the circulation process for FSS induction was initiated. In brief, after 24 h of incubation at 37 °C and 5% CO_2 concentration, cells adhered to under side of the glass panel and the glass panel was incorporated into the device as described above. The circulation process (speed level = 200 rpm) started for 24 h under sterile incubation conditions (37 °C and 5% of CO_2). Via repeated computational simulations, a rotational speed level of 200 rpm was found as adequate to provide 10 dyn/cm^2 of shear force at the plates' peripheral region. Lastly, light microscopic examination was conducted (Leica DC480°, Leica Microsystems, Wetzlar, Germany) to verify the cell orientation (after 24 h with and without rotation), followed by phallacidin fluorescence staining according to the manufacturer's protocol (Appendix 3) (BODYPY° FL Phallacidin, ThermoFisher Scientific, MA, USA) and fluorescence microscopy with Leica/Leitz DM RBE° (Leica Microsystems, Wetzlar, Germany). The cell body and its longitudinal actin fibre orientation was put in relation to the total-force-vector (Fig. 5) (resulted from the flow velocity-vector and the centrifugal force-vector) which was calculated by formula 3. For differentiation into an oriented and non-oriented cell formation, an angle of 90° was set as threshold value.

Results

Our analysis was focused on two main aspects:

1. Simulation of the fluid flow characteristics as well as quantification of the arising shear forces at the plate/plate flow chamber with reliable reproducibility
2. Assessment of the impact of fluid shear stress on osteoblast cells in terms of altered cell morphology and intracellular structural changes

Evaluation of the fluid flow characteristics by computerised simulations and quantification of the resulting forces

The computational fluid dynamic analysis and the quantification of the occurring shear forces within the plate/plate flow chamber were central part of this investigation. The cellular-fluid flow setup was based on the fact that osteoblast cells show responses at 10 dyn/cm^2 at a speed level of 200 rpm.

On the topside of the upper plate (rotating glass panel), the computerised simulations demonstrated a gradient increased flow with shear forces from the centre (1 dyn/cm^2) to the periphery (10 dyn/cm^2). Minor effects of shear forces (0–2 dyn/cm^2) were recorded on the surface of the bottom plate. It could be demonstrated that a bigger radius of rotation correlates with higher shear forces as

expressed in formula 1. Further simulations aimed to verify the pattern of fluid flow (laminar versus turbulent flow). For this purpose, the conditions on the upper and lower surface of the upper plate as well as in the area in between the two plates were of particular interest. The simulations revealed a strong turbulent flow on the entire top surface of the upper plate, especially in the centre and the area around the circumferential edges (Fig. 2). The flow from the peripheral region turned backward and amplified the turbulent flow on the top surface. The development of two opposite flow directions was observed within the area in between the plates. The flow along the lower plates' surface was directed from the periphery to the centre whereas the fluid movement along the underside of the upper plate was inversely orientated (Fig. 2). Regarding the upper compartment, peripheral turbulent flow along the outer edges was similar to the fluid movements within the area in between the plates. At the top, the turbulent flow directed from the centre to the periphery whereas the turbulences at the bottom were orientated in reverse to that. Moreover, the effect of the shear forces on the osteoblast cells was also influenced by the centrifugal force. This force can be calculated using formula 3:

$$F = \rho \cdot h \cdot \varpi^2 \cdot r$$

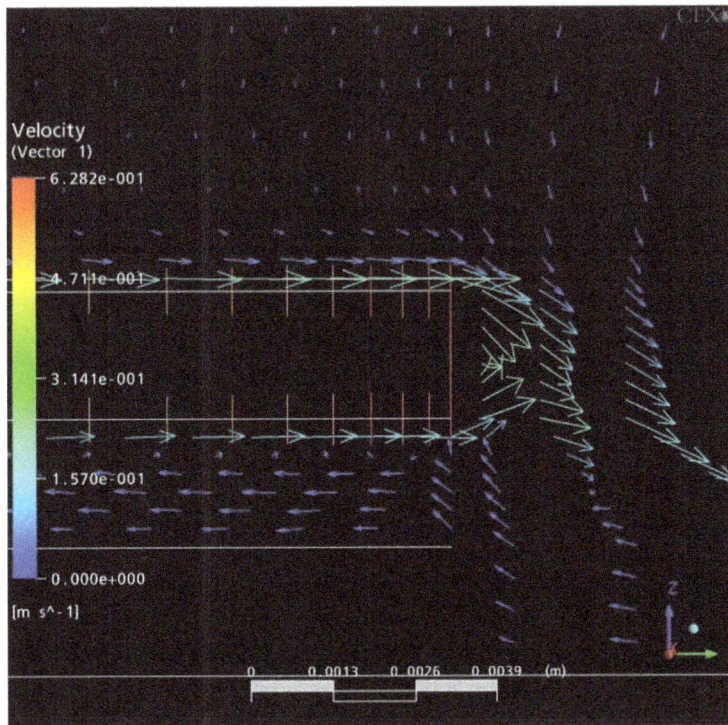

Fig. 2 Side view of a computerized simulation, showing the flow chambers' lower compartment and the flow profile in between the two plates; shearing gap and bottom plate are shown on the *left* side; rotation speed = 200 rpm; colour code bar (*left edge*) showing shear force values [Pa] [1 Pa = 10 dyn/cm^2]; flow direction presented by *arrows*

in which ρ = density, h = height, ω = angular velocity and r = radius.

Figure 3 shows the respective physical force and its dependence on a bigger radius and higher rotational speed. The results of this study indicate that the centrifugal force represents only a little proportion of effective forces. Hence, the centrifugal forces' impacts on the tested cells are considered to be insignificant.

Morphological changes of osteoblast cell clusters and individual cells

Cells were subjected to 24 h of fluid flow rotations at a speed level of 200 rpm. The exposed test cells within the new FSS chamber changed their orientation in accordance with the flow direction. Microscopic evaluation was conducted via a random screening at the peripheral site (2.5-cm radial distance) within a predefined area of interest (0.2 cm × 0.2 cm) through cell counting (at least $n = 40$ cells/region of interest) and morphological cell characterisation. The FSS-triggered effect was demonstrated as cells realigned themselves towards the flow direction, whereby only cells with an aspect ratio greater than 2:1 were included. To assess the alterations taking place inside the cell body, osteoblast cells were treated with a fluorescence stain to visualise actin fibres. In addition, the cells were split into two groups; the first group ($n = 5$) remained untreated, without any impact of shear stress (Fig. 4) while the cells in the second group ($n = 5$) underwent a 24-h rotational impact with 8.35 dyn/cm² shear force. All tests and analysis were repeated at least six times. The cells

showed a reproducible ($n > 6$) realignment of the actin cytoskeleton towards the fluid flow direction (Fig. 5), whereas the actin fibres of the untreated group showed random orientations. Findings were termed a trend if more than 50% of all screened cells ($n > 21$ cells) underwent reorientation.

Discussion

The aim of this study was to establish a new FSS model that is easy to use as well as simple to assemble in order to create reproducible fluid shear forces on cells close to implant material surfaces. Todays' commonly used commercial flow devices differ in geometry and function, which makes comparisons between experiments difficult [4, 10, 26, 27]. The benefits of this novel testing device are reproducible laminar flows under controlled conditions (regulated temperature as well as steady partial pressure of CO_2). Due to its reproducibility, the stimulation of osteoblast cells by shear forces becomes assessable.

In this FSS chamber, osteoblasts were cultured on the bottom of a rotating round glass panel that moves within a resting liquid. Computerised simulations determined a value of 200 rpm as the optimal system configuration in which a constant laminar flow occurs without pulsatile character. When creating laminar flows, induction of turbulences at boundary surfaces results in flow instability. To reduce this negative effect occurring in frequently used stationary devices, cells were cultured on a carrier plate, which is placed within the lower petri dish. In this context, the direct contact between the carrier plate and another interface was omitted.

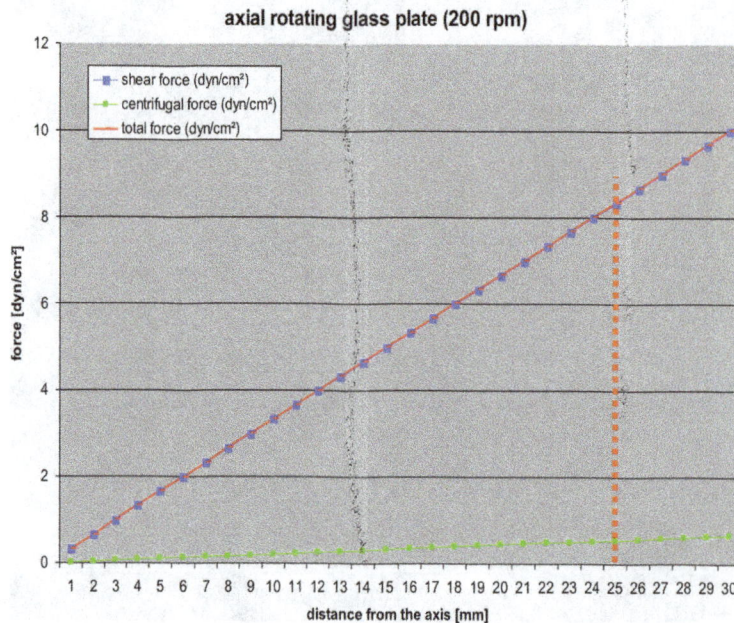

Fig. 3 Diagram for visualisation of the calculation of shear stress rates taking into account the centrifugal force and the glass plates' dimensions. For example, at a distance of 25 mm from the centre of the upper plate, the shear forces' value is 8.33 dyn/cm², together, with an additional centrifugal force that has a value of 0.55 dyn/cm²

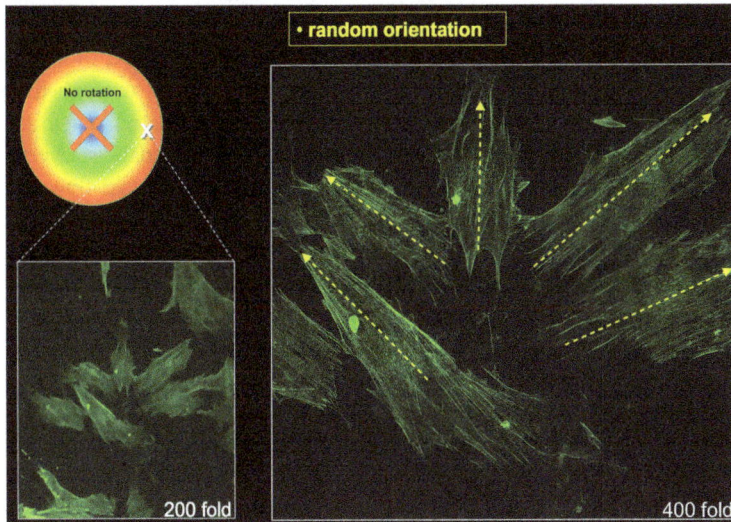

Fig. 4 Randomly orientated osteoblasts without influence of rotation (phallacidin fluorescence staining). On the *left side* with 200× and on the *right side* with 400× magnification. The *white* X on the *coloured circle* marks the location upon the plate where the osteoblasts were located. The *red* X marks the centre of the plate

Laminar flows were chosen to achieve a good reproducibility. This required a flow profile that is characterised by parallel moving liquid layers [26] that are present in the area in between the upper and lower plate. To define the most favourable position of the cell-bearing surface, computerised simulations were performed. Herein, it could be demonstrated that rising shear forces along the plate surfaces' ($0-2$ dyn/cm^2) are too low for osteoblast test cell stimulation, which occurs at about 10 dyn/cm^2 [28, 29].

The bottom of the glass plate generated enough shear forces (10 dyn/cm^2 in the periphery) to meet the requirements of an osteoblast-stimulating laminar flow chamber. Further on, the simulations indicated that the flow profile in between the two plates was not influenced by peripheral turbulences alongside the peripheral regions. To verify a cellular realignment towards the shear direction, cells were microscopically examined prior and after exposure to shear forces for 24 h upon a spinning disc at a speed level of

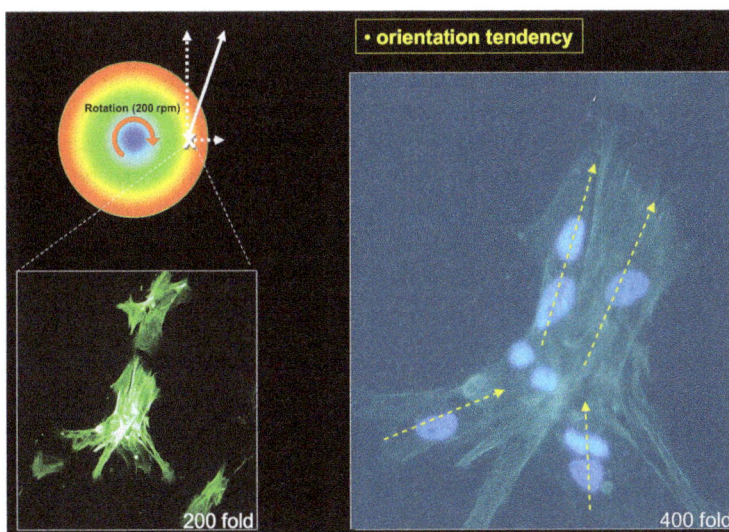

Fig. 5 Osteoblasts with an orientation tendency after 24 h of rotation (phallacidin fluorescence staining). On the *left side* with 200× and on the *right side* with 400× magnification. The *yellow arrows* show the orientation of the cells. The *red arched arrow* within the *coloured circle* shows the direction of rotation. The *dashed white line* oriented to the *right* stands for the resulting centrifugal force. The dashed *white line* pointing *upwards* shows the direction of the resulting flow resistance. The *solid white arrow* stands for the vectorial sum of the abovementioned forces

200 rpm. Even if not sufficiently meaningful alone, observing changes in osteoblast cell morphology are still appropriate methods to verify the good usability of a flow chamber for the generation of reproducible FSS. Although not statistically significant, a tendency of cellular realignment towards the liquid flow direction was demonstrated. Similarly, several studies have revealed characteristic changes of osteoblast morphology triggered by fluid shear stress, which depends on exposure time and strength [22, 30]. Likewise to our findings, these changes are characterised by the formation of actin stress fibres, which in turn align towards the longitudinal cell axis and mainly appear near the nucleus [8, 31]. However, the manual approach of analysing the actin fibres' orientation has to be stated as a drawback of the present study, since it does not meet the requirements of a valid measurement. Immunofluorescence microscopy is largely a qualitative, or semiquantitative, approach with a limited capability of precise fibre differentiation and/or quantification since standard binary thresholds failed to exhaustively segment all fibres because of their wide variations in intensity and background levels [32]. Hence, more objective measurements could be provided by the use of an automated software-assisted processing. In this context, the FibreScore Algorithm by Lichtenstein et al. presents a potential solution for quantification, since it allows the reliable segmentation of each actin fibre. The procedure itself is based on the acquisition of different pixel intensities, whereby it works through the correlation of pixel adjacent regions with synthetic fibre templates at different orientations and their assignment for the central pixel with the highest correlation coefficient among all orientations [32].

Due to the fact that constant flows were generated within the parallel flow chamber only, the situations of in vitro experiments differ from in vivo setting where dynamic flow profiles are particular [33]. As the constant laminar flow profile is not physiological in bones [34], vessels and other tissues [35], the informative value of the experimental setting is limited but it could be used for various cell proliferation and differentiation modulations. In accordance with this, constant laminar flows were rated to have more impact on target cells than pulsatile and oscillating flow profiles. With regard to these findings, the flow profile generated within the reported device meets the requirements to induce cell morphology changes by FSS.

In addition, when using the new flow chamber, an additive effect of FSS and centrifugal forces on the cells could be seen. Other flow chambers did not reveal this phenomenon due to the fact that the liquid flow moves along a stationary cell surface only [4, 10, 22].

When comparing this new fluid flow chambers with other reported devices [4, 10], several differences are seen. Commonly, test cells are placed on a fixed surface with the culture medium flowing along. According to the method of flow generation, they can be classified into open and sealed systems. Open systems, which are hydrostatically driven, are characterised by a fluid flow that passes the stationary phase once only [36]. In sealed models, the culture medium recirculates pump driven through the system [22]. Due to their inherent system-related drawbacks such as turbulent flow generation on boundary surfaces, those flow chambers are inappropriate for laminar flow creation. However, open systems have benefits of allowing the use of different culture media in a row without ceasing the fluid shear stress. Therefore, one can easily enable or disable different stimuli by exchanging the culture medium to evaluate its cellular impact. Sealed systems such as reported in this study do not provide this option. Initially added substances within the culture medium cannot be eliminated during the experimental process. Instead, stopping the flow and draining the cells would be necessary which would cause another unwanted influence to the test cells.

Besides, in the model reported in this study, microscopic examinations are possible after completing the experiment only. Nevertheless, an advantage of the new flow chamber is the possibility of testing different cell colonies simultaneously in one single experiment by placing cells in different radial locations on the spinning disc. Due to the current flow gradient from the centre to the periphery, different cell colonies are exposed to various levels of shear forces. To simplify the process of cell reaction examination, the use of a larger sized glass panel could be considered.

Biomaterial researchers are constantly looking for innovative materials like surface-binding ligands and implant materials, pursuing the aim of improving biocompatibility and healing into host tissues. For this purpose, this new developed flow chamber could provide an easy, as well as economic way to investigate material qualities in combination with tissue cells affected by FSS. A specific material to be tested could replace the cell-bearing glass panel. Alternatively, the glass panel could be coated with surface ligands in different ways [37]. A potential use for evaluation of stem cell differentiation and/or proliferation with fluid shear stress as a mechanical stimulus may be assumed as well.

Conclusions

To create fluid shear stress under in vitro conditions, several flow chambers have been developed in the past. The experimental setup of the flow chamber in the centre of this study offers advantages such as simplicity to assemble and ease of use as well as the creation of reproducible fluid shear forces on cells. Due to the new design, different cell types could be simultaneously analysed under reproducible conditions, by placing them in different radial positions. As a result of an increasing flow gradient from the centre to the periphery, different shear forces become available in one single experiment without changing the rotational speed level. Besides, cellular changes in osteoblast morphology and orientation using this model of fluid shear stress were proven.

Appendix 1

Table 1 Listing of the single components of the flow chamber together with manufacturers' data

Component	Manufacturer	Order no.
Large petri dish	Becton Dickinson, Franklin Lakes, NJ, USA	353025
Titanium gear shaft	Custom made	
Glass panel	Custom made	
Gear wheels	Custom made	
Electric motor	MFA Como Drills, Kent, UK	941D Series
Transformer	Voltcraft, Wollerau, Switzerland	PS 152 A

Appendix 2

Table 2 Listing of the culture media and additives together with manufacturers' data

Culture medium/additives	Manufacturer	Order no.	Concentration
Dulbecco's modified Eagle medium (DMEM) with L-glutamine, plus 4.5 g glucose, without NaHCO$_3$, without Natriumpyruvate	Life Technology, Carlsbad, USA	11966-025	
Penicillin/streptomycin	Life Technology, Carlsbad, USA	15640-055	100 IU penicillin/ 100 µg streptomycin/ml
Ca^{2+}/Mg^{2+} free Hanks' balanced salt solution (HBSS)–buffer	Life Technology, Carlsbad, USA	14170-070	
Fetal calf serum (FCS)	Life Technology, Carlsbad, USA	10270-098	10%
L-Glutamate	Life Technology, Carlsbad, USA	25030-024	1%
Ethylenediaminetetraacetic acid (EDTA) solution	Sigma Aldrich, St. Louis, USA	E7889	0.5 M
L-Ascorbic acid 2-phosphate	Sigma Aldrich, St. Louis, USA	A-8960	1 mmol/l ASC (affinity isolated antibody)
Dexamethasone	Serva Bioproducts, Heidelberg, Germany	18660	100 nmol/l

Appendix 3
Phallacidin fluorescence staining

- Fixation in 4% paraformaldehyde with room temperature (10 min)
- Washing with PBS (2× 10 min)
- 0.1% Triton x-100 within PBS for cell membrane permeabilization (3–5 min)
- Washing with PBS (2× 10 min)
- Incubation with 1% PBS-BSA to avoid unspecific bindings (20–30 min)
- Incubation with Phallatoxin-solution [12.5 µl stock solution (Phallacidin B-607, Mobitec) + 500 µl PBS] (20 min)
- Washing with PBS (2× 20 min)
- Air drying of the microscope slides then covering with fluorescence mounting-medium

Abbreviations
FSS: Fluid shear stress

Acknowledgements
The authors thank the Department of Hydraulic Machines, Faculty of Mechanical Engineering, Technical University of Munich, Germany, for helping with the computerised simulations.

Funding
Nothing to declare

Availability of data and materials
The datasets supporting the conclusions of this article are available at the repository of the University Medical Centre Mainz, Germany, and can be provided on request.

Authors' contributions
PK had substantial contribution to both conception and study design and acquisition of data and played a leading role in coordinating and drafting the manuscript. DT participated in both the statistical analysis and interpretation of data and played a major role in drafting the manuscript. AA helped to draft the manuscript by critically revising it for intellectual content. WG participated in the acquisition of data and helped to draft the

manuscript. BR was involved in drafting the manuscript by revising it critically for intellectual content. A-NB and KM have made substantial contribution to conception and study design and played a leading role in drafting the manuscript by revising it critically for intellectual content. KM has given final approval of the version to be published. All authors read and approved the final manuscript.

Competing interests

The authors Kämmerer P.W., Thiem D.G.E., Alshihri A., Wittstock G.H., Bader R., Al-Nawas B. and Klein M.O. declare that they have no conflict of interest.

Author details

[1]Department of Oral and Maxillofacial Surgery, Facial Plastic Surgery, University Medical Centre Rostock, Schillingallee 35, 18057 Rostock, Germany. [2]Department of Prosthetic and Biomaterial Sciences, King Saud University, Riyadh, Saudi Arabia. [3]Harvard School of Dental Medicine, Boston, MA, USA. [4]Department of Oral and Maxillofacial Surgery, Plastic Surgery, University Medical Centre Mainz, Mainz, Germany. [5]Department of Orthopedics, University Medical Centre Rostock, Rostock, Germany.

References

1. Ehrlich PJ, Lanyon LE. Mechanical strain and bone cell function: a review. Osteoporos Int. 2002;13(9):688–700.
2. Vaughan TJ, Haugh MG, Mcnamara LM. A fluid-structure interaction model to characterize bone cell stimulation in parallel-plate flow chamber systems. J R Soc Interface. 2013;10(81):20120900.
3. Weinbaum S, Cowin SC, Zeng Y. A model for the excitation of osteocytes by mechanical loading-induced bone fluid shear stresses. J Biomech. 1994;27(3):339–60.
4. Anderson EJ, Falls TD, Sorkin AM, Knothe Tate ML. The imperative for controlled mechanical stresses in unraveling cellular mechanisms of mechanotransduction. Biomed Eng Online. 2006;5:27.
5. Bancroft GN, Sikavitsas VI, van den Dolder J, Sheffield TL, Ambrose CG, Jansen JA, et al. Fluid flow increases mineralized matrix deposition in 3D perfusion culture of marrow stromal osteoblasts in a dose-dependent manner. Proc Natl Acad Sci U S A. 2002;99(20):12600–5.
6. Datta N, Pham QP, Sharma U, Sikavitsas VI, Jansen JA, Mikos AG. In vitro generated extracellular matrix and fluid shear stress synergistically enhance 3D osteoblastic differentiation. Proc Natl Acad Sci U S A. 2006;103(8):2488–93.
7. Yu X, Botchwey EA, Levine EM, Pollack SR, Laurencin CT. Bioreactor-based bone tissue engineering: the influence of dynamic flow on osteoblast phenotypic expression and matrix mineralization. Proc Natl Acad Sci U S A. 2004;101(31):11203–8.
8. Pavalko FM, Chen NX, Turner CH, Burr DB, Atkinson S, Hsieh YF, et al. Fluid shear-induced mechanical signaling in MC3T3-E1 osteoblasts requires cytoskeleton-integrin interactions. Am J Physiol. 1998;275(6 Pt 1):C1591–601.
9. Astrof NS, Salas A, Shimaoka M, Chen J, Springer TA. Importance of force linkage in mechanochemistry of adhesion receptors. Biochemistry. 2006; 45(50):15020–8.
10. Bakker DP, van der Plaats A, Verkerke GJ, Busscher HJ, van der Mei HC. Comparison of velocity profiles for different flow chamber designs used in studies of microbial adhesion to surfaces. Appl Environ Microbiol. 2003;69(10):6280–7.
11. Bannister SR, Lohmann CH, Liu Y, Sylvia VL, Cochran DL, Dean DD, et al. Shear force modulates osteoblast response to surface roughness. J Biomed Mater Res. 2002;60(1):167–74.
12. Becker J, Kirsch A, Schwarz F, Chatzinikolaidou M, Rothamel D, Lekovic V, et al. Bone apposition to titanium implants biocoated with recombinant human bone morphogenetic protein-2 (rhBMP-2). A pilot study in dogs. Clin Oral Investig. 2006;10(3):217–24.
13. Hung CT, Allen FD, Pollack SR, Brighton CT. What is the role of the convective current density in the real-time calcium response of cultured bone cells to fluid flow? J Biomech. 1996;29(11):1403–9.
14. Ryder KD, Duncan RL. Parathyroid hormone enhances fluid shear-induced [Ca2+](i) signaling in osteoblastic cells through activation of mechanosensitive and voltage-sensitive Ca2+ channels. J Bone Miner Res. 2001;16(2):240–8.

15. Rath AL, Bonewald LF, Ling J, Jiang JX, Van Dyke ME, Nicolella DP. Correlation of cell strain in single osteocytes with intracellular calcium, but not intracellular nitric oxide, in response to fluid flow. J Biomech. 2010;43(8):1560–4.
16. Klein-Nulend J, van der Plas A, Semeins CM, Ajubi NE, Frangos JA, Nijweide PJ, et al. Sensitivity of osteocytes to biomechanical stress in vitro. FASEB J. 1995;9(5):441–5.
17. Klein-Nulend J, Semeins CM, Ajubi NE, Nijweide PJ, Burger EH. Pulsating fluid flow increases nitric oxide (NO) synthesis by osteocytes but not periosteal fibroblasts—correlation with prostaglandin upregulation. Biochem Biophys Res Commun. 1995;217(2):640–8.
18. Mcgarry JG, Klein-Nulend J, Mullender MG, Prendergast PJ. A comparison of strain and fluid shear stress in stimulating bone cell responses—a computational and experimental study. FASEB J. 2005;19(3):482–4.
19. Nauman EA, Satcher RL, Keaveny TM, Halloran BP, Bikle DD. Osteoblasts respond to pulsatile fluid flow with short-term increases in PGE(2) but no change in mineralization. J Appl Physiol. 2001;90(5):1849–54.
20. Galbraith CG, Yamada KM, Sheetz MP. The relationship between force and focal complex development. J Cell Biol. 2002;159(4):695–705.
21. Orr AW, Ginsberg MH, Shattil SJ, Deckmyn H, Schwartz MA. Matrix-specific suppression of integrin activation in shear stress signaling. Mol Biol Cell. 2006;17(11):4686–97.
22. Chen NX, Ryder KD, Pavalko FM, Turner CH, Burr DB, Qiu J, et al. Ca(2+) regulates fluid shear-induced cytoskeletal reorganization and gene expression in osteoblasts. Am J Physiol Cell Physiol. 2000;278(5):C989–97.
23. Hughes-Fulford M. Signal transduction and mechanical stress. Sci STKE. 2004;2004(249):RE12.
24. Ruel J, Lemay J, Dumas G, Doillon C, Charara J. Development of a parallel plate flow chamber for studying cell behavior under pulsatile flow. ASAIO J. 1995;41(4):876–83.
25. Kazakidi A, Sherwin SJ, Weinberg PD. Effect of Reynolds number and flow division on patterns of haemodynamic wall shear stress near branch points in the descending thoracic aorta. J R Soc Interface. 2009;6(35):539–48.
26. Brown DC, Larson RS. Improvements to parallel plate flow chambers to reduce reagent and cellular requirements. BMC Immunol. 2001;2:9.
27. Usami S, Chen HH, Zhao Y, Chien S, Skalak R. Design and construction of a linear shear stress flow chamber. Ann Biomed Eng. 1993;21(1):77–83.
28. Sikavitsas VI, Bancroft GN, Holtorf HL, Jansen JA, Mikos AG. Mineralized matrix deposition by marrow stromal osteoblasts in 3D perfusion culture increases with increasing fluid shear forces. Proc Natl Acad Sci U S A. 2003;100(25):14683–8.
29. Mcgarry JG, Klein-Nulend J, Prendergast PJ. The effect of cytoskeletal disruption on pulsatile fluid flow-induced nitric oxide and prostaglandin E2 release in osteocytes and osteoblasts. Biochem Biophys Res Commun. 2005;330(1):341–8.
30. Carvalho RS, Scott JE, Yen EH. The effects of mechanical stimulation on the distribution of beta 1 integrin and expression of beta 1-integrin mRNA in TE-85 human osteosarcoma cells. Arch Oral Biol. 1995;40(3):257–64.
31. Malone AM, Batra NN, Shivaram G, Kwon RY, You L, Kim CH, et al. The role of actin cytoskeleton in oscillatory fluid flow-induced signaling in MC3T3-E1 osteoblasts. Am J Physiol Cell Physiol. 2007;292(5):C1830–6.
32. Lichtenstein N, Geiger B, Kam Z. Quantitative analysis of cytoskeletal organization by digital fluorescent microscopy. Cytometry A. 2003;54(1):8–18.
33. Jacobs CR, Yellowley CE, Davis BR, Zhou Z, Cimbala JM, Donahue HJ. Differential effect of steady versus oscillating flow on bone cells. J Biomech. 1998;31(11):969–76.
34. Srinivasan S, Agans SC, King KA, Moy NY, Poliachik SL, Gross TS. Enabling bone formation in the aged skeleton via rest-inserted mechanical loading. Bone. 2003;33(6):946–55.
35. Papadaki M, Eskin SG. Effects of fluid shear stress on gene regulation of vascular cells. Biotechnol Prog. 1997;13(3):209–21.
36. James NL, Harrison DG, Nerem RM. Effects of shear on endothelial cell calcium in the presence and absence of ATP. FASEB J. 1995;9(10):968–73.
37. Kämmerer PW, Lehnert M, Al-Nawas B, Kumar VV, Hagmann S, Alshihri A, et al. Osseoconductivity of a specific streptavidin-biotin-fibronectin surface coating of biotinylated titanium implants—a rabbit animal study. Clin Implant Dent Relat Res. 2015;17 Suppl 2:e601–12.

22

Significance of mandibular molar replacement with a dental implant: a theoretical study with nonlinear finite element analysis

Masazumi Yoshitani[1]* , Yoshiyuki Takayama[2] and Atsuro Yokoyama[1]

Abstract

Background: Dental implants are frequently applied to unilateral defects in the mandible. However, implant placement in the molar region of the mandible can be difficult due to anatomical structure. The aim of this study was to evaluate the distribution of occlusal force in a mandibular shortened dental arch (SDA) with implants.

Methods: Three-dimensional finite element (FE) models of the mandible with varying numbers of teeth and implants were constructed. Models Im6 and Im67 contained one and two implants in the defect of the left molar region, respectively. Models Im456 and Im4567 contained three and four implants in the defect of the left premolar and molar regions, respectively. Model MT67 contained a defect in the molar region with no implant placed. Model MT7 represented natural dentition without a left second molar, as a control. Modification of the condition of occlusal contacts assuming the intercuspal position was performed before analysis under load 400 N; therefore, the load condition as total force on the occlusal surface was 400 N. FE analyses were subsequently performed under load conditions of loads 100, 200, and 800 N. The distribution of reaction forces on the occlusal surface and the mandibular condyle was investigated.

Results: Force distribution in models Im67 and Im4567 appeared to be symmetrical under all load conditions. Occlusal force distribution in models Im6 and Im456 was similar to that in model MT7. However, the occlusal force at the second premolars on the defect side in those models was larger under loads 100 and 200 N. Conversely, the occlusal force on the first molars was much larger than that in model MT7 under load 800 N.

Conclusions: Within the limitations of this theoretical study, we demonstrated that restoration with the same number of implants as missing teeth will show almost symmetric occlusal force distribution, and it will produce less biomechanically stress for a unilateral defect of the mandible. However, if restoration of a missing second molar with an implant is impossible or difficult, then an SDA with implants may also be acceptable except for individuals with severe bruxism.

Keywords: Dental implant, SDA, Occlusal force distribution, Finite element analysis

* Correspondence: zumi@jade.dti.ne.jp
[1]Division of Oral Functional Science, Department of Oral Functional Prosthodontics, Graduate School of Dental Medicine, Hokkaido University, Kita-13, Nishi-7, Kita-ku, Sapporo 060-8648, Japan
Full list of author information is available at the end of the article

Background

Dental implant treatment has been frequently applied in dental practice as the most important prosthodontic procedure with long-term predictability to restore oral function, maintain occlusion, and improve the quality of life (QoL) of a patient [1]. Clinically, dental implants are mainly applied to correct mandibular distally extended edentulism [2]. However, implant placement in the molar region of a mandible occasionally has some anatomical difficulties, such as lingual concavity of a mandible, small distance to the mandibular canal, insufficient space between the alveolar ridge and opposing teeth, and lack of keratinized mucosa. Especially, lingual concavities in an edentulous mandible appear to be related to risk of perforation in the lingual cortical bone during dental implant insertion, which may lead to hemorrhages or infections in the parapharyngeal space [3, 4]. Lingual concavities have a prevalence of 68% in the molar region and occur at a significantly higher rate in the second molar (90%) than in the first molar (56%) [5]. To avoid these risks, implants may not always be suitable to repair second molar defects.

Dental implant treatment is also associated with higher initial costs in general [6, 7]. Therefore, a cost-effective treatment is desired. Removable partial dentures with a single posterior implant could be a possible treatment option in the case of inappropriate implant placement in the second molar region. However, the least amount of Oral Health Impact Profile improvement was observed in patients with removable partial dentures compared with patients with implant-supported fixed prostheses [8]. Thus, patients who desire a fixed prosthesis may not be satisfied with a removable overdenture.

The shortened dental arch (SDA) is known as an acceptable concept in natural dentition for its lower cost than restoration of missing teeth. Kayser et al. found no significant differences between subjects with SDA of three to five occlusal units (OUs) and those with complete dental arches with regard to masticatory ability, signs, and symptoms of temporomandibular disorders, migration of remaining teeth, periodontal support, and oral comfort [9–11]. Therefore, according to this concept, second molar defects may not need to be replaced. Fueki et al. identified that only 3% of subjects missing just the second molar(s) sought prosthetic treatment compared with 58% of subjects missing first and second molars [12]. Baba et al. investigated the relationship between patterns of missing OUs and oral health-related QoL in subjects with SDA and reported that a significant difference was observed between groups with and without first molar occlusal contact [13]. Although these studies have examined SDA in natural dentition, there are few studies on SDA including dental implants.

From the viewpoint of occlusal force distribution, when a second molar defect remains without prosthesis, the force might concentrate in the implant, residual teeth, or temporomandibular joints (TMJs). Therefore, the aim of this study was to investigate occlusal force distribution in SDA in the mandible with/without an implant using a three-dimensional (3D) finite element model (FEM).

Methods

Finite element models

The 3D FEMs were constructed based on those reported by Kasai et al. [14], Kayumi et al. [15] and consisted of a mandible, natural teeth with the periodontal ligament (PDL), and titanium implant(s) with superstructures in the left premolar and molar regions.

The surface of the mandible was generated using measurements of a commercially available model (QS7, SOMSO) of the dentate mandible with a 3D laser scanner (LPX-250, Roland DG). Appropriate thickness of the cortical bone was determined according to the anatomical findings [16, 17] and given with computer-aided design software (Rhinoceros, AppliCraft). The mass/volume and shape of the mandible were assumed to be 2 and B, respectively, according to the classification of Lekholm and Zarb [18]. The dimensions of the natural teeth and PDL were based on previous literature [19, 20]. The PDL had approximately the same surface area as the anatomical value, with uniform thickness of 0.25 mm at all sites [20]. The diameter and the length of the implants measured 3.75 and 10 mm, respectively. All materials were assumed to be linear and isotropic except for the PDL, which had biphasic properties as previously described [21–24]. The properties of other materials were based on previous studies [25–29] (Table 1).

The occlusal surfaces of the implants and the teeth were simplified and flattened in agreement with Monson's sphere (10 cm diameter) and included two condyle points and the incisal point. Six models with varying numbers of teeth and implants were constructed. Model Im67 contained two implants placed in the left molar region (Fig. 1a). Model Im6 contained one implant placed in the left molar region (Fig. 1b). Model Im4567 contained four implants placed in the left premolar and molar regions (Fig. 1c). Model Im456 contained three implants placed in the left premolar and molar regions (Fig. 1d). Model MT67 contained no implant placed in the molar defect (Fig. 1e). Model MT7 represented natural dentition without the second molar as a control (Fig. 1f).

Validation of models

Nonlinear characteristics according to the load displacement curve of teeth [21–24] and cartilage [30] were given to the springs for the opposing teeth and TMJs, respectively (Fig. 2). The nonlinear elasticity of the springs on the teeth and implants simulated

Table 1 Material properties

Material	Modulus of elasticity (MPa)	Poisson ratio	References
Cortical bone	140,000	0.3	Kunavisarut et al. [26]
Cancellous bone	7900	0.3	Kunavisarut et al. [26]
Enamel	80,000	0.3	Korioth and Hannan [24]
Dentin	17,600	0.25	Korioth and Hannan [24]
Implant (titan)	117,000	0.32	Kunavisarut et al. [26]
Superstructure (gold alloy)	94,000	0.3	Van Zyl et al. [25], Kitamura et al. [28], Kobayashi et al. [27]
PDL phase1	0.33	0.3	Kim et al. [23], Misch [22], Perfitt et al. [20], Miura et al. [21]
PDL phase 2	16	0.45	Kim et al. [23], Misch [22], Perfitt et al. [20], Miura et al. [21]

displaceability of opposing natural teeth at compression and separation of the occlusal surface from opposing teeth at tension.

The PDLs of natural teeth and the springs corresponding to opposing teeth demonstrated a two-stage displaceability corresponding to the measurement of the load displacement curve of real teeth [21, 22] (Fig. 3).

Kumagai et al. [31] investigated occlusal force distribution in human using the Dental Prescale System. They described that the distribution of the occlusal force was greatest at molar region followed by the premolar and anterior region. Our theoretical model was based on Kasai [14] and Kayumi's [15] reports. The theoretical model with natural teeth and no defect in Kayumi's report and the occlusal force distribution in this model under load 400 N described later are shown in Figs. 4 and 5, respectively. This distribution was similar to the measurement in human body by Kumagai et al. [31].

Boundary conditions of models

The boundary conditions are shown in Fig. 1a–f. To simplify the FEM, TMJs and maxillary teeth were replaced with appropriate springs (Fig. 6). The springs for the maxillary teeth, except for the anterior teeth, were directed perpendicular to the occlusal plane, which was defined using Monson's sphere. The apical end of each spring was restrained in all directions. The other end of the spring was attached to the node corresponding to the occlusal central pit on a mandibular tooth, which allowed displacement perpendicular to the occlusal plane. The springs for TMJs linked an external restricted node to the top of the mandibular condyle [14, 29].

Loading conditions

The loading conditions simulated intercuspal clenching. With the assumption that occlusal force was generated by the contractile force of four bilateral masticatory muscles, masseter, temporalis, and medial and lateral pterygoids, loading points and directions of the loads were generated based on previous literature [19, 25] (Fig. 6). The summation of the reaction force at the occlusal surfaces of the teeth and superstructures was used as a standard for the load amount. For example, the load condition that resulted in a total reaction force of 400 N in the preliminary FEM with natural dentition was designated as "load 400 N."

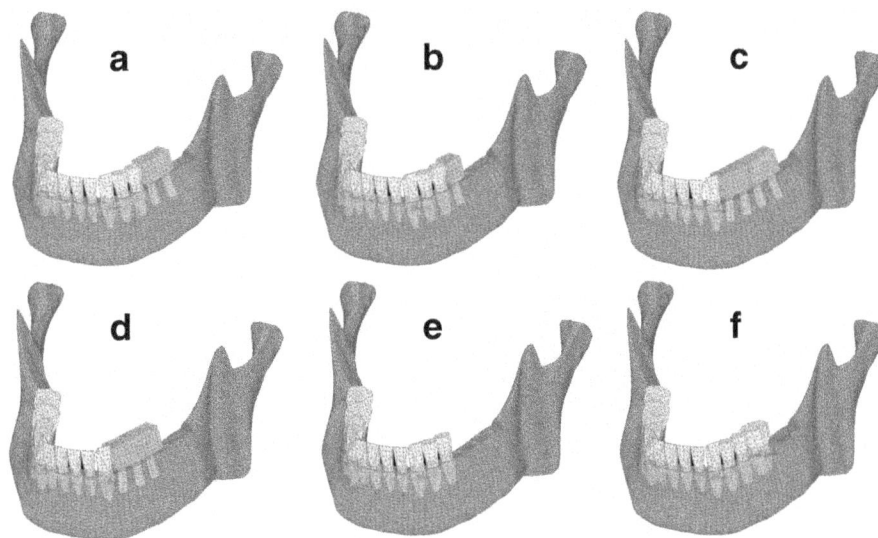

Fig. 1 Three-dimensional finite element model. The tooth roots and implant bodies are displayed with permeability. **a** Im67, **b** Im6, **c** Im4567, **d** Im456, **e** MT67, and **f** MT7

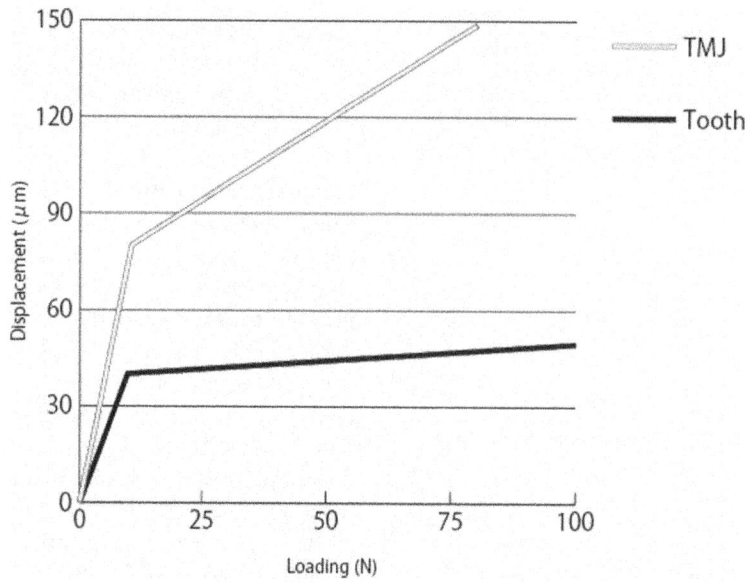

Fig. 2 Load displacement curves of springs

Analysis

Analysis was performed according to the report by Kayumi et al. [15]. In linear finite element analysis (FEA), all teeth maintain perfect contact with antagonists with no stress on occlusal surfaces before loading. However, there must be some occlusal force on the occlusal surface when a mandible is in the intercuspal position. Since the displaceabilities of osseointegrated implants, natural teeth with PDLs, and TMJs are quite different from one another, the results of linear FEA under some occlusal loads should not correspond to real biomechanical conditions.

To verify the similarity of the FE models to the real stomatognathic system, "initializing" of models, i.e., modification of the condition of occlusal contact assuming the intercuspal position, was performed before analysis. This procedure was performed by modifying occlusal contacts on the implants so that the distribution of occlusal force was symmetrical under load 400 N [15]. The occlusal contacts were modified by altering the load displacement curves of the springs on the implants. The load displacement curve was shifted so that the spring provided little resistance to compressive forces until the gap closed, i.e., occlusal surface came in contact with antagonists (Fig. 7). The size of the gap was determined by trial and error, such that the occlusal force, namely, the reaction force of the springs on the occlusal surface, was distributed with approximate symmetry [14, 15] in models Im6, Im67, Im456, and Im4567. This size

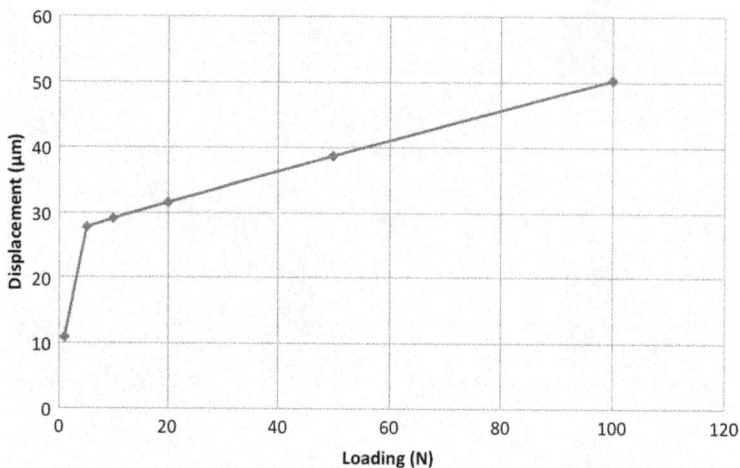

Fig. 3 Load displacement curves of natural teeth in FE model

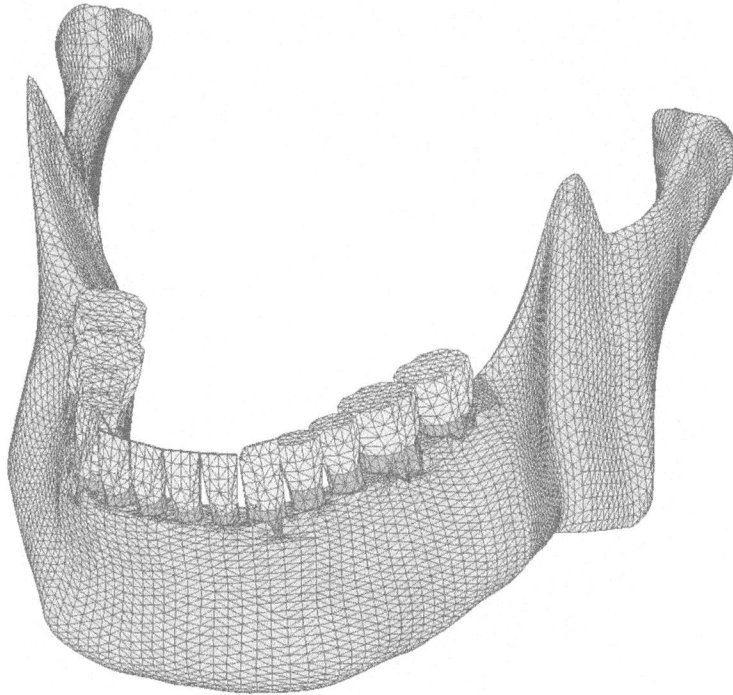

Fig. 4 Three-dimensional finite element model with natural teeth and no defect

was determined so that the amount of reaction force on the most posterior teeth on both sides became as equal as possible. After initializing was completed, symmetric distribution of the reaction force on the teeth and the superstructures was confirmed in each model. Thereafter, the FEA was performed under the load conditions of loads 100, 200, and 800 N using the software package MSC.Marc2010 (MSC Software). The distribution of the reaction forces on the occlusal surface and the mandibular condyle, which were regarded as the occlusal force and the load on the TMJ, respectively, was investigated.

Results

The distributions of occlusal force are shown in Fig. 8. In model MT67 (Fig. 8e), the occlusal force at the first premolar on the defect side was 10.0–86.5 N, which was 1.2–15.0-fold larger than that on the natural dentition side. The occlusal force at the second premolar on the defect side was 24.6–190.1 N, which was 2.6–8.3-fold larger than on the natural dentition side. The occlusal force at the TMJ on the defect side was 26.8–214.6 N, which was 1.2–1.5-fold larger than that on the natural dentition side. The occlusal force was concentrated at the second premolar on the defect side and

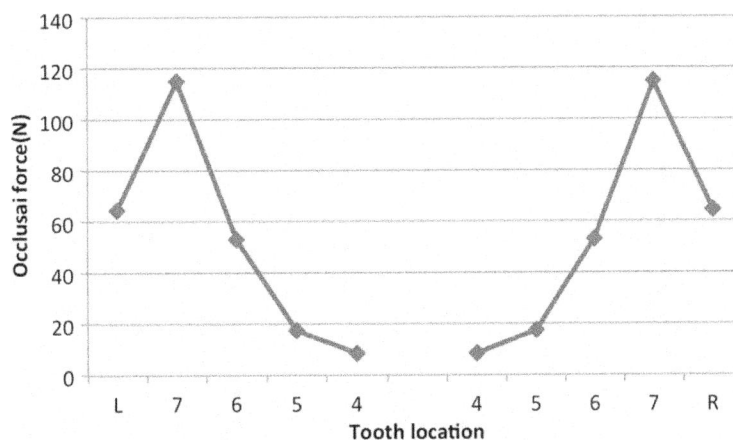

Fig. 5 Distribution of occlusal force in the natural teeth model displayed in Fig.4

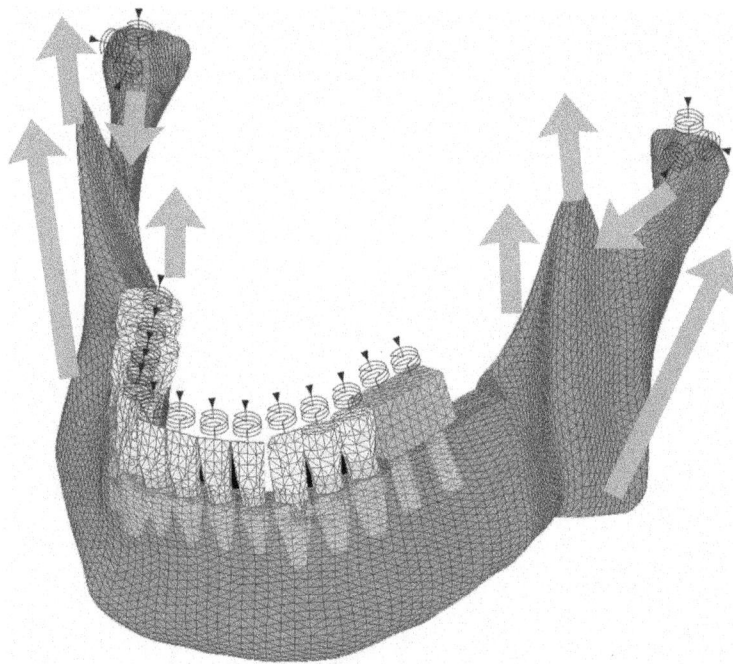

Fig. 6 Springs for opposing teeth and TMJs and load directions. Arrows indicate loads, arrowheads indicate restricted nods, and spiral lines indicate springs

approximately equivalent to that at the second molar on the natural dentition side.

In model MT7 (Fig. 8f), the occlusal force at the first premolar on the defect side was almost equivalent to that on the natural dentition side. The occlusal forces at the second premolar under loads 100, 200, 400, and 800 N were 8.6, 21.0, 43.2, and 84.5 N, respectively. These forces were 1.1–3.8-fold larger on the defect side than that on the natural dentition side. Additionally, the occlusal forces at the first molar under loads 100, 200, 400, and 800 N were 18.5, 47.2, 110.7, and 239.0 N, respectively. These forces were 1.5–2.1-fold larger on

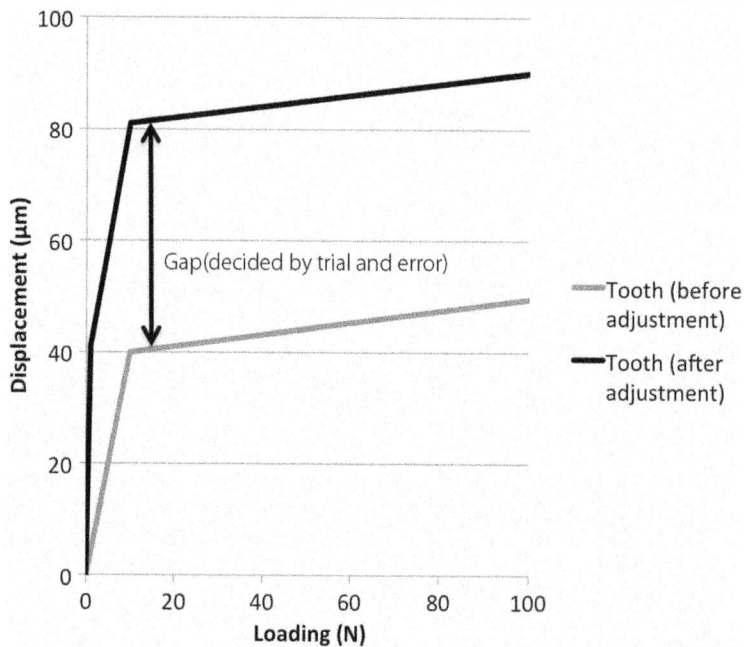

Fig. 7 Initializing models altering the load displacement curves of springs

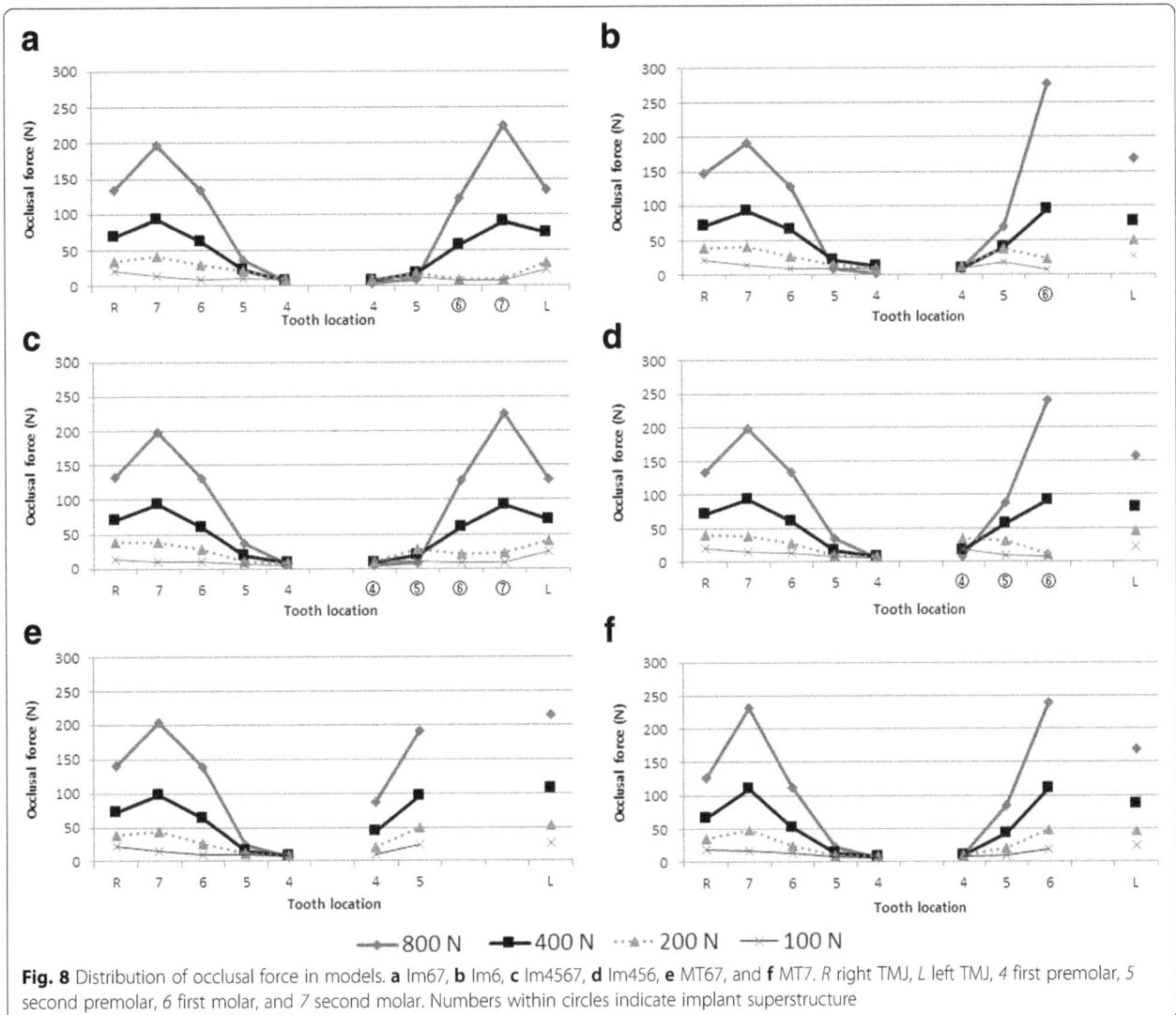

Fig. 8 Distribution of occlusal force in models. **a** Im67, **b** Im6, **c** Im4567, **d** Im456, **e** MT67, and **f** MT7. *R* right TMJ, *L* left TMJ, *4* first premolar, *5* second premolar, *6* first molar, and *7* second molar. Numbers within circles indicate implant superstructure

the defect side than that on the natural dentition side. The occlusal force at the TMJ on the defect side was 24.9–169.1 N, which was 1.1–1.3-fold larger than that on the natural dentition side. The occlusal force was concentrated at the first molar on the defect side and approximately equivalent to that at the second molar on the natural dentition side.

In model Im67 (Fig. 8a), the occlusal force at the premolars and the TMJ on the defect side was smaller than that in model MT67 (shown in Fig. 8e). The occlusal force at the second premolar and TMJ in model Im67 was 9.7–18.3 and 23.7–134.3 N, respectively. Compared with model MT67, the occlusal force at the second premolar and left TMJ in model Im67 was reduced by 0.005–0.5-fold and 0.6–0.9-fold, respectively. Under loads 100 and 200 N, the occlusal force at the implants was slightly smaller than that on the natural dentition side. Under load 800 N, the occlusal force at the first and second molars was 122.7 and 224.9 N, respectively. The occlusal force at the implants

was slightly larger than that at natural teeth on the contralateral side. However, occlusal force distribution in model Im67 was considered to be almost symmetrical.

In model Im6 (Fig. 8b), the occlusal force at the second premolar under loads 100, 200, 400, and 800 N were 18.3, 37.0, 38.8, and 70.2 N, respectively. The occlusal force was larger than that in model Im67 (shown in Fig. 8a), while it was approximately equivalent to that in model MT7 (shown in Fig. 8f). Under loads 100 and 200 N, the occlusal force at the second premolar on the defect side was larger than that at the implant. However, it was smaller than that at the right second molar (most posterior tooth on the natural dentition side). Under load 800 N, the occlusal force at the implant was 276.9 N, which was 1.4-fold larger than that at the most posterior tooth on the natural dentition side. Compared with model MT67, the occlusal force concentration at the second premolar was reduced but remained 2.0–8.3-fold larger than that on the contralateral side.

Comparing model Im6 with model MT7, the occlusal force at the second premolar on the defect side was 1.9-fold larger under load 100 N and 2.8-fold larger under load 200 N. Under load 800 N, the occlusal force at the implant was much larger than that at the first molars on both sides in model MT7. However, occlusal force distribution in model Im6 was similar to that in model MT7.

In model Im4567 (Fig. 8c), under loads 100 and 200 N, the occlusal force at the premolars on the defect side was slightly larger than that on the natural dentition side. Conversely, the occlusal force at the molars on the defect side was slightly smaller than that on the natural dentition side. Under load 800 N, the occlusal force at the second premolar on the defect side was reduced and that at the second molar on the defect side was increased. However, occlusal force distribution in model Im4567 was considered to be almost symmetrical. The occlusal force at the TMJ was symmetrical under every load condition.

In model Im456 (Fig. 8d), under loads 100 and 200 N, the occlusal force at the premolars on the defect side was larger than that in model Im4567 (shown in Fig. 8c). The occlusal force was also larger than that in model MT7 (shown in Fig. 6f). However, the occlusal force at the second premolar under load 200 N was 34.5 N, which was slightly smaller than the occlusal force at the second molar on the natural dentition side. Under load 800 N, the occlusal force at the first molar was increased to 240 N. However, it was almost equivalent to that in model MT7 (shown in Fig. 6f). The occlusal force at the TMJ was slightly increased compared with that in model Im4567 (shown in Fig. 8c).

Discussion

FEM

FEA is useful for mechanical simulations of a living body and has been used in implant dentistry research under careful consideration of the analysis conditions [32, 33]. Although some reports have demonstrated that bone density varies according to bone type and location, the material properties of the mandible were homogenous and isotropic in this study. However, the effect of this difference was considered to be negligible under the confirmation of the displacement of teeth and implants because of its far larger elastic modulus and far smaller strain than those of soft tissues, such as TMJs and PDL. Since the purpose of the present study was to examine the distribution of occlusal forces on the occlusal surface, occlusal forces should be mainly affected by the displaceability of TMJs and teeth, not by that of osseointegrated implants.

The FEMs in this study were based on those reported by Kasai et al. [14] and Kayumi et al. [15]. The displaceability of TMJs was regarded as that of the cartilage [30]

because it has a far smaller elastic modulus than that of the TMJ disc [34, 35]. Therefore, the elastic modulus of the springs corresponding to TMJs was determined based on the thicknesses of the TMJ disc [36] and articular cartilage [35], the stress-strain curve of the intervertebral discs [30], and the displacement of the condyle [37, 38] in intercuspal clenching by indirect measurement. Although the material properties of the human body vary on an individual basis, the models used in this study were therefore considered to be appropriate to investigate the distribution of occlusal forces on the teeth, implants, and TMJs.

Loading condition

Based on previous literature [31, 39], occlusal loading of 200 N was considered to correspond with hard clenching. However, a previous study indicated that the maximum biting force (400 N) was better for occlusal adjustment with intercuspal clenching. Therefore, this study was performed with the assumption that the maximum functional force was 400 N. Occlusal loading of 100 N was considered to correspond with light clenching while loading of 200 N was considered to correspond with middle clenching. Calculations were also performed under a load of 800 N, which was assumed to be the maximum nonfunctional occlusal force, such as that exerted in nocturnal bruxism. Because of the difficulty of controlling nocturnal bruxism, this value was considered to be sufficient to include as the condition under maximum force [40]. However, Hattori et al. [41] described that neuromuscular regulatory systems control maximum clenching strength under various occlusal conditions. Therefore, the large force used in this study may not occur clinically in the SDA except in the case of nocturnal bruxism.

Occlusal force distribution in dentition

Occlusal adjustment is usually performed to obtain symmetrical occlusal force distribution in natural dentition. However, occlusal force distribution among natural teeth and implants depends on occlusal force because of the difference of displaceability between a natural tooth and an implant [14, 15]. Therefore, we evaluated the result of the analysis from viewpoints of symmetry of occlusal force distribution and existence of harmful load on implants, residual teeth, and TMJs.

In this study, occlusal force distribution under load 400 N was adjusted to maintain symmetry. In models Im67 and Im4567, occlusal load on premolars did not show large asymmetry even in lower and higher loading conditions. Thus, restoration with implants of the same number of missing teeth was recommended for unilateral defect(s) of the mandibular premolar and molar regions. In models Im6 and Im456, occlusal force distribution was altered more than in models Im67 and Im4567. However, occlusal force distribution in models Im6 and Im456 was similar to that in model MT7. Since most patients missing only second molars do not always receive replacements, as described above [12], restoring mandibular distally extended edentulism with a second molar defect might be acceptable, similar to receiving no prosthetic treatment for a second molar defect in natural dentition. However, a much larger occlusal force on the superstructure of the first molar was observed compared with the first molar on the natural dentition side of model Im6, the first molar on the natural dentition side of model Im456, and the first molar on the defect side of model MT7 under load 800 N. These finding might indicate a risk of damage to implants and surrounding bone tissue.

Effect on TMJs

In this study, force distribution on the left TMJ (defect side) was similar to that on the right TMJ (natural dentition side) under not only load 100 N but also other loading conditions. Hattori et al. [41] did not find evidence that the SDA causes overloading of the joints or the teeth, which suggests that neuromuscular regulatory systems control maximum clenching strength under various occlusal conditions. Reissmann et al. [42] also demonstrated no significant difference between SDA patients and removable dental prosthesis patients. Therefore, apprehension concerning overloading of TMJs in an SDA with implants is considered to be negligible.

Limitations of this study

It should be noted that our results were obtained under conditions of vertical loading by bilaterally balanced muscle activity with tight intercuspation in the correct mandibular position because the horizontal displacement of the premolars and molars was restrained. The actual distribution of occlusal forces may differ due to individual differences in the material properties of the soft tissue. Additionally, the lateral load, which may occur in lateral movement of the mandible during mastication, was not considered. Furthermore, this study investigated only the biomechanical aspect of the SDA using implants. The function and QoL of real patients with SDA should be investigated in future studies. Moreover, it is unclear whether the occlusal force of each tooth and implant observed in this study is harmful in human. Further investigation should include analysis of bone strain.

Conclusions

Within the limitations of this theoretical study, we demonstrated that restoration with the same number of implants as missing teeth shows almost symmetric occlusal force distribution, and it produced less biomechanically stress for a unilateral defect of the mandible. However, if restoration of a missing second molar with an implant is impossible or difficult, then an SDA with implants may also be acceptable except for individuals with severe bruxism.

Authors' contributions

MY designed the study, constructed FE models, performed final calculations, and wrote the manuscript. YT constructed FE models and programming for nonlinear FE models. AY constructed FE models. All authors read and approved the final manuscript.

Competing interests

Author Masazumi Yoshitani, Yoshiyuki Takayama, and Atsuro Yokoyama state that there are no competing interests.

Author details

[1]Division of Oral Functional Science, Department of Oral Functional Prosthodontics, Graduate School of Dental Medicine, Hokkaido University, Kita-13, Nishi-7, Kita-ku, Sapporo 060-8648, Japan. [2]Removable Prosthodontics, Hokkaido University Hospital, Hokkaido University, Kita-14, Nishi-5, Kita-Ku, Sapporo 060-8648, Japan.

References

1. Chappuis V, Buser R, Bragger U, Bornstein MM, Salvi GE, Buser D. Long-term outcomes of dental implants with a titanium plasma-sprayed surface: a 20-year prospective case series study in partially edentulous patients. Clin Implant Dent Relat Res. 2013;15:780–90.
2. Bural C, Bilhan H, Cilingir A, Geckili O. Assessment of demographic and clinical data related to dental implants in a group of Turkish patients treated at a university clinic. J Adv Prosthodont. 2013;5:351–8.
3. Leong DJ, Chan HL, Yeh CY, Takarakis N, Fu JH, Wang HL. Risk of lingual plate perforation during implant placement in the posterior mandible: a human cadaver study. Implant Dent. 2011;20:360–3.
4. Chan HL, Benavides E, Yeh CY, Fu JH, Rudek IE, Wang HL. Risk assessment of lingual plate perforation in posterior mandibular region: a virtual implant placement study using cone-beam computed tomography. J Periodontol. 2011;82:129–35.
5. Nickenig HJ, Wichmann M, Eitner S, Zoller JE, Kreppel M. Lingual concavities in the mandible: a morphological study using cross-sectional analysis determined by CBCT. J Craniomaxillofac Surg. 2015;43:254–9.
6. Vogel R, Smith-Palmer J, Valentine W. Evaluating the health economic implications and cost-effectiveness of dental implants: a literature review. Int J Oral Maxillofac Implants. 2013;28:343–56.
7. Beikler T, Flemmig TF. EAO consensus conference: economic evaluation of implant-supported prostheses. Clin Oral Implants Res. 2015;26(Suppl 11):57–63.
8. Swelem AA, Gurevich KG, Fabrikant EG, Hassan MH, Aqou S. Oral health-related quality of life in partially edentulous patients treated with removable, fixed, fixed-removable, and implant-supported prostheses. Int J Prosthodont. 2014;27:338–47.
9. Kayser AF. Shortened dental arches and oral function. J Oral Rehabil. 1981;8:457–62.
10. Witter DJ, de Haan AF, Kayser AF, van Rossum GM. A 6-year follow-up study of oral function in shortened dental arches. Part I: occlusal stability. J Oral Rehabil. 1994;21:113–25.
11. Witter DJ, Creugers NH, Kreulen CM, de Haan AF. Occlusal stability in shortened dental arches. J Dent Res. 2001;80:432–6.
12. Fueki K, Igarashi Y, Maeda Y, Baba K, Koyano K, Sasaki K, Akagawa Y, Kuboki T, Kasugai S, Garrett NR. Effect of prosthetic restoration on oral health-related quality of life in patients with shortened dental arches: a multicentre study. J Oral Rehabil. 2015;42:701–8.
13. Baba K, Igarashi Y, Nishiyama A, John MT, Akagawa Y, Ikebe K, Ishigami T, Kobayashi H, Yamashita S. Patterns of missing occlusal units and oral health-related quality of life in SDA patients. J Oral Rehabil. 2008;35:621–8.

14. Kasai K, Takayama Y, Yokoyama A. Distribution of occlusal forces during occlusal adjustment of dental implant prostheses: a nonlinear finite element analysis considering the capacity for displacement of opposing teeth and implants. Int J Oral Maxillofac Implants. 2012;27:329–35.

15. Kayumi S, Takayama Y, Yokoyama A, Ueda N. Effect of bite force in occlusal adjustment of dental implants on the distribution of occlusal pressure: comparison among three bite forces in occlusal adjustment. Int J Implant Dent. 2015;1:14.

16. Kasai K, Enomoto Y, Ogawa T, Kawasaki Y, Kanazawa E, Iwasawa T. Morphological characteristics of vertical sections of the mandible obtained by CT scanning. Anthropol Sci. 1996;104:187–98.

17. Lim JE, Lee SJ, Kim YJ, Lim WH, Chun YS. Comparison of cortical bone thickness and root proximity at maxillary and mandibular interradicular sites for orthodontic mini-implant placement. Orthod Craniofac Res. 2009;12:299–304.

18. Zarb GA, Bolender CL. Implant prosthodontics for edentulous patients: current and future directions. In: Elsubeihi ES, Attard N, Zarb GA, editors. Prosthodontic treatment for edentulous patients: complete denture and implant-supported prostheses. 12th ed. St. Louis: Mosby; 2004.

19. Sicher H, DuBrul EL. The musculature. The dentition and occlusion. In: Sicher H, DuBrul EL, editors. Sicher and DuBrul's Oral Anatomy. 8th ed. St. Louis. Ishiyaku EuroAmerica: Tokyo; 1988.

20. Schroeder HE. Development, structure, and function of periodontal tissues. In: Schroeder HE, editor. The Periodontium. Berlin: Springer-Verlag; 1986.

21. Parfitt GJ. Measurement of the physiological mobility of individual teeth in an axial direction. J Dent Res. 1960;39:608–18.

22. Miura H, Hasegawa S, Okada D, Ishihara H. The measurement of physiological tooth displacement in function. J Med Dent Sci. 1998;45:103–15.

23. Misch CE. Occlusal considerations for implant-supported prostheses: implant protective occlusion and occlusal materials. In: Misch CE, Bidez MW, editors. Contemporary implant dentistry. 2nd ed. St Louis: Mosby; 1999.

24. Kim Y, Oh TJ, Misch CE, Wang HL. Occlusal considerations in implant therapy: clinical guidelines with biomechanical rationale. Clin Oral Implants Res. 2005;16:26–35.

25. Korioth TW, Hannam AG. Deformation of the human mandible during simulated tooth clenching. J Dent Res. 1994;73:56–66.

26. van Zyl PP, Grundling NL, Jooste CH, Terblanche E. Three-dimensional finite element model of a human mandible incorporating six osseointegrated implants for stress analysis of mandibular cantilever prostheses. Int J Oral Maxillofac Implants. 1995;10:51–7.

27. Kunavisarut C, Lang LA, Stoner BR, Felton DA. Finite element analysis on dental implant-supported prostheses without passive fit. J Prosthodont. 2002;11:30–40.

28. Kobayashi K, Yorimoto T, Hikita K, Maida T. Abutment forms and restorative materials in adhesive prosthesis: a finite element analysis. Dent Mater J. 2004;23:75–80.

29. Kitamura E, Stegaroiu R, Nomura S, Miyakawa O. Influence of marginal bone resorption on stress around an implant––a three-dimensional finite element analysis. J Oral Rehabil. 2005;32:279–86.

30. Martinez JB, Oloyede VO, Broom ND. Biomechanics of load-bearing of the intervertebral disc: an experimental and finite element model. Med Eng Phys. 1997;19:145–56.

31. Kumagai H, Suzuki T, Hamada T, Sondang P, Fujitani M, Nikawa H. Occlusal force distribution on the dental arch during various levels of clenching. J Oral Rehabil. 1999;26:932–5.

32. Iplikcioglu H, Akca K, Cehreli MC, Sahin S. Comparison of non-linear finite element stress analysis with in vitro strain gauge measurements on Morse taper implant. Int J Oral Maxillofac Implants. 2003;18:258–65.

33. Eser A, Akca K, Eckert S, Cehreli MC. Nonlinear finite element analysis versus ex vivo strain gauge measurement on immediately loaded implants. Int J Oral Maxillofac Implants. 2009;24:439–46.

34. Tanaka E, van Eijden T. Biomechanical behavior of the temporomandibular joint disc. Crit Rev Oral Biol Med. 2003;14:138–50.

35. Singh M, Detamore MS. Biomechanical properties of the mandibular condylar cartilage and their relevance to the TMJ disc. J Biomech. 2009; 42:405–17.

36. Hansson T, Nordstrom B. Thickness of the soft tissue layers and articular disk in temporomandibular joints with deviations in form. Acta Odontol Scand. 1977;35:281–8.

37. Minagi S, Ohmori T, Sato T, Matsunaga T, Akamatsu Y. Effect of eccentric clenching on mandibular deviation in the vicinity of mandibular rest position. J Oral Rehabil. 2000;27:175–9.

38. Yamazaki M, Yugami K, Baba K, Ohyama T. Effect of clenching level on mandibular displacement in Kennedy Class II partially edentulous patients. Int J Prosthodont. 2003;16:183–8.

39. Gibbs CH, Mahan PE, Lundeen HC, Brehnan K, Walsh EK, Holbrook WB. Occlusal forces during chewing and swallowing as measured by sound transmission. J Prosthet Dent. 1981;46:443–9.

40. Nishigawa K, Bando E, Nakano M. Quantitative study of bite force during sleep associated bruxism. J Oral Rehabil. 2001;28:485–91.

41. Hattori Y, Satoh C, Seki S, Watanabe Y, Ogino Y, Watanabe M. Occlusal and TMJ loads in subjects with experimentally shortened dental arches. J Dent Res. 2003;82:532–6.

42. Reissmann DR, Heydecke G, Schierz O, Marre B, Wolfart S, Strub JR, Stark H, Pospiech P, Mundt T, Hannak W, Hartmann S, Wostmann B, Luthardt RG, Boning KW, Kern M, Walter MH. The randomized shortened dental arch study: temporomandibular disorder pain. Clin Oral Investig. 2014;18:2159–69.

23

The influence of surface texture and wettability on initial bacterial adhesion on titanium and zirconium oxide dental implants

Torsten Wassmann[1][*] ⓘ, Stefan Kreis[2], Michael Behr[2] and Ralf Buergers[1,2]

Abstract

Background: This study aims to investigate bacterial adhesion on different titanium and ceramic implant surfaces, to correlate these findings with surface roughness and surface hydrophobicity, and to define the predominant factor for bacterial adhesion for each material.

Methods: Zirconia and titanium specimens with different surface textures and wettability (5.0 mm in diameter, 1.0 mm in height) were prepared. Surface roughness was measured by perthometer (R_a) and atomic force microscopy, and hydrophobicity according to contact angles by computerized image analysis. Bacterial suspensions of *Streptococcus sanguinis* and *Staphylococcus epidermidis* were incubated for 2 h at 37 °C with ten test specimens for each material group and quantified with fluorescence dye CytoX-Violet and an automated multi-detection reader.

Results: Variations in surface roughness (R_a) did not lead to any differences in adhering *S. epidermidis*, but higher R_a resulted in increased *S. sanguinis* adhesion. In contrast, higher bacterial adhesion was observed on hydrophobic surfaces than on hydrophilic surfaces for *S. epidermidis* but not for *S. sanguinis*. The potential to adhere *S. sanguinis* was significantly higher on ceramic surfaces than on titanium surfaces; no such preference could be found for *S. epidermidis*.

Conclusions: Both surface roughness and wettability may influence the adhesion properties of bacteria on biomaterials; in this context, the predominant factor is dependent on the bacterial species. Wettability was the predominant factor for *S. epidermidis* and surface texture for *S. sanguinis*. Zirconia did not show any lower bacterial colonization potential than titanium. Arithmetical mean roughness values R_a (measured by stylus profilometer) are inadequate for describing surface roughness with regard to its potential influence on microbial adhesion.

Keywords: Zirconia, Titanium, Bacterial adhesion, Hydrophobicity, Roughness

Background

Dental implants are one of the most frequently used treatment options for the replacement of missing teeth. The oral microflora and its dynamic interactions with the implant substrata seem to crucially influence the long-term success or failure of dental implants [1–6]. As soon as implant surfaces are exposed to the human oral cavity, they are immediately colonized by microorganisms [7, 8].

The initial bacterial adhesion on implants is the first and essential step in the geneses of complex peri-implant biofilms, which, in turn, may result in peri-implantitis and loss of the supporting bone [3].

The type of implant material and its specific texture and physico-chemical surface properties influence the quantity and quality of microbial colonization [1, 9–12]. In modern biomaterial research, implant surfaces are mainly modified to increase osseous integration into the alveolar bone; recently however, implant surfaces are also modified to reduce biofilm formation after exposure to the oral cavity. Innovative implant materials or

* Correspondence: torsten.wassmann@med.uni-goettingen.de
[1]Present address: Department of Prosthodontics, University Medical Center Goettingen, Robert-Koch-Strasse 40, 37075 Goettingen, Germany
Full list of author information is available at the end of the article

surface modifications with reduced adhesion properties or even with antibacterial properties are of pertinent clinical interest [13, 14]. Up to now, monolithic titanium has been the most frequently used base material and gold standard for the construction of implant systems. Titanium is known for its excellent biocompatibility and outstanding mechanical properties [15]. Zirconia implant materials (ZrO_2) were introduced as an alternative to titanium implants, mainly because of their supposedly reduced potential to adhere microorganisms [1, 16–19]. Surface roughness, texture, and wettability are regarded as the most significant surface factors influencing microbial accumulation on implants [9, 10, 12, 20]. Increased surface roughness on implant surfaces correlates with faster and firmer integration into the surrounding bone [21]. On the other hand, however, most studies indicate a positive correlation between surface roughness and the amount of adhering bacteria [1, 9–11, 19, 20, 22, 23]. For titanium implant surfaces, Bollen et al. found a threshold R_a value of 0.2 μm, and lower values did not further influence the quantity of bacterial adhesion [24]. In almost every corresponding investigation, the arithmetical mean roughness R_a—which is measured by stylus profilometer—is used as a parameter to describe implant surface roughness. Rupp et al. showed that surfaces with very different morphologies may share the same R_a value. Furthermore, R_a values alone may be inadequate to describe "surface roughness" in respect to its potential influence on microbial adhesion [25]. For this reason, we additionally applied atomic force microscopy (AFM) for a three-dimensional assessment of the surface topography of the tested materials. AFM, which was developed to obtain fine details of a surface on a molecular scale, was found to be the most suitable instrument for surface roughness measurements [11, 26]. Furthermore, the crucial influence of surface wettability on bacterial adhesion is widely accepted, but there is still conflicting evidence if substrata with hydrophobic properties reduce or enhance the quantity of adhering microorganisms [9, 10, 27–31]. Although most studies describe surface roughness rather than wettability as the dominant factor for bacterial adhesion, the data on this matter is somewhat ambiguous [9–11, 20, 32–37]. So far, no study has yet varied surface roughness and hydrophobicity in well-defined patterns to define the crucial surface factor for different bacterial species.

The aim of the present in vitro study was to investigate bacterial adhesion (by means of the test species *Streptococcus sanguinis* and *Staphylococcus epidermidis*) on ten different titanium and zirconia implant surfaces. Surface texture and wettability were modified in well-defined patterns to correlate these surface properties with the amount of initially adhering bacteria and to define the predominant factor for each material and bacterial species.

Methods

Characterization of implant materials

In this study, we assessed two different implant materials in the form of round specimens (each measuring 5.0 mm in diameter and 1.0 mm in thickness, see Table 1). Half of the specimens were made of grade 1 pure titanium (Mechanische Werkstatt Biologie, University of Regensburg, Germany) and the other half of zirconia ceramic (IPS e.max ZirCAD; Ivoclar Vivadent, Ellwangen, Germany). The grade of the titanium used is the purest commercially available alloy. In comparison to other titanium grades, it is ductile and soft; however, there are very low amounts of impurities (≤1625%) and thus the lowest interferences caused by contained trace elements. The zirconia ceramic is a high-strength yttrium-stabilized zirconium oxide ceramic and as such a metal oxide ceramic. Due to its excellent mechanical properties, this ceramic is used in a wide range of indications.

Twenty specimens of each experimental implant material were subjected to one of the following surface treatments to modify surface roughness and surface free energy. The surface of some specimens was polished to high gloss with a polishing machine (Motopol 8; Buehler, Düsseldorf, Germany) and wet abrasive paper discs (Buehler, Lake Bluff, IL) with a grit of 1000, 2000, and 4000. Other specimens were sandblasted either with 50 or 250 μm aluminum trioxide at 2.5 bar for 20 s (both; Korox, Bego, Bremen, Germany). In the second part of the investigation, we additionally modified surface free energy values on the material surfaces of the rough and smooth substrata by applying n-propylsilane; hydrophilic conditions were altered by the application of aminosilane. As a result of various surface finishes (roughness and surface free energy) and the two starting materials (titanium and ceramic), there were finally ten different groups of test specimen with unique properties.

Surface roughness values of three specimens of each of the ten material groups were determined at three different sites with a stylus instrument (Perthometer S6P; Perthen, Göttingen, Germany) and shown as the arithmetic average peak-to-valley value (R_a). Water contact angles (hydrophobicities) were calculated from automated contact angle measurements (OCA 15 plus; Dataphysics Instruments, Filderstadt, Germany) with deionized water. Nine drops of the liquid (one drop 1 μl) were examined on each substratum, and the contact angle was measured exactly 15 s after the positioning of the drop.

Three-dimensional images of rough and smooth implant surfaces were obtained by means of atomic force microscopy (AFM) using the tapping mode scan of an AFM VEECO machine (Plainview, USA); this method was also used to determine the surface topography. We scanned several randomly selected areas measuring either 3 μm × 3 μm or 30 μm × 30 μm for each of the

Table 1 Arithmetic average of surface roughness R_a (means and standard deviations [μm]) and wettability (means and standard deviations [°]) of the ten tested material

Implant material	Roughness	R_a [μm]	Wettability	[°]
Ceramic	Rough	1.32 ± 0.10	Hydrophobic	83.6 ± 2.0
			Hydrophilic	47.3 ± 2.4
	Medium	0.49 ± 0.03		60.7 ± 2.6
	Smooth	0.05 ± 0.02	Hydrophobic	72.0 ± 10.5
			Hydrophilic	41.4 ± 2.5
Titanium	Rough	2.98 ± 0.31	Hydrophobic	107.6 ± 3.2
			Hydrophilic	76.2 ± 1.9
	Medium	0.83 ± 0.06		86.1 ± 3.0
	Smooth	0.09 ± 0.02	Hydrophobic	96.8 ± 2.8
			Hydrophilic	65.2 ± 2.3

test groups and sterilized all titanium specimens with UV light for 1 h before use.

Microbial adhesion

We isolated a *S. epidermidis* strain culture (AC-Acession: AF270147) from the skin of one of the authors; the sample was identified and confirmed by 16S rDNA—nucleotide comparison (IDNS® version v3.1.63r14 © Smart-Gene 2005 Molecular Mycobacteriology). After isolation, *S. epidermidis* was proliferated in BHI—culture medium (Bacto™ Brain Heart Infusion, BD Becton, Dickinson and Company Sparks, MD, USA). Glycerine was added, and bacterial cultures were stored at −80 °C. Prior to testing, cultures were defrosted and incubated at 37 °C overnight. We cultivated *S. sanguinis* (strain 20068; DSMZ) in sterile trypticase soy broth (Tryptic Soy Broth; BD Diagnostics, Sparks, MD, USA) supplemented with yeast extract (Sigma-Aldrich, St. Louis, Mo, USA). For both types of bacteria, cells were harvested by centrifugation, washed twice in phosphate-buffered saline (PBS) (Sigma-Aldrich, St. Louis, Mo, USA), and resuspended in normal saline. After that, we adjusted the cells by densitometry (Genesys 10S; Thermo Spectronic, Rochester, NY, USA) at 600 nm to a MacFarland 0.4 standard optical density that equalled the bacterial concentration of approximately 5×10^9 cfu (colony forming units)/ml.

We determined the quantity of bacterial adhesion with a fluorescence dye, i.e., the CytoX-Violet Cell Proliferation Kit (Epigentek Group Inc., New York, USA), and recorded fluorescence intensities with an automated multi-detection reader (Fluostar optima; BMG labtech, Offenburg, Germany) at wavelengths of 560 nm excitation and 590 nm emission. High relative fluorescence intensities indicate high numbers of viable adhering bacteria. For simulating the influence of a salivary pellicle, we incubated specimens in 48-well plates with 1 ml of artificial saliva for 2 h prior to adhesion testing [2]. We then removed the saliva, added 1 ml of bacterial

suspension to each well, and incubated the well plates at 37 °C for 120 min on an orbital shaker. After biofilm formation, we extracted the bacterial solution by suction and washed the specimens once with PBS to remove non-adherent bacteria. All specimens were transferred to a new 48-well plate. For each well, we added 200 μl PBS and 20 μl CytoX-Violet (indicator solution) and incubated the well plates at 37 °C for 120 min in darkness; 190 μl of the indicator solution from each well was transferred to sterile black 96-well plates, and fluorescence intensities were recorded.

Ten specimens of each material group tested were investigated. As control references, we used the fluorescence values of pure phosphate-buffered saline (0-control), buffer and CytoX-Violet (dye-control), and pure bacterial solution (bacteria-control).

Statistical analysis

All calculations and graphic displays were done with SPSS 16.0 for Windows (SPSS Corporation, Chicago, IL, USA). Means and standard deviations for R_a, water contact angles, and relative fluorescence intensities were calculated. We used three-way analysis of variance (ANOVA) to analyze the influence of R_a and hydrophobicity on the adherence of *S. sanguinis* and *S. epidermidis* to the titanium and ceramic specimens. The Tukey–Kramer multiple comparison test was applied for post hoc analysis, and the level of significance was set at $\alpha = 0.05$.

Results
Characterization of implant material groups

The median surface roughness values (R_a) of each material group ($n = 10$) tested are shown in Table 1. The differences in R_a between rough, medium, and smooth specimens were statistically significant for ceramic as well as for titanium ($p < 0.01$ for all comparisons). The roughness values of rough and medium ceramic specimens (1.32 μm/0.49 μm) were significantly lower than those of titanium specimens (2.98 μm/0.83 μm; $p < 0.01$ for both comparisons). No significant difference was found between the R_a of smooth titanium and smooth ceramic specimens (0.09 μm/0.05 μm; $p = 0.983$).

The median water contact angles (wettability) of each specimen are given in Table 1. All four hydrophobic surfaces showed significantly higher contact angles than the corresponding hydrophilic surfaces ($p < 0.01$ for rough ceramic, smooth ceramic, rough titanium, and smooth titanium). Roughness values did not change after hydrophilization or hydrophobization (data not shown).

Examples of the atomic force micrographs are given in Fig. 1a–d (30 μm × 30 μm = 900 μm² scan area), e–h (3 μm × 3 μm = 9 μm² scan area). Considerably higher roughness values could be observed on the sandblasted ceramic and titanium surfaces than on the corresponding polished surfaces. Neither the 900 μm² scan areas nor the corresponding AFM roughness profiles showed any well-defined differences between ceramic and titanium for smooth and rough specimens (Fig. 2a). On closer examination (9 μm² scan areas), small grooves (measuring approximately 0.5 μm in diameter and 0.08 μm in height) could be observed on the smooth ceramic substrata (Fig. 1g), whereas the smooth titanium surfaces seemed to be totally plane (Fig. 1h). Furthermore, the microstructure of rough titanium appeared to be significantly more irregular than the smooth titanium surface and both ceramic surfaces (Fig. 2b).

Influence of surface roughness on bacterial adhesion

The relative fluorescence intensities (rfi) for *S. epidermidis*, indicating the quantity of adhering staphylococci, narrowly varied between 2931 and 2697 relative fluorescence units (rfu) (Fig. 3a). Except for smooth titanium (2931 ± 99 rfu), on which significantly more adhering bacteria were found than on medium titanium (2697 ± 127 rfu; $p = 0.002$) and rough titanium (2734 ± 145 rfu; $p = 0.014$), variations in surface roughness did not lead to any differences in adhering *S. epidermidis*. The differences in staphylococcal adhesion on smooth (2908 ± 74 rfu), medium (2789 ± 143 rfu), and rough (2749 ± 162 rfu) ceramic specimens were not statistically significant ($p > 0.05$ for all comparisons).

In general, significantly more *S. sanguinis* adhered to ceramic surfaces than to titanium surfaces ($p < 0.05$ for all comparisons, except for smooth ceramic compared with rough titanium: $p = 0.244$) (Fig. 3b). Titanium specimens (smooth titanium 3263 ± 475 rfu; medium titanium 3331 ± 641 rfu; rough titanium 3656 ± 855 rfu) tended to show higher streptococcal adhesion on rough surfaces in comparison to medium and smooth surfaces, but the differences between the tested material groups were not statistically significant ($p > 0.05$ for all comparisons). On ceramic surfaces (smooth ceramic 4668 ±

1562 rfu; medium ceramic 5590 ± 1493 rfu, rough ceramic 6875 ± 428 rfu), higher surface roughness led to increased *S. sanguinis* adhesion ($p < 0.05$ for all comparisons, except for smooth ceramic compared with medium ceramic: $p = 0.244$).

Influence of surface wettability (hydrophobicity) on bacterial adhesion

S. epidermidis (Fig. 4a) tended to show higher bacterial adhesion on hydrophobic surfaces (titanium smooth 5337 ± 1511 rfu, titanium rough 5916 ± 2472 rfu, ceramic smooth 3395 ± 1738 rfu, and ceramic rough 2676 ± 1476 rfu) than on hydrophilic surfaces (titanium smooth 3897 ± 985 rfu, titanium rough 5662 ± 1884 rfu, ceramic smooth 2522 ± 775 rfu, and ceramic rough 1644 ± 1225 rfu), but these differences were not statistically significant ($p > 0.05$ for all comparisons). A comparison of rough and smooth specimens did not show any differences in staphylococcal adhesion ($p > 0.05$ for all comparisons).

In general, the potential to adhere *S. sanguinis* was significantly higher for all ceramic surfaces—hydrophobic and hydrophilic—than for titanium specimens ($p < 0.05$ for all 16 comparisons) (Fig. 4b). A comparison of hydrophobic and hydrophilic surfaces did not show any statistically significant differences (for smooth titanium: $p = 0.997$; for rough titanium: $p = 0.999$; for smooth ceramic: $p = 0.723$; and for rough ceramic: $p > 0.999$). Hydrophilic titanium and hydrophilic ceramic surfaces did not show any statistically significant differences between rough and smooth surfaces ($p > 0.05$ for both comparisons).

Discussion

The problems involved in osseous healing of dental implants appear to be largely solved. Biofilm formation on exposed implant and abutment surfaces, however, is a fortiori crucial for the long-term therapeutic success of an implant, because biofilms are the most frequent cause of peri-implantitis and implant loss [3–7]. Consequently, new implant surface modifications with reduced properties to accumulate microorganisms or even with antibacterial properties are of pertinent clinical interest [8, 9]. In general, the physico-chemical surface properties of an implant—influenced by the type of material, its surface morphology, and surface coatings—define the potential to adhere oral microorganisms [4, 10, 11]. In this context, surface roughness and hydrophobicity seem to be the main material-linked factors influencing microbial adhesion and biofilm formation on implant surfaces [12, 13]. Therefore, the main object of the present study was to investigate bacterial adhesion on different titanium and ceramic implant surfaces, to correlate these findings with surface roughness and surface hydrophobicity, and to

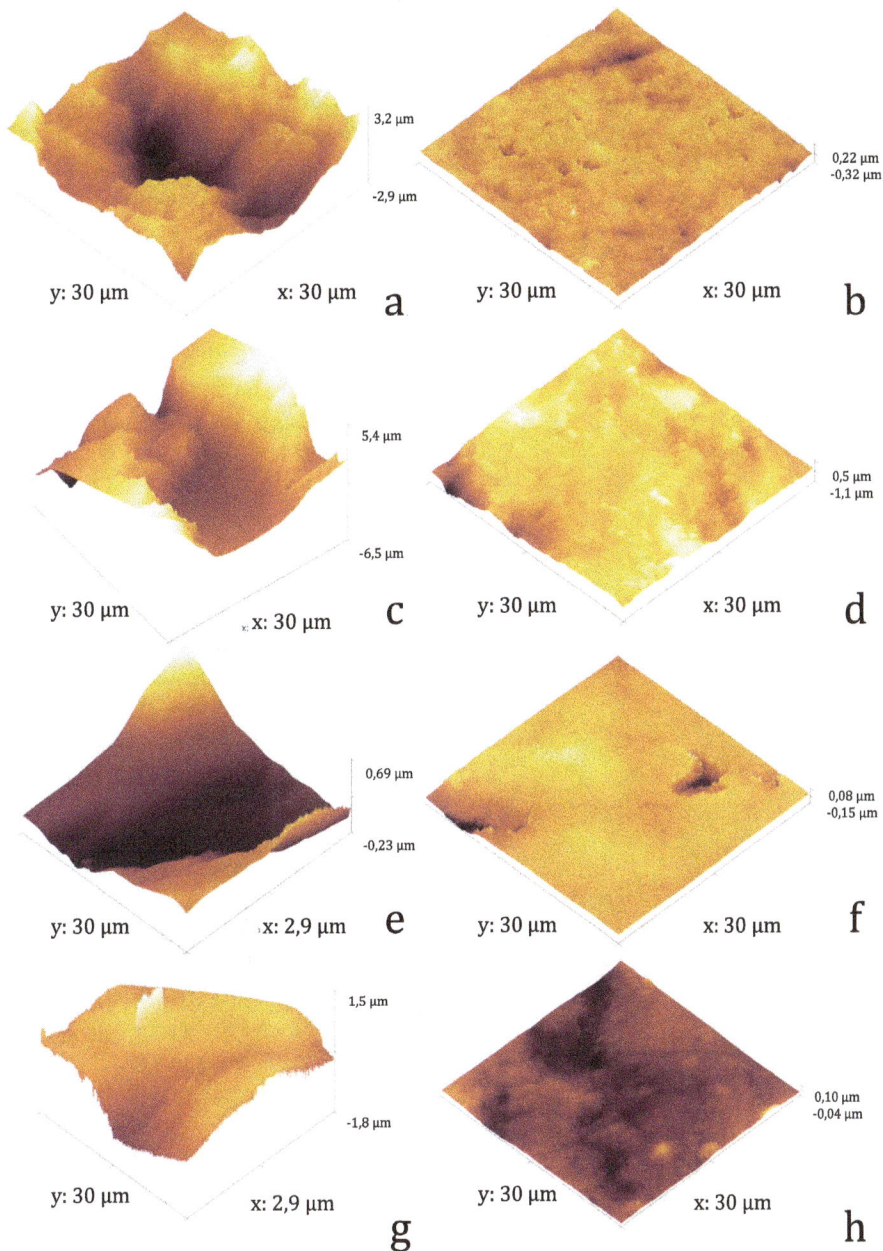

Fig. 1 AFM images for 30 μm × 30 μm (**a–d**) and 3 μm × 3 μm scan areas (**e–h**) of rough ceramic (**a, e**), smooth ceramic (**b, f**), rough titanium (**c, g**), and smooth titanium (**d, h**)

define the predominant factor for bacterial adhesion for each material group.

Implant materials and biological potentials

In dental implantology, titanium is the most frequently and most successfully used "gold standard" material because of its biocompatibility and excellent mechanical properties. The surface structure of titanium can be modified very easily by sandblasting, acid etching, plasma spraying, etc. to optimize integration into the surrounding bone [14]. Recently, high-strength zirconia implant materials (ZrO_2) have been invented as an alternative to titanium because of their resistance to corrosion and their enhanced esthetics in case of exposure and because dental ceramics are generally regarded as biomaterial with low potential to accumulate biofilms [15–18]. In fact, very little information is available on the microbial performance of zirconium implant materials. Some recent studies about biofilm formation on implant surfaces have concluded that zirconium oxide may have lower bacterial colonization potential than titanium [4, 18], an effect that is attributed to the specific

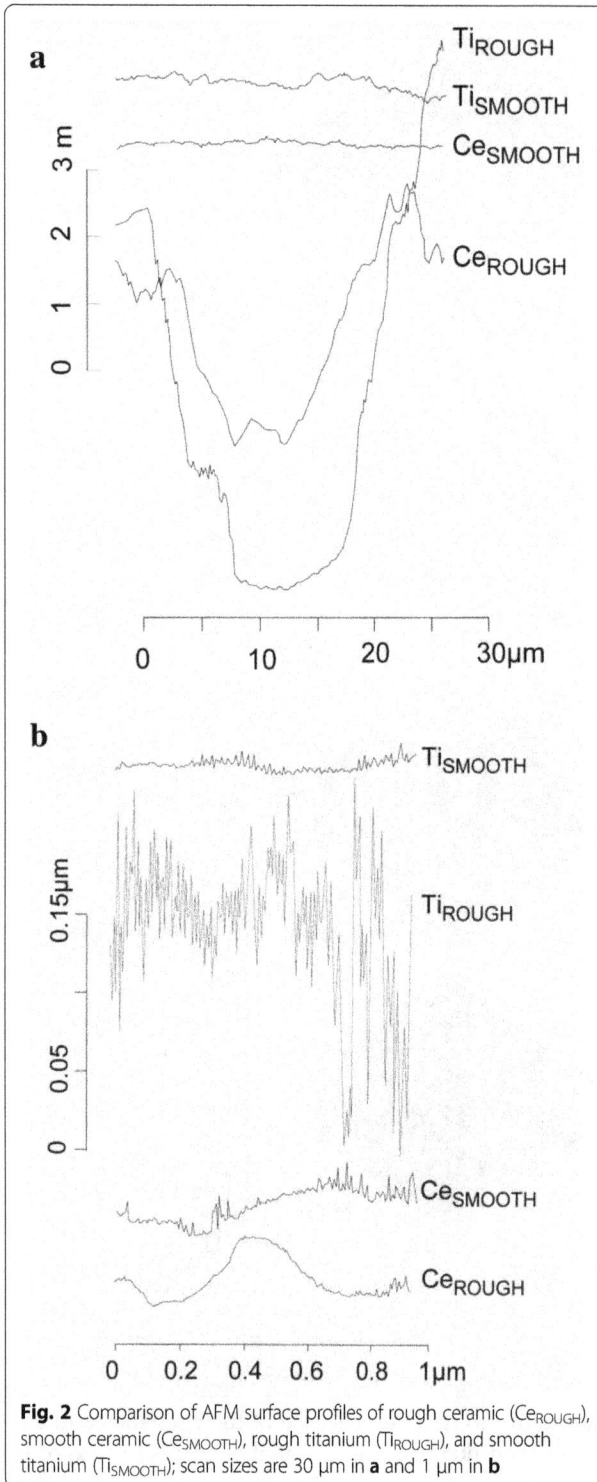

Fig. 2 Comparison of AFM surface profiles of rough ceramic (Ce$_{ROUGH}$), smooth ceramic (Ce$_{SMOOTH}$), rough titanium (Ti$_{ROUGH}$), and smooth titanium (Ti$_{SMOOTH}$); scan sizes are 30 μm in **a** and 1 μm in **b**

are not unambiguous with regard to the influence of the substratum material (titanium vs. zirconia) on bacterial adhesion. We could not find any difference between the bacterial accumulation on titanium and ceramic for *S. epidermidis*, but the potential to adhere *S. sanguinis* was significantly higher on ceramic than on titanium. Some authors reported antibacterial effects for titanium, which may be a further explanation for the rather low amounts of adhering bacteria on titanium [22, 23]. Furthermore, titanium is coated by a layer of surface oxide, which physical and mechanical characteristics are more closely related to ceramic than to metal. This phenomenon may explain why similar protein-binding properties on titanium and zirconium oxide have been reported and why zirconia did not show any reduced bacterial adhesion in the present study [20].

Surface roughness and shear forces

Besides, the surface material itself and its chemical composition, surface roughness, and hydrophobicity have a crucial influence on the accumulation of microorganisms. In most previous studies on bacterial adhesion on titanium and ceramic surfaces, the quantity of bacterial adhesion showed a direct positive correlation with surface roughness [4, 10, 18, 24–26]. In case of interacting surface roughness and hydrophobicity, roughness seems to be dominant in in vitro settings [11, 25, 27]. This phenomenon is enhanced in vivo because of the sheltering effect of rough surfaces against the removal forces present in the oral cavity [10, 28–30]. These observations were confirmed by one of our own studies, in which in vivo and in vitro initial bacterial adhesion followed the circular surface irregularities, consisting of the grinding tracks generated by the machine manufacturing of the specimen with a lathe [25]. Nevertheless, two in vivo studies reported contradictory observations on the impact of surface roughness on bacterial adhesion. Gatewood et al. [31] and Wennerberg et al. [32] worked with volunteers who carried specimens in their periodontal pockets respectively modified implant abutments for a test period up to 4 weeks and could not find any different amounts of adhering oral biofilms, neither on rough nor on smooth titanium surfaces.

In most in vivo studies on this matter, specimens are mounted on individual splints and thus exposed to shear forces related to salivary flow, muscles, and chewing activity [4, 10, 25, 33]. With regard to the "real in situ situation," no corresponding removal forces are present in the peri-implant region, which is protected from such forces by the adjacent peri-implant mucosa. The tight contact between the peri-implant soft tissues and the implant abutment surface protects implant surfaces from extensive shear forces. Therefore, shear forces and the influence of surface roughness may be overestimated in

chemical structure and the resulting electric conductivity of zirconia [4, 10, 19]. In contrast, other studies have not indicated such superiority of zirconia with regard to its microbial performance but have shown that the development of biofilm is not influenced by the type of material surface [9, 10, 20, 21]. The results of the present study

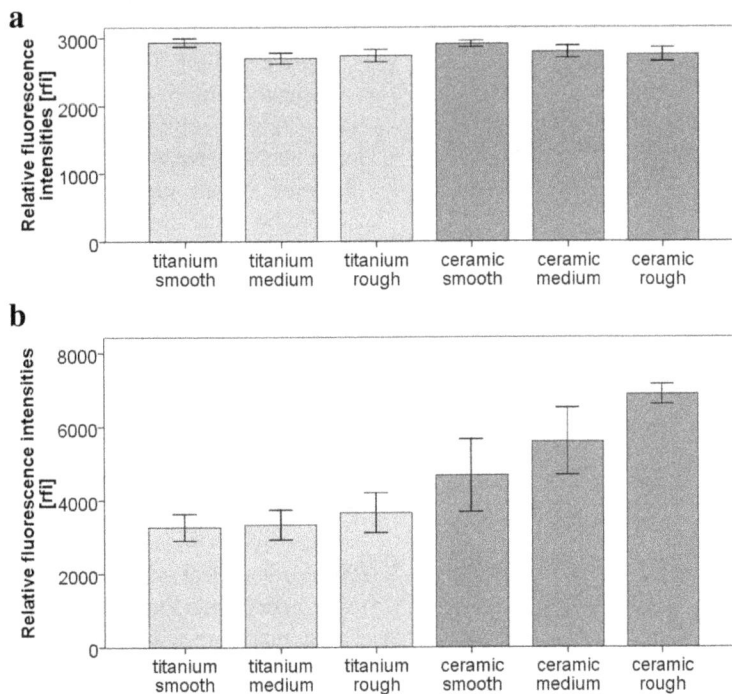

Fig. 3 Relative fluorescence intensities (rfi) of *S. epidermidis* (**a**) and *S. sanguinis* (**b**) on titanium and ceramic implant surfaces with different grades of roughness (means and standard deviations)

these specific settings. As a result, we choose a semi-static experimental setup, in which specimens were placed in an orbital shaker to simulate fluid movements in the peri-implant sulcus. This consideration was approved by the findings of Elter et al. who investigated supra- and subgingival biofilm formation on implant abutments with different roughness values. Biofilm accumulation in supragingival areas was shown to be significantly increased by higher R_a values, whereas this correlation was not found in subgingival areas [5].

In the present study, sandblasting (with 50 or 250 μm aluminum trioxide) resulted in significant increases of R_a on titanium and ceramic surfaces. These R_a values were higher than those for commercially available implant abutments (observed to range from 0.10 to 0.30 μm) [35]. According to the classification by Albrektsson and Wennerberg, smooth ceramic and titanium materials and the medium ceramic material were classified as "smooth" ($R_a < 0.5$ μm), the medium titanium material as "minimally rough" (R_a 0.5–1.0 μm), the rough ceramic material as "moderately rough" (R_a 1.1–2.0 μm), and the rough titanium material as "rough" ($R_a > 2.0$ μm) [36]. Although titanium and zirconia had the same treatment, polishing and sandblasting resulted in significantly higher R_a values on the titanium specimens than on the zirconia specimens. For titanium, Bollen et al. and Quirynen et al. evaluated a threshold R_a of 0.2 μm; below this threshold, a change in roughness

did not significantly affect the quantity of plaque accumulation [27, 37]. The medium and rough surfaces in the present study showed R_a values above the threshold of 0.2 μm; therefore, a correlation between R_a and bacterial adhesion should be expected. Surprisingly, in the present study, surface roughness (R_a) did not influence the quantity of adhering *S. epidermidis*, neither on titanium nor on zirconia. For *S. sanguinis*, such correlation was observed for zirconia but not for titanium. A possible explanation for this phenomenon can be found in the AFM observations. On closer examination (9 μm² scan areas, see Fig. 2b) and from a bacterial point of view (a single cell measures approximately 1 μm in diameter), no significant differences in surface profile or morphology could be found between all surfaces tested (except for rough titanium). From a microscopic or an AFM viewpoint, most surfaces are rough no matter how fine the finish; therefore, all types of surfaces provide adequate adhesion conditions for microbial accumulation [1]. The large-scale surface irregularities (>30 μm) on the sandblasted titanium and zirconia specimens, which were observed during the examination of the 900 μm² scan areas (Fig. 2a) and which were indicated by high R_a values, did not influence bacterial adhesion in the present semi-static experimental setup. However, these irregularities will probably increase microbial adhesion in an in vivo testing with supragingival exposition of specimens, when the influence of intraoral shear forces

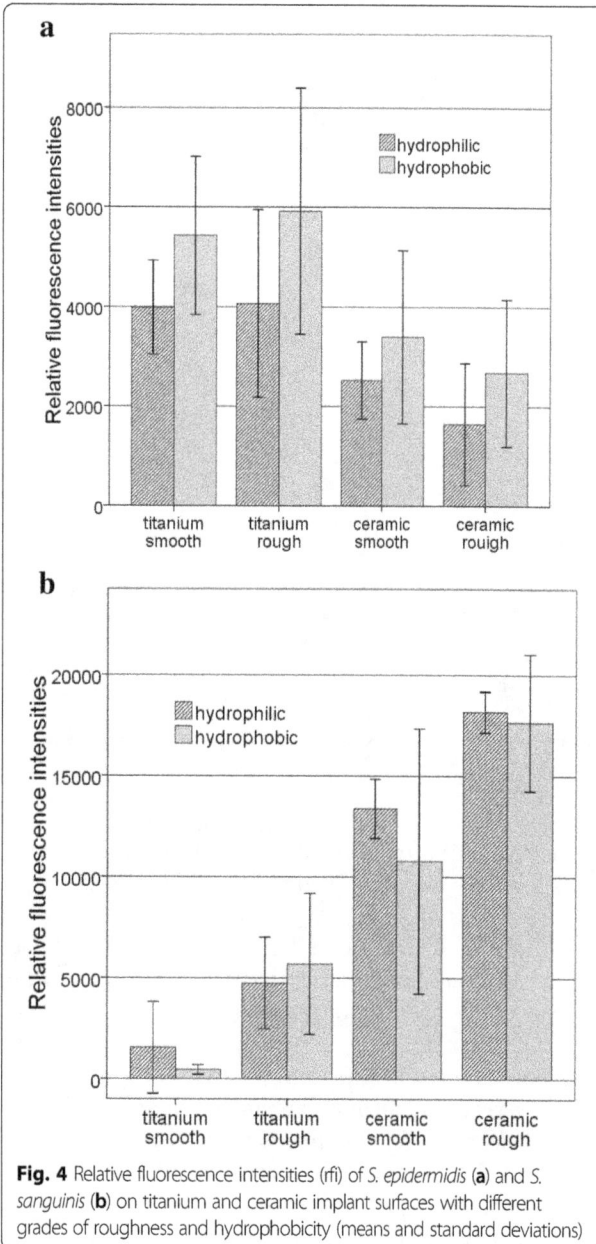

Fig. 4 Relative fluorescence intensities (rfi) of *S. epidermidis* (**a**) and *S. sanguinis* (**b**) on titanium and ceramic implant surfaces with different grades of roughness and hydrophobicity (means and standard deviations)

who observed different bacterial coverage on surfaces of the same roughness but different detailed surface morphology [40]. The different adhesion properties of *S. epidermidis* and *S. sanguinis* with regard to the influence of surface morphology may result from morphologic differences between the bacterial species. Accordingly, Barbour et al. observed that *Actinomyces naeslundi* adhere better to smooth surfaces than to rough surfaces, whereas *Streptococcus mutans* prefer rough substrata [40]. In addition, Taylor et al. could not clearly relate surface roughness of PMMA surfaces to the amount of adhering *S. epidermidis*, which supports the results of the present study [41].

Surface free energy and hydrophobicity

Besides surface roughness and morphology, the hydrophobicity and surface free energy (SFE) of an implant surface are known to influence bacterial adhesion [42, 43]. Physico-chemical interactions (non-specific) are composed of van der Waals forces, electrostatic interactions, and acid-based interactions, which in turn define the surface free energy of a substratum [44]. The surface free energy can be calculated by contact angle measurement of different liquids with differing hydrophobicities [25] or by measuring the wettability by determining water contact angles [45]. Results from different studies that relate surface free energy and hydrophobicity to microbial adhesion are conflicting [44, 46]. However, it has become apparent that, according to the thermodynamic model of microbial adhesion, hydrophobic materials are preferentially colonized by hydrophobic bacteria and vice versa [39, 44, 47–49]. Consequently, the adhesion properties of different bacteria are affected by the hydrophobicity of the bacterial cell surface [11, 44]. Both *S. epidermidis* and *S. sanguinis* are known to be rather hydrophobic; therefore, hydrophobic surfaces are preferable [44, 49]. Accordingly, Drake et al. reported that titanium samples with hydrophobic surfaces have higher levels of bacterial colonization of *S. sanguinis* than titanium samples with hydrophilic surfaces [50]. Surface roughness itself is known to influence hydrophobicity [51], but many studies have also clearly shown that minor variations in surface roughness do not significantly affect hydrophobicity values [12]. In the present study, different specimens with varying hydrophobicity but similar surface roughness were selected to eliminate the influence of surface roughness. To our knowledge, this is the first in vitro study to vary surface roughness and hydrophobicity in well-defined patterns to define the predominant factor for the two single-species biofilms tested. For *S. sanguinis*, no significant difference could be found with regard to bacterial adhesion between the hydrophobic and hydrophilic surfaces of zirconia and titanium. In contrast, *S. epidermidis* showed higher initial adhesion on hydrophobic than on hydrophilic surfaces; this finding can be attributed to the hydrophobic properties of

becomes apparent [25, 28, 29]. In contrast, the small grooves (measuring approximately 0.5 μm in diameter) on smooth zirconia surfaces in AFM may possibly explain the enhanced potential to adhere bacteria in contrast to totally plane titanium surfaces, because initial microbial colonization has been shown to start from very small—and not from large-scale—pits and gullies [25, 26, 38, 39]. In summary, characterizing the influence of surface morphology on initial bacterial adhesion (in the semi-static and static environment such as the peri-implant) by surface roughness values such as R_a alone is rather inadequate because of the requirement of an additional three-dimensional analysis of the microstructure. These observations were confirmed by Barbour et al.

S. epidermidis and explained by the thermodynamic model of microbial adhesion.

Biofilm models

In vivo biofilm models with multi-species biofilms offer the opportunity to evaluate materials in simulated clinical conditions including composite plaque, salivary pellicle, and removal forces [18]. Although the understanding of oral biofilms and the influence of surface characteristics on microbial accumulation has increased, significant gaps in the fundamental knowledge about the formation and establishment of such microbial communities still exist. Furthermore, the most essential processes in oral biofilm formation are not yet fully understood [52]. Therefore, it is necessary to examine the correlation between bacterial adhesion—including differences between different species—and modifications of surface characteristics in simplified, reproducible, and manageable in vitro systems to transfer the knowledge on fundamental in vitro matters to new clinical biomaterial implementations. Additionally, we indicated in a previous study the possibility of a correlation between in vivo and semi-static in vitro findings in respect to microbial adhesion on surfaces with different surface properties [25]. Even in a simplified in vitro setting, the quantity and quality of bacterial accumulation are influenced by many factors; in vitro relationships between surface characteristics and bacterial adhesion depend on experimental conditions, such as preconditioning protein films and the simulation of shear forces [8, 53]. For example, salivary proteins mediate the initial accumulation of microorganisms in the human oral cavity [54]. For simulating the influence of the salivary pellicle in vitro, specimens may be incubated in various saliva solutions before bacterial adhesion testing. In the present study, all specimens were pre-incubated with artificial saliva [2], which was chosen to exclude the influence of inter-individual variations in salivary protein content and the composition of human saliva so that reproducible results could be achieved [26, 55]. Two different single-species biofilms, *S. epidermidis* and *S. sanguinis*, were used as test microorganisms to investigate the potential of differently treated implant surfaces to adhere these bacteria. *S. epidermidis* and *S. sanguinis* are not usually associated with active peri-implantitis, but they are amongst the main early colonizers of oral tissues and artificial biomaterials, paving the way for more pathogenic species [56–58]. *S. epidermidis* and *S. sanguinis* represent two dominant but very different bacterial families, i.e., Streptococcaceae and Staphylococcaceae, which are members of the human oral microbiome; these bacteria normally reside on the mucous membranes of humans and can bind to hard surfaces in the oral cavity [57]. *S. sanguinuis* is commonly present in the human oral cavity and known as a pioneer bacterium of oral biofilms [10, 18, 56, 58, 59]. *S. epidermidis*, normally a commensal bacterium of the skin, is a major concern for

patients with surgical implants, causing the growth of pathogenic biofilms on various implant devices, such as breast and hip implants, which may result in implant failure [60]. In some recent studies, *S. epidermidis* has also been detected in pathogenic biofilms on failing dental implants [43]. Fluorometric techniques offer the opportunity to quantitatively investigate a high number of specimens in a short period of time and, at the same time, provide reproducible and significant data [25]. In this study, the CytoX-Violet Cell Proliferation Assay Kit was used to simply measure the amount of viable bacteria adhering to the test specimens. The fluorometric change of the indicator solution shows the activity of the cellular dehydrogenases and is directly proportional to the cell viability of adhering bacteria. It should be mentioned that this specific method fails to indicate vital adhering bacteria and cannot differentiate between cultivable vital cells and non-cultivable vital cells. This is important because large amounts of dead bacteria (up to 40%) have already been found after short incubation times [25].

Conclusions

Within the limitations of an in vitro study, our results indicate that surface roughness as well as wettability may influence the adhesion properties of bacteria on implant surfaces. Furthermore, the predominant factor for adhesion depends on the bacterial species itself. Zirconia implant material did not show any lower bacterial colonization potential than titanium. The influence of substratum material, surface texture, and wettability of implant surfaces on microbial adhesion does not exactly follow universal rules and differs between bacterial species. Additionally, arithmetical mean roughness values R_a (measured by stylus profilometer) are inadequate for describing surface roughness in respect to its potential influence on microbial adhesion. Future studies may use more sophisticated techniques such as confocal microscopy, wide-angle confocal microscopy or laser scanning microscopy in order to gain precise three-dimensional topographical values and to evaluate their influence on microbial adhesion.

Acknowledgements
The great support of Juri Allerdings and the skilled technical assistance of Gerlinde Held and Marlene Rosendahl are gratefully acknowledged.

Funding
The study has been funded solely by the institutions of the authors.

Authors' contributions
TW participated in the design of the study, carried out the statistical analysis, and drafted the manuscript. SK designed and manufactured the specimen and carried out the microbial trials. MB and RB conceived of the study and participated together in its design and coordination. MB helped to draft the manuscript, so did RB. All authors read and approved the final manuscript.

Author details
[1]Present address: Department of Prosthodontics, University Medical Center Goettingen, Robert-Koch-Strasse 40, 37075 Goettingen, Germany.
[2]Department of Prosthetic Dentistry, Regensburg University Medical Centre, Regensburg, Germany.

References

1. Poon CY, Bhushan B. Comparison of surface roughness measurements by stylus profiler, AFM and non-contact profiler. Wear. 1995;190:76–88.

2. Hahnel S, Rosentritt M, Handel G, Bürgers R. Surface characterization of dental ceramics and initial streptococcal adhesion in vitro. Dent Mater. 2009;25:969–75.

3. Abrahamsson I, Berglundh T, Lindhe J. Soft tissue response to plaque formation at different implant systems. A comparative study in the dog. Clin Oral Implants Res. 1998;9:73–9.

4. Scarano A, Piattelli M, Caputi S, Favero GA, Piattelli A. Bacterial adhesion on commercially pure titanium and zirconium oxide disks: an in vivo human study. J Periodontol. 2004;75:292–6.

5. Elter C, Heuer W, Demling A, Hannig M, Heidenblut T, Bach FW, et al. Supra- and subgingival biofilm formation on implant abutments with different surface characteristics. Int J Oral Maxillofac Implants. 2008;23:327–34.

6. Oh TJ, Yoon J, Misch CE, Wang HL. The causes of early implant bone loss: myth or science? J Periodontol. 2002;73:322–33.

7. Zitzmann NU, Abrahamsson I, Berglundh T, Lindhe J. Soft tissue reactions to plaque formation at implant abutments with different surface topography. An experimental study in dogs. J Clin Periodontol. 2002;29:456–61.

8. Busscher HJ, Rinastiti M, Siswomihardjo W, van der Mei HC. Biofilm formation on dental restorative and implant materials. J Dent Res. 2010;89: 657–65.

9. Van Brakel R, Cune MS, Van Winkelhoff AJ, De Putter C, Verhoeven JW, Van Der Reijden W. Early bacterial colonization and soft tissue health around zirconia and titanium abutments: an in vivo study in man. Clin Oral Implants Res. 2010. doi:10.1111/j.1600-0501.2010.02005.

10. Al-Ahmad A, Wiedmann-Al-Ahmad M, Faust J, Bachle M, Follo M, Wolkewitz M, et al. Biofilm formation and composition on different implant materials in vivo. J Biomed Mater Res B Appl Biomater. 2010;95:101–9.

11. Teughels W, Van Assche N, Sliepen I, Quirynen M. Effect of material characteristics and/or surface topography on biofilm development. Clin Oral Implants Res. 2006;17:68–81.

12. Quirynen M, Bollen CM. The influence of surface roughness and surface-free energy on supra- and subgingival plaque formation in man. A review of the literature. J Clin Periodontol. 1995;22:1–14.

13. An YH, Friedman RJ. Concise review of mechanisms of bacterial adhesion to biomaterial surfaces. J Biomed Mater Res. 1998;43:338–48.

14. Palmquist A, Omar OM, Esposito M, Lausmaa J, Thomsen P. Titanium oral implants: surface characteristics, interface biology and clinical outcome. J R Soc Interface. 2010;7:515–27.

15. Hannig C, Hannig M. The oral cavity—a key system to understand substratum-dependent bioadhesion on solid surfaces in man. Clin Oral Investig. 2009;13:123–39.

16. Kawai K, Urano M. Adherence of plaque components to different restorative materials. Oper Dent. 2001;26:396–400.

17. Piconi C, Maccauro G. Zirconia as a ceramic biomaterial. Biomaterials. 1999; 20:1–25.

18. Rimondini L, Cerroni L, Carrassi A, Torricelli P. Bacterial colonization of zirconia ceramic surfaces: an in vitro and in vivo study. Int J Oral Maxillofac Implants. 2002;17:793–8.

19. Poortinga AT, Bos R, Busscher HJ. Measurement of charge transfer during bacterial adhesion to an indium tin oxide surface in a parallel plate flow chamber. J Microbiol Methods. 1999;38:183–9.

20. Lima EM, Koo H, Vacca Smith AM, Rosalen PL, Del Bel Cury AA. Adsorption of salivary and serum proteins and bacterial adherence on titanium and zirconia ceramic surfaces. Clin Oral Implants Res. 2008;19:780–5.

21. Tanner A, Maiden MF, Lee K, Shulman LB, Weber HP. Dental implant infections. Clin Infect Dis. 1997;25:213–7.

22. Bundy KJ, Butler MF, Hochman RF. An investigation of the bacteriostatic properties of pure metals. J Biomed Mater Res. 1980;14:653–63.

23. Leonhardt A, Dahlen G. Effect of titanium on selected oral bacterial species in vitro. Eur J Oral Sci. 1995;103:382–7.

24. Rimondini L, Fare S, Brambilla E, Felloni A, Consonni C, Brossa F, et al. The effect of surface roughness on early in vivo plaque colonization on titanium. J Periodontol. 1997;68:556–62.

25. Bürgers R, Gerlach T, Hahnel S, Schwarz F, Handel G, Gosau M. In vivo and in vitro biofilm formation on two different titanium implant surfaces. Clin Oral Implants Res. 2010;21:156–64.

26. Burgers R, Hahnel S, Reichert TE, Rosentritt M, Behr M, Gerlach T, et al. Adhesion of Candida albicans to various dental implant surfaces and the influence of salivary pellicle proteins. Acta Biomater. 2010;6:2307–13.

27. Quirynen M, Bollen CM, Papaioannou W, Van Eldere J, van Steenberghe D. The influence of titanium abutment surface roughness on plaque accumulation and gingivitis: short-term observations. Int J Oral Maxillofac Implants. 1996;11:169–78.

28. Hannig M. Transmission electron microscopy of early plaque formation on dental materials in vivo. Eur J Oral Sci. 1999;107:55–64.

29. Quirynen M, van der Mei HC, Bollen CM, Schotte A, Marechal M, Doornbusch GI. An in vivo study of the influence of the surface roughness of implants on the microbiology of supra- and subgingival plaque. J Dent Res. 1993;72:1304–9.

30. Nyvad B, Fejerskov O. Scanning electron microscopy of early microbial colonization of human enamel and root surfaces in vivo. Scand J Dent Res. 1987;95:287–96.

31. Gatewood RR, Cobb CM, Killoy WJ. Microbial colonization on natural tooth structure compared with smooth and plasma-sprayed dental implant surfaces. Clin Oral Implants Res. 1993;4:53–64.

32. Wennerberg A, Sennerby L, Kultje C, Lekholm U. Some soft tissue characteristics at implant abutments with different surface topography. A study in humans. J Clin Periodontol. 2003;30:88–94.

33. Grossner-Schreiber B, Teichmann J, Hannig M, Dorfer C, Wenderoth DF, Ott SJ. Modified implant surfaces show different biofilm compositions under in vivo conditions. Clin Oral Implants Res. 2009;20:817–26.

34. Rupp F, Scheideler L, Rehbein D, Axmann D, Geis-Gerstorfer J. Roughness induced dynamic changes of wettability of acid etched titanium implant modifications. Biomaterials. 2004;25:1429–38.

35. Quirynen M, Bollen CM, Willems G, van Steenberghe D. Comparison of surface characteristics of six commercially pure titanium abutments. Int J Oral Maxillofac Implants. 1994;9:71–6.

36. Albrektsson T, Wennerberg A. Oral implant surfaces: part 1—review focusing on topographic and chemical properties of different surfaces and in vivo responses to them. Int J Prosthodont. 2004;17:536–43.

37. Bollen CM, Papaioanno W, Van Eldere J, Schepers E, Quirynen M, van Steenberghe D. The influence of abutment surface roughness on plaque accumulation and peri-implant mucositis. Clin Oral Implants Res. 1996;7:201–11.

38. Quirynen M, De Soete M, van Steenberghe D. Infectious risks for oral implants: a review of the literature. Clin Oral Implants Res. 2002;13:1–19.

39. Weerkamp AH, Uyen HM, Busscher HJ. Effect of zeta potential and surface energy on bacterial adhesion to uncoated and saliva-coated human enamel and dentin. J Dent Res. 1988;67:1483–7.

40. Barbour ME, O'Sullivan DJ, Jenkinson HF, Jagger DC. The effects of polishing methods on surface morphology, roughness and bacterial colonisation of titanium abutments. J Mater Sci Mater Med. 2007;18:1439–47.

41. Taylor RL, Verran J, Lees GC, Ward AJ. The influence of substratum topography on bacterial adhesion to polymethyl methacrylate. J Mater Sci Mater Med. 1998;9:17–22.

42. Quirynen M, Van der Mei HC, Bollen CM, Van den Bossche LH, Doornbusch GI, van Steenberghe D, et al. The influence of surface-free energy on supra- and subgingival plaque microbiology. An in vivo study on implants. J Periodontol. 1994;65:162–7.

43. Subramani K, Jung RE, Molenberg A, Hammerle CH. Biofilm on dental implants: a review of the literature. Int J Oral Maxillofac Implants. 2009;24: 616–26.

44. Grivet M, Morrier JJ, Benay G, Barsotti O. Effect of hydrophobicity on in vitro streptococcal adhesion to dental alloys. J Mater Sci Mater Med. 2000;11: 637–42.

45. Bürgers R, Schneider-Brachert W, Rosentritt M, Handel G, Hahnel S. Candida albicans adhesion to composite resin materials. Clin Oral Investig. 2009;13: 293–9.

46. Nassar U, Meyer AE, Ogle RE, Baier RE. The effect of restorative and prosthetic materials on dental plaque. Periodontol. 2000;1995;8,114–124.

47. Mabboux F, Ponsonnet L, Morrier JJ, Jaffrezic N, Barsotti O. Surface free energy and bacterial retention to saliva-coated dental implant materials—an in vitro study. Colloids Surf B Biointerfaces. 2004;25:199–205.

48. Weerkamp AH, van der Mei HC, Busscher HJ. The surface free energy of oral streptococci after being coated with saliva and its relation to adhesion in the mouth. J Dent Res. 1985;64:1204–10.

49. Verran J, Taylor RL, Lees GC. Bacterial adhesion to inert thermoplastic surfaces. J Mater Sci Mater Med. 1996;7:597.

50. Drake DR, Paul J, Keller JC. Primary bacterial adhesion of implant surfaces. Int J Oral Maxillofac Implants. 1999;14:226–32.

51. Lim YJ, Oshida Y. Initial contact angle measurements on variously treated dental/medical titanium materials. Biomed Mater Eng. 2001;11:325–41.

52. Steinberg D, Sela MN, Klinger A, Kohavi D. Adhesion of periodontal bacteria to titanium and titanium alloy powders. Clin Oral Implants Res. 1998;9:67–72.

53. Bakker DP, Postmus BR, Busscher HJ, van der Mei HC. Bacterial strains isolated from different niches can exhibit different patterns of adhesion to substrata. Appl Environ Microbiol. 2004;70:3758–60.

54. Carlen A, Rudiger SG, Loggner I, Olsson J. Bacteria-binding plasma proteins in pellicles formed on hydroxyapatite in vitro and on teeth in vivo. Oral Microbiol Immunol. 2003;18:203–7.

55. Edgerton M, Lo SE, Scannapieco FA. Experimental salivary pellicles formed on titanium surfaces mediate adhesion of streptococci. Int J Oral Maxillofac Implants. 1996;11:443–9.

56. Grossner-Schreiber B, Griepentrog M, Haustein I, Muller WD, Lange KP, Briedigkeit H, et al. Plaque formation on surface modified dental implants. An in vitro study. Clin Oral Implants Res. 2001;12:543–51.

57. Dewhirst FE, Chen T, Izard J, Paster BJ, Tanner AC, Yu WH, et al. The human oral microbiome. J Bacteriol. 2010;192:5002–17.

58. Kolenbrander PE, Ganeshkumar N, Cassels FJ, Hughes CV. Coaggregation: specific adherence among human oral plaque bacteria. FASEB J. 1993;7: 406–13.

59. Del Curto B, Brunella MF, Giordano C, Pedeferri MP, Valtulina V, Visai L, et al. Decreased bacterial adhesion to surface-treated titanium. Int J Artif Organs. 2005;28:718–30.

60. Freedman AM, Jackson IT. Infections in breast implants. Infect Dis Clin North Am. 1989;3:275–87.

24

Osteogenesis ability of CAD/CAM porous zirconia scaffolds enriched with nano-hydroxyapatite particles

Moustafa N. Aboushelib[1][*] and Rehab Shawky[2]

Abstract

Background: The aim of this study was to evaluate osteogenesis ability of CAD/CAM porous zirconia scaffolds enriched with hydroxy apatite used to augment large boney defects in a dog model.

Methods: Surgical defects were made bilaterally on the lower jaw of 12 Beagle dogs. Cone beam CT images were used to create three dimensional images of the healed defects. Porous zirconia scaffolds were fabricated by milling custom made CAD/CAM blocks into the desired shape. After sintering, the pores of half of the scaffolds were filled with a nano-hydroxy apatite (HA) powder while the other half served as control. The scaffolds were inserted bilaterally in the healed mandibular jaw defects and were secured in position by resorbable fixation screws. After a healing time of 6 weeks, bone-scaffold interface was subjected to histomorphometric analysis to detect the amount of new bone formation. Stained histological sections were analyzed using a computer software ($n=12$, $a=0.05$). Mercury porosimetery was used to measure pore sizes, chemical composition was analyzed using energy dispersive x-ray analysis (EDX), and the crystal structure was identified using x-ray diffraction micro-analysis (XRD).

Results: HA enriched zirconia scaffolds revealed significantly higher volume of new bone formation (33% ± 14) compared to the controls (21% ± 11). New bone deposition started by coating the pore cavity walls and proceeded by filling the entire pore volume. Bone in-growth started from the surface of the scaffold and propagated towards the scaffold core. Islands of entrapped hydroxy apatite particles were observed in mineralized bone matrix.

Conclusions: Within the limitations of this study, hydroxy apatite enhanced osteogenesis ability of porous zirconia scaffolds.

Keywords: Nano-porous, Hydroxyapatite coating, Zirconia, Scaffold

Background

Principles of tissue engineering are used today in an attempt to reconstruct damaged human tissue. In the dental field, several types of bone grafting materials are currently available which could be directly used to augment atrophic jaws before implant placement. However, the main drawback of these grafts is related to difficulty of preserving the required shape of the graft during the healing time [1]. Protecting the grafting material using titanium meshes or other temporary devices may not be applicable in non-accessible areas. Nevertheless, using autogenous bone blocks may not be an acceptable option for many patients due to the expected morbidity of the donor site [2].

Today, different types of pre-shaped bone grafting materials are currently available for augmenting atrophic ridges. One of the greatest challenges facing successful ridge augmentation is to maintain the desired shape after soft tissue closure [3]. Several studies reported a high rate of bone resorption after insertion of implants in bone augmented ridges [4, 5]. On the other hand, porous non resorbable scaffolds have the advantage of maintaining ridge shape and dimensions during healing time.

Yttrium partially stabilized tetragonal zirconia polycrystalline material, known commercially in the dental field as zirconia, was first used in orthopedic surgery as a hip joint prosthesis [6]. Soon the material gained diverse applications in the dental field as a core and framework material,

* Correspondence: moustafaaboushelib@gmail.com
[1]Dental Biomaterials Department, Faculty of Dentistry, Alexandria University, Champollion st, Azarita, Alexandria, Egypt
Full list of author information is available at the end of the article

implant abutment, implant fixture, and a bone scaffold as well. Using computer-assisted design and milling technology (CAD/CAM), the fabrication of accurate and precise restorations became a simple procedure [3, 7].

One of the desired features of a bone scaffold is to resist functional loads as well [8]. Several studies evaluated bone reaction against optimized zirconia scaffold surfaces [9]. Studies ranging from cell culture to full scale animal models have indicated that osteointegration observed on optimized zirconia surfaces was equal if not superior to different materials, namely titanium alloy. These studies either focused on optimizing the surface structure of zirconia scaffolds controlling its porosity, geometric structure, and micro-roughness, or by coating the surface with a bioactive layer to enhance the process of osteogenesis ability [10–13]. Porous zirconia scaffolds could also be used as a drug delivery vehicle to enhance bone response as well [14]. A recent study attributed enhanced cell viability to the internal structure of the scaffold rather than to the type of coating material used [15].

Modern radiographic imaging techniques in combination with advanced computer designing software could reconstruct a three-dimensional image of large boney defects [16]. Designing the shape of the required scaffold could easily be performed to accurately fit the available defect size using advanced imaging and designing software [17]. Finally, the required shape could be directly milled from different materials using CAD/CAM technology and the milled scaffold could be inserted in the exposed boney defect.

The aim of this study was to evaluate osteogenesis ability of customized CAD/CAM porous zirconia scaffolds inserted in healed boney defects in the mandible of a dog model. The proposed hypothesis of this study was that hydroxyapatite-enriched zirconia scaffolds would enhance osteogenesis ability compared to the controls.

Methods

Preparation of the scaffold

Zirconia powder (50 µm, 3 mol YTZP, E grade, Tosoh, Japan) was mixed with 50 wt.% resin beads (50 µm polymethyl methacrylate powder) added to create microscopic pore sizes. Thirty weight percent coarse sodium chloride particles (500–700 µm) were added to the mix to create large interconnected pores. The powder was mixed in a rotating cylinder for 24 h to insure homogenous powder distribution. A binder material (1 wt.% polyvinyl glycol) was added to the mix, and the powder was isostatically pressed into cylinders (40 mm in diameter and 80 mm in length) to create the required dimensions of the CAD/CAM milling blocks. The blocks were partially sintered at 1250 °C for 30 min then soaked in deionizer water for 24 h to dissolve the salt particles.

Jaw defect and scaffold design

The ethics committee of Alexandria University approved the working protocol used in this study (STDF reintegration grant 489) according to the university code of conduct regarding using animals in scientific studies. After approval of the ethics committee on publishing parts of the obtained data, 2-year-old healthy male Beagle dogs (weighing 10–12 kg) were generally anesthetized by administration of subcutaneous injection of atropine (0.05 mg/kg; Kwangmyung Pharmaceutical, Seoul, Korea) and an intravenous injection of a mixed xylazine (Rompun, Bayer Korea, Seoul, Korea) and zoletil (Virbac, Carros, France) and maintained by inhalation anesthesia (Gerolan, Choongwae Pharmaceutical, Seoul, Korea). Surgical flap was reflected to expose the premolar-molar region of the lower jaw with minimum amount of trauma, afterwards the involved teeth were removed and a surgical block 2 cm long × 2 cm deep was cut using a surgical guide to demarcate the wound boundaries. Finally, the surgical flap was repositioned and sutured and the dogs received an antibiotic (20 mg/kg of cefazoline sodium, intramuscularly; Yuhan, Seoul, Korea) for 3 days, given soft diet, and the surgical site was sprayed with topical 0.2% chlorhexidine solution. After 3-month healing time, three-dimensional images of the boney defect was performed using cone beam CT radiographic imaging (I cat, Imaging science international, Hatfield, PA). The images were transferred to an open access CAD/CAM software (CAMworks, Geometric Americas INC, Scottsdale, AZ) and the design of the required zirconia scaffold was reconstructed to accurately fit the modeled boney defect putting in account the expected sintering shrinkage of the material (25 vol.% shrinkage). The scaffold was designed to restore normal contour of the resected ridge. Five axes dry milling unit (DWX-51D 5, Roland, Parkway, Irvin, Cal) was used to mill the prepared blocks into the required shape and the scaffold was sintered at 1350 °C for 4 h.

Enriching with nano-hydroxyapatite

Nano-hydroxyapatite particles were prepared using sol gel chemical precipitation method. The sol was thermally aged at low temperature at 50 °C for 2 h. Upon drying the sol particles agglomerated into a dry gel through van der Waals forces composed of 10–14-nm particles. A crystalline apatite is achieved after sintering at 450 °C resulting in a gained structure of 25–55 nm in diameter. Twenty-five weight percent suspension of nano-hydroxyapatite particles were added to 80% ethyl alcohol and stirred to achieve a homogenous suspension, and the right scaffold of each dog was immersed in the prepared suspension for 15 min under vacuum to insure adequate filling of all pores. Scaffolds were dried at 120 °C for 180 min and the process was repeated two times. Finally, the coated scaffolds were heated at 900 °C for 30 min to ensure proper drying of the particles without changing the chemistry of the particles or the supporting scaffold.

Characterization of the prepared scaffolds

Mercury porosimetery was performed for evaluate pore size and distribution and to measure the total porosity percent of the scaffolds. Pore sizer (Porosimeter, Micromeritics 9320, USA) was used for testing the produced porosity on the nanoscale covering pore diameter in range from 360 to 0.006 μm.

Energy dispersive X-ray analysis (EDX) (INCA Penta FETX3, OXFORD Instruments, Model 6583, England) and X-ray diffraction analysis (XRD) (PANalytical, X Pert PRO, The Netherlands) with Cu target ($\lambda = 1.54$ Å), 45 kV, 40 mA, and 2θ (10°–80°) were used to analyze elemental surface composition and crystal structure of the scaffolds. Density of the prepared scaffolds was compared to theoretical density of fully sintered zirconia.

Surgical phase

Twelve weeks after healing of the resected ridges, the animals were exposed to the second stage surgery where the created defect size was exposed using the same procedures described previously and each scaffold was seated in its final position. Resorbable collagen membrane (Biomend, Zimmer Inc, CA, USA) was used to cover the exposed surface of the scaffold and soft tissue was gently expanded and sutured to secure proper wound closure using resorbable suture material (Vicryl Rapide 5; Ethicon Inc., Somerville, NY). To increase primary retention, the scaffolds were fixed using resorbable polylactic acid fixation screws (Rapidsorb, Deput Synthes, PA, USA).

Histomorphometric analysis

Six weeks after insertion of the scaffolds, the animals were given an over dose of an anesthetic injection and section blocks were obtained by cutting the mandible maintaining 10 mm of sound bone around the scaffolds. Cut sections were immediately fixed in 4% buffered formaldehyde and dehydrated in graded ethanol solutions using a dehydration system under agitation and vacuum, and the specimens were then defatted in xylene solution. Finally, the specimens were embedded in transparent chemically polymerized methyl methacrylate resin (methyl methacrylate 99%, Sigma-Aldrich, Steinheim, Germany). After polymerization, the specimens were cut along the long axis of the scaffolds using a diamond-coated disc rotating in a micro-sectioning system (Micracut 150 precision cutter, Metkon, Bursa, Turkey) followed by polishing using 800 grit silicon carbide paper. One hundred-micrometer-thick cut sections were stained using Stevenel's blue and van Gieson picrofuchsin. Histomorphometric analysis was performed using

digital images obtained using a light stereomicroscope (Olympus BX 61, Hamburg, Germany) equipped with a high-resolution digital camera (E330, Olympus, Imaging Corp, Beijing, China).

Measurements were made by first calculating the pore volume on the images using digital tracing option of the software (white pores on the images), and the amount of new bone formation (mineralized tissue stained red) was calculated as a percent of the total pore volume (Olympus CellM & CellR, version 3.3, Olympus Soft Imaging Solutions).

Examiner reliability was cross checked by re-evaluating randomly selected digital images by another expert examiner. The recorded correlation coefficient ranged from 0.83 to 0.92, indicating high reliability for all measured parameters. The data obtained were expressed as mean and standard deviation values and were analyzed using Student's t test (SPSS 15.0, SPSS, Chicago, IL).

Results

Mercury porosimetery revealed comparable ($F = 0.057$, $P < 0.92$) average pore diameter (85 ± 24 μm) for all the prepared scaffolds. Smallest pore diameter was 34 ± 2 μm and the largest pore diameter was 720 ± 13 μm. After filling the pores with hydroxyapatite, there was a significant ($F = 16.1$, $P < 0.01$) reduction in total porosity percent from 83 to 44 wt.% indicating that the nano-particles filled almost half of the available pores. There was also a significant reduction in average pore diameter from 85 ± 24 to 46 ± 29 μm. Amount of measured porosity was directly related to the measured bulk density of the scaffold structure. Agglomerates of hydroxyapatite particles were observed filling the porous structure (Fig. 1a, b).

EDX analysis of the enriched scaffolds revealed that Ca/P ratio was 1.67 indicating the presence of pure hydroxyapatite in the enriched scaffolds. XRD pattern revealed the characteristic peaks specific for the hexagonal HA crystal phase represented by (211), (112), and (300) peaks. Peaks of tetragonal yttrium zirconium oxide were detected for all specimens.

Histomorphometric analysis revealed that hydroxyapatite-enriched scaffolds had significantly ($F = 14$, $P < 0.02$) higher amount of new bone formation ($33\% \pm 14$) compared to the controls ($21\% \pm 11$). Amount of new bone formation was calculated as a percent of the total pore volume measured on each image. New bone growth started by lining pore cavity and propagated to gradually fill the entire pore volume (Fig. 2a). Bone ingrowth proceeded from the periphery of the scaffold and propagated towards its center (Fig. 2b). The surface under the guided tissue membrane was filled with unmineralized connective tissue. Regional areas of entrapped hydroxyapatite were observed inside the pore

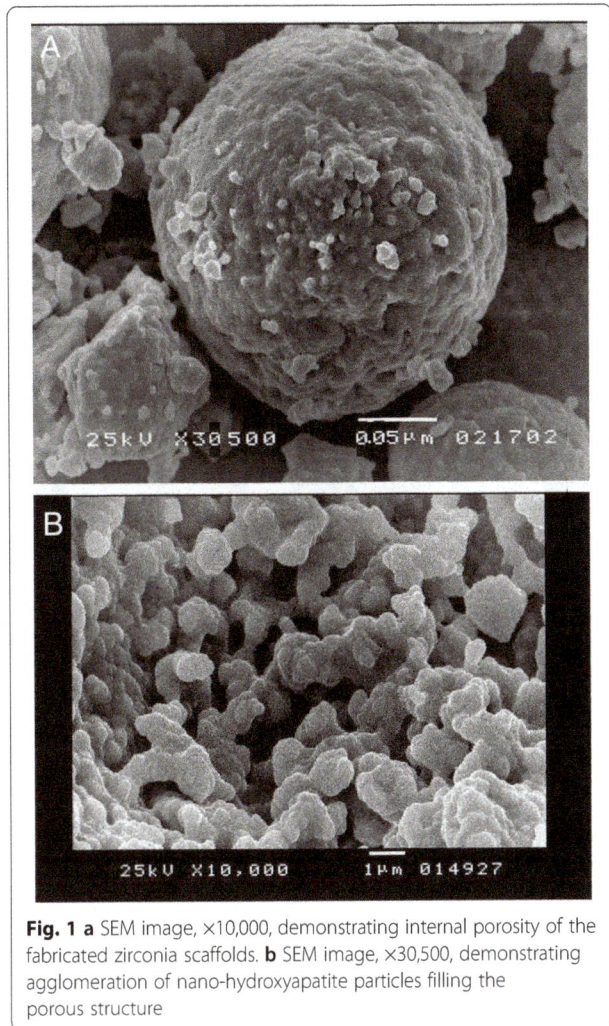

Fig. 1 a SEM image, ×10,000, demonstrating internal porosity of the fabricated zirconia scaffolds. **b** SEM image, ×30,500, demonstrating agglomeration of nano-hydroxyapatite particles filling the porous structure

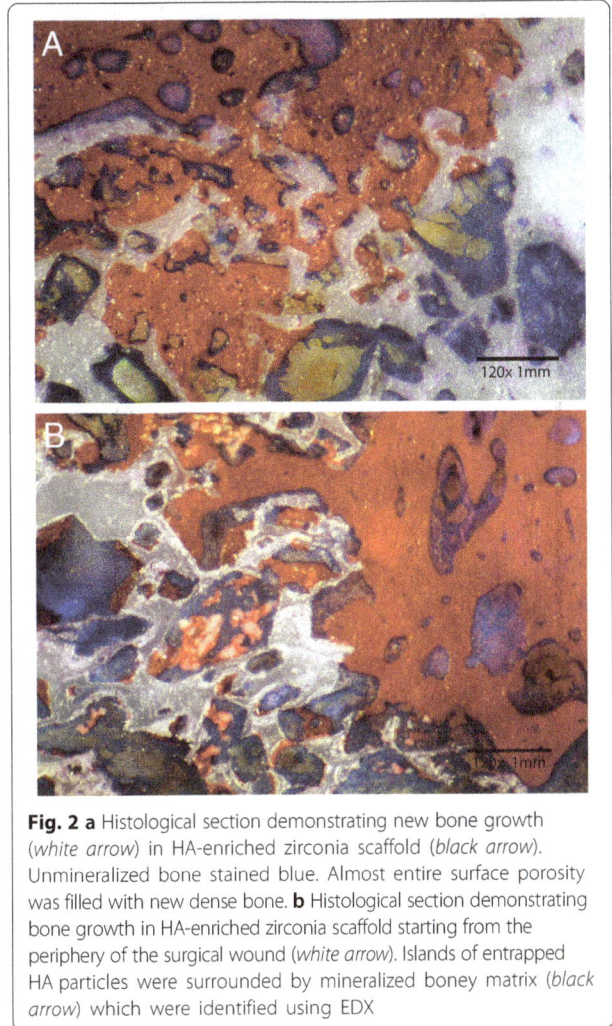

Fig. 2 a Histological section demonstrating new bone growth (*white arrow*) in HA-enriched zirconia scaffold (*black arrow*). Unmineralized bone stained blue. Almost entire surface porosity was filled with new dense bone. **b** Histological section demonstrating bone growth in HA-enriched zirconia scaffold starting from the periphery of the surgical wound (*white arrow*). Islands of entrapped HA particles were surrounded by mineralized boney matrix (*black arrow*) which were identified using EDX

cavity of the enriched scaffolds (Fig. 2b). Entrapped islands of hydroxyapatite were surrounded by mineralized tissue. Lower amount of mineralized bone was observed for uncoated scaffolds (Fig. 3a, b).

Radiographic examination revealed clear margins separating newly inserted scaffolds from surrounding bone defect (Fig. 4a). After completion of healing time, the margins between the scaffold and bone defect became less demarcated due to deposition and ingrowth of new bone (Fig. 4b).

Discussion

Porous scaffolds are designed to allow ingrowth of the surrounding bone within the internal porosity of the solid matrix. Different types of bioactive materials were mixed with zirconia to enhance bone formation. Two sizes of pores were incorporated in the structure of the fabricated scaffolds. Micro-pores in range of 50 μm constituted the majority of the entire pore volume (50 wt.%) of the fabricated scaffolds (Fig. 1a).

This pore volume was expected to provide adequate housing for osteoblasts and provide a mechanism of cell attachment on a microscopic level. Larger pore sizes (500–700 μm) reduced the density (30 wt.%) of the prepared scaffolds and created internal channels that connected different surfaces together creating a pathway for blood circulation [12, 15].

Previous research studies concerned with osteointegration of zirconia material reported comparable if not superior performance compared to different types of titanium alloys. This behavior was attributed to several factors related to the mechanical, physical, and chemical properties of zirconia [18]. With optimization of surface structure and geometry using a different technique, zirconia became available today as one piece dental implant [19].

Reconstruction of atrophic alveolar ridges could be achieved using a wide variety of grafting materials. However, maintaining the required shape of the graft represents a great challenge for the surgeon especially in regions subjected to functional loads. In the field of

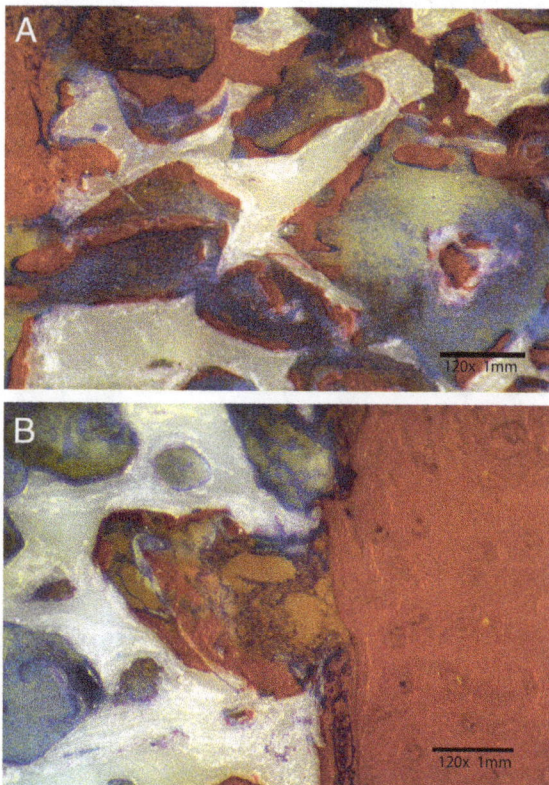

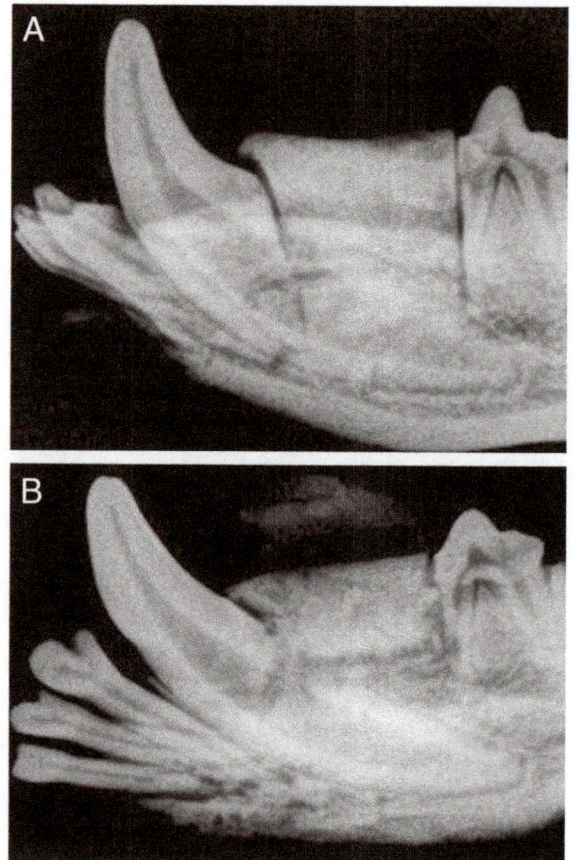

Fig. 3 a Histological section demonstrating bone growth in control zirconia scaffold (*white arrow*). Mineralized bone formation (*black arrow*) was less dense compared to HA-enriched scaffolds. **b** Histological section showing different sizes of pores present in porous zirconia scaffolds (Control specimen). Mineralization started by lining pore walls (*white arrow*). Unmineralized bone stained blue

Fig. 4 a Peri-apical X-ray of zirconia scaffold immediately placed in bone defect. Margins between scaffold and bone are clearly demarcated. **b** Peri-apical X-ray of zirconia scaffold after completion of healing time. Margins between bone defect and scaffold are less demarcated due to new bone growth

maxillofacial and cosmetic surgery, the graft must be mechanically strong to maintain its shape when placed in the surgical site and it must resist resorption and degradation to prevent collapse of the supported tissue [11].

Customized CAD/CAM porous zirconia scaffolds could easily be fabricated with high precision to fit the demands of the required surgical site. It could be used to augment atrophic alveolar ridges, replace bone loss in the maxillofacial region, and in cosmetic surgery as well. The scaffold is designed to be osteointgrated with the surrounding boney tissue thus it could perform mechanical function as well. The internal design of the scaffold enhanced blood circulation to ensure that the structure of the scaffold does not interrupt the biology of the surrounding tissue [15]. In combination with optimized nano-porous surface produced by selective infiltration etching, the scaffold could be enriched with different bioactive agents to enhance healing and osteogenesis ability with the surrounded tissue.

Histomorphometric analysis revealed that bone growth start to develop as early as 6 weeks by lining pore cavity walls. Mineralized bone matrix was observed to penetrate 1–2 mm under the surface of the scaffolds thus providing

mechanical stability of the inserted prosthesis. Healing continued by filling the entire pore volume (Fig. 2a, b). The presence of nano-hydroxyapatite particles enhanced bone growth and deposition compared to uncoated surfaces (Fig. 3a, b). Hydroxyapatite enhanced osteogenesis ability of zirconia scaffolds, and the proposed hypothesis was accepted.

Kim et al. used coated zirconia scaffolds to augment calvarial defects in a rabbit model and reported closely matching values regarding porosity and density of the prepared scaffolds and regarding the amount of newly measured bone formation [20]. However, in this study, hydroxyapatite particles were not fused to the structure of the scaffold but were used to fill the pores resulting in much quicker release once in contract with body fluid which explains the superior performance of the enriched scaffolds.

Islands of hydroxyapatite particles were observed entrapped in the mineralized bone lining the internal pores of the enriched scaffold. Similar observation regarding the solubility of hydroxyapatite was reported in a cell culture study on porous zirconia surfaces [21]. In a clinical study, micro-porous-coated zirconia scaffolds demonstrated four times higher bone ingrowth and seven times higher bone-scaffold contact compared to uncoated scaffolds inserted in the maxilla of human patient [5].

Several trials used porous titanium scaffolds as a matrix for repair of large boney defects. Enriching these scaffolds with various growth factors enhanced clinical outcome [22–24]. However, the design of these scaffolds remains basically a network of interconnected wire structure that acts as a matrix filling the boney defect. CAD/CAM technology allows fabrication of custom-made zirconia scaffolds with full control over the distribution, size, and percentage of the created porosity.

In this study, the scaffolds were inserted in healed wounds in the alveolar ridge of dogs. The external surface of the scaffolds was protected by a resorbable-guided tissue membrane to prevent soft tissue migration which could compete with deposition of the required boney matrix. Traces of the collagen matrix of the membrane were observed on the free surface of the scaffolds. Being CAD/CAM fabricated from special milling blocks, the design of the scaffold could easily be tailored to meet the demands of different fields. In the field of implant dentistry, the future site of dental implant could be considered in the design of the scaffold to facilitate easier placement which will be considered in further studies.

Conclusions

Within the limitations of this study, hydroxyapatite enhanced osteogenesis ability of porous zirconia scaffolds.

Acknowledgements

Part of this study was supported by STDF reintegration grant number 489 and was performed in collaboration with the Oral Surgery Department, Faculty of Dentistry, Alexandria University, Egypt.

Authors' contributions

MNA prepared the specimens and performed the characterization process. He participated in preparation of histological section, data collection and analysis, and in preparation of the manuscript. RS performed the surgical phase of the study, provided animal care, looked after housing facilities, and participated in drafting the manuscript. Both authors read and approved the final manuscript.

Competing interests

Moustafa Aboushelib and Rehab Shawky declare that they have no competing interests.

Author details

[1]Dental Biomaterials Department, Faculty of Dentistry, Alexandria University, Champollion st, Azarita, Alexandria, Egypt. [2]Oral Surgery Department, Faculty of Dentistry, Alexandria University, Alexandria, Egypt.

References

1. Chiapasco M, Casentini P, Zaniboni M. Bone augmentation procedures in implant dentistry. Int J Oral Maxillofac Implants. 2009;24:237–59.
2. Rocchietta I, Fontana F, Simion M. Clinical outcomes of vertical bone augmentation to enable dental implant placement: a systematic review. J Clin Periodontol. 2008;35:203–15.
3. Louis PJ, Gutta R, Said-Al-Naief N, Bartolucci AA. Reconstruction of the maxilla and mandible with particulate bone graft and titanium mesh for implant placement. J Oral Maxillofac Surg. 2008;66:235–45.
4. Riachi F, et al. Influence of material properties on rate of resorption of two bone graft materials after sinus lift using radiographic assessment. Int J Dent. 2012;2012:737262.
5. Malmstrom J, Slotte C, Adolfsson E, Norderyd O, Thomsen P. Bone response to free form-fabricated hydroxyapatite and zirconia scaffolds: a histological study in the human maxilla. Clin Oral Implants Res. 2009;20:379–85.
6. Stewart TD, et al. Severe wear and fracture of zirconia heads against alumina inserts in hip simulator studies with microseparation. J Arthroplasty. 2003;18:726–34.
7. Aboushelib, MN. Fatigue and Fracture Resistance of Zirconia Crowns Prepared with Different Finish Line Designs. J Prosthodont 2012; e publication ahead of print:
8. Yang JZ, Hu XZ, Sultana R, Edward Day R, Ichim P. Structure design and manufacturing of layered bioceramic scaffolds for load-bearing bone reconstruction. Biomed Mater. 2015;10:045006.
9. Teimouri A, Ebrahimi R, Emadi R, Beni BH, Chermahini AN. Nano-composite of silk fibroin-chitosan/Nano ZrO2 for tissue engineering applications: fabrication and morphology. Int J Biol Macromol. 2015;76:292–302.
10. An SH, et al. Porous zirconia/hydroxyapatite scaffolds for bone reconstruction. Dent Mater. 2012;28:1221–31.
11. Alizadeh A, et al., Synthesis of calcium phosphate-zirconia scaffold and human endometrial adult stem cells for bone tissue engineering. Artif Cells Nanomed Biotechnol 2014;44:66–73.
12. Mondal D, et al. Fabrication of multilayer ZrO(2)-biphasic calcium phosphate-poly-caprolactone unidirectional channeled scaffold for bone tissue formation. J Biomater Appl. 2012;28:462–72.
13. Pattnaik S, et al. Chitosan scaffolds containing silicon dioxide and zirconia nano particles for bone tissue engineering. Int J Biol Macromol. 2011;49:1167–72.
14. Naleway SE, Fickas KC, Maker YN, Meyers MA, McKittrick J. Reproducibility of ZrO2-based freeze casting for biomaterials. Mater Sci Eng C Mater Biol Appl. 2016;61:105–12.
15. Song YG, Cho IH. Characteristics and osteogenic effect of zirconia porous scaffold coated with beta-TCP/HA. J Adv Prosthodont. 2014;6:285–94.
16. Okano T, et al. Absorbed and effective doses from cone beam volumetric imaging for implant planning. Dentomaxillofac Radiol. 2009;38:79–85.
17. Anssari Moin D, Hassan B, Wismeijer D. A novel approach for custom three-dimensional printing of a zirconia root analogue implant by digital light processing. Clin Oral Implants Res. 2016; 25.a head of print.
18. Yamashita D, et al. Effect of surface roughness on initial responses of osteoblast-like cells on two types of zirconia. Dent Mater J. 2009;28:461–70.
19. Aboushelib M, Salem N, Abotaleb A, Abd El Moniem N. Influence of surface nano-roughness on osseointegration of zirconia implants in rabbit femur heads using selective infiltration etching technique. J Oral Implantol 2012;39:583–90.
20. Kim HW, et al. Porous ZrO2 bone scaffold coated with hydroxyapatite with fluorapatite intermediate layer. Biomaterials. 2003;24:3277–84.
21. Kim HW, Kim HE, Salih V, Knowles JC. Dissolution control and cellular responses of calcium phosphate coatings on zirconia porous scaffold. J Biomed Mater Res A. 2004;68:522–30.
22. Zhu W, Zhao Y, Ma Q, Wang Y, Wu Z, Weng X. 3D-printed porous titanium changed femoral head repair growth patterns: osteogenesis and vascularisation in porous titanium. J Mater Sci Mater Med. 2017;28:62–5.
23. Arifvianto B, Leeflang MA, Zhou J. Diametral compression behavior of biomedical titanium scaffolds with open, interconnected pores prepared with the space holder method. J Mech Behav Biomed Mater. 2017;68:144–54.
24. Chen H, Wang C, Yang X, Xiao Z, Zhu X, Zhang K, Fan Y, Zhang X. Construction of surface HA/TiO coating on porous titanium scaffolds and its preliminary biological evaluation. Mater Sci Eng C Mater Biol Appl. 2017;70:1047–56.

25

ISQ calculation evaluation of in vitro laser scanning vibrometry-captured resonance frequency

Stijn Debruyne[1†], Nicolas Grognard[2,3*†], Gino Verleye[4], Korneel Van Massenhove[5], Dimitrios Mavreas[3] and Bart Vande Vannet[3]

Abstract

Background: Implant stability testing at various stages of implant therapy by means of resonance frequency analysis is extensively used. The overall measurement outcome is a function of the resulting stiffness of three entities: surrounding bone, bone-implant complex, and implant-Smartpeg complex. The influence of the latter on the overall measurement results is presently unknown. It can be investigated in vitro by use of imbedded implants with mounted Smartpegs. This enables to keep the influence of the two other entities constant and controlled.

The purpose of this study is to verify if a laboratory laser Doppler vibrometry technology-based procedure results in comparable ISQ results after calculation of captured resonance frequency spectra by aid of the Osstell algorithm with direct Osstell IDX device measurements.

Methods: A laboratory procedure was engineered to record frequency spectra of resin-imbedded test implants with mounted Smartpegs, after electromagnetic excitation with the Osstell IDX device and laser Doppler vibrometry response detection. Fast Fourier transformation data processing of resonance frequency data resulted in determination of a maximum resonance frequency values allowing calculation of implant stability quotient (ISQ) values using the Osstell algorithm.

Results: Laboratory-based ISQ values were compared to Osstell IDx device-generated ISQ values for Straumann tissue level, Ankylos, and 3i Certain implant systems. For both systems, a correlation coefficient $r = 0.99$ was found. Furthermore, a clinically rejectable mean difference of 0.09 ISQ units was noted between both datasets.

Conclusions: The proposed laboratory method with the application of the Osstell algorithm for ISQ calculation is appropriate for future studies to in vitro research aspects of resonance frequency analysis implant stability measurements.

Keywords: Implant stability, RFA, ISQ, Osstell Mentor, Osstell IDx, Laser Doppler vibrometry, Straumann tissue level implants, Ankylos implants

* Correspondence: nicolas.kliniekroyal@gmail.com
†Equal contributors
[2]Kliniek Royal, Koningstraat 41, 8400 Ostend, Belgium
[3]CHIR-Unit Dentistry–ORHE, Department of Orthodontics, Faculty of Medicine and Pharmacy, Vrije Universiteit Brussel, Laarbeeklaan 103, 1090 Brussels, Belgium
Full list of author information is available at the end of the article

Background

At present, multiple implant stability assessment methodologies are used, both of invasive and non-invasive nature, including percussion test [1], X-ray evaluation [2], cutting resistance during implant insertion (e.g., electronic insertion torque determination) [3], turn-out or reverse torque test [4], Periotest® [5, 6], and resonance frequency analysis ("RFA"), e.g., the Osstell method [7, 8]. The validity of those methods can be evaluated to their sensitivity to detect small changes in stability that are not detectable with clinical and/or radiographical methods. Electronic devices such as insertion torque devices, Periotest, and Osstell Mentor devices are commercially available instruments that allow quantitative implant stability analysis at a level that is not feasible with traditional clinical or radiographical methods [9]. The Osstell device methodology is based on quantitative assessment of (micro) deflection of the implant—by aid as a transducer—in the surrounding jawbone, induced by controlled appliance of electromagnetic excitation. The properties of a transducer (e.g., stiffness and screw properties), the stiffness of the "implant-transducer" complex, the properties and stiffness of "implant-bone" complex, e.g., the effective height of the coronal implant part above the bone crest [7, 8], and the stiffness of the bone itself are measurement influencing factors (Integration Diagnostics Company®, Osstell mathematical explanation, 2009).

In the past, various versions of the Osstell device have been developed and marketed. The original version consisted of a wired version of the transducer. The transducer consisted of two built-in piezoceramic elements. One piezoceramic element served as the transmittor element, receiving an electrically generated sine wave with varying frequency. The response signal was analyzed by an oscilloscope with the resonance frequency in kilohertz as the outcome unit.

The launch of the Osstell Mentor® in 2004 included the introduction of a less voluminous, much more user-friendly, non-cabled transducer, called Smartpeg. Smartpegs are small aluminum rods with three different parts: a coronal part with an implant system-specific screw fitting into the individual implant, a hexagon part enabling easy tightening/un-tightening, and a magnet serving as the electromagnetic puls captor. The apparatus itself was a compact device with an incorporated microcomputer and electromagnetic signal emitting and receiving tipped probe. Excitation of the implant-mounted Smartpeg is performed by four electromagnetic pulses with different frequencies inducing Smartpeg vibration in mostly two directions perpendicular to each other. The vibration directions correspond to a low and a high resonance frequency. The manufacturer recommends performing at least two measurements, in order to

identify these possible different stabilities. Furthermore, in order to suppress electromagnetic environmental noise, the working principle is refined by four times repeated emission of each excitation frequency. In summary, 16 pulses are emitted for each single measurement. The captured outcome of each in fourfold emitted signal is converted by the built-in microcomputer into a frequency spectrum by a "fast Fourier transformation" (FFT) method, ending up to detect among the four calculated spectra the two highest peaks representing the resonance frequencies of the implant. The latter will be used to calculate the so-called implant stability quotients (ISQ) by aid of a mathematical algorithm. ISQ is a unitless number, ranging between 0 and 100. If the difference between the two peaks is less than 3 ISQ units, or in case of only one peak detection, only 1 ISQ value will be displayed by the microcomputer. The 2009 Osstell ISQ version and the present Osstell IDx® version do make use of the same algorithm.

The computed ISQ value is based on the following calculation formulae:

$$\text{ISQ} = (f4 \times e) + (f3 \times d) + (f2 \times c) + (f \times b) + a$$

Hereby, f denotes the measured maximum resonance frequency (RF). Coefficients a, b, c, d, and e are property information of Osstell (Osstell AB, Gothenburg, Sweden). The coefficients were provided for internal use under the agreement of no publication. From clinical reports [10–16] listed in Table 1, it can be concluded that ISQ values for one specific implant system, inserted in comparable jawbone regions, differ considerably between outcomes obtained by the original wired Osstell device and the more recent Osstell Mentor device. These findings were confirmed in both a clinical trial with an approximate difference of 9 ISQ units [16] and in vitro on human cadaver jawbone with an approximate difference of 10 ISQ units [17]. This means that the comparison of clinical studies reporting implant stability outcomes generated by different versions of Osstell devices in (systematic) reviews needs caution and correction.

Purpose

The purpose of this in vitro study was to develop a laboratory method, intended for future research of aspects of implant-Smartpeg complex stiffness and its possible influence on the overall RFA-based implant stability determination. For this, a combination of laser Doppler vibrometry for measurement and signal processing by aid of fast Fourier transformation analysis was used. Laser Doppler vibrometry technology permits to determine both the resonance frequency and deflection behavior of a mounted Smartpeg. The latter can be of interest since different implant types possess different

Table 1 Published secondary implant stability values for Straumann tissue level RN SLA surfaced implants (Ø = 4.1 mm)

Author and study	Implant position (implant number)	Mean ISQ values at given time-point post-insertion	Type of Osstell device used
Barewal et al. 2003 [10]	UJP (10) LJP (17)	8 W: 58 8 W: 62.5	Wired Osstell transducer
Bisschof et al. 2003 [11]	UJP (54) LJP (36)	12 W: 57.1 12 W: 64.7	Wired Osstell transducer
Huwiler et al., 2006 [12]	UJP + LJP (17)	8 W: 62.8	Wired Osstell transducer
Han et al. 2009 [13]	LJP + LJP (10)	8 W: 75.2 12 W: 78.8	Osstell Mentor
Bornstein et al. 2009 [14]	LJP (56)	7 W: 81.1 12 W: 83.3	Osstell Mentor
Guler et al. 2013 [15]	UJP + LJP (108)	8 W: 71.2	Osstell Mentor

prosthetic connections that suit different types of Smart-pegs. In vitro research enables to control and simulate in a standardized way the stiffness of the surrounding bone and the stiffness of the implant-bone complex by imbedding implants in self-curing resin. Complete imbedding of the implant to the most coronal level simulates a normal clinical situation of total osseointegration. Incomplete imbedding allows to both measure the deflection mode of the Smartpeg and the implant itself when different vertical points are used to execute the measurement (Fig. 1).

Laser Doppler vibrometry possesses a working principle based on the so-called Doppler effect and allows non-contact quantitative measurement of vibration (https://en.wikpedia.org/wiki/Laser_scanning_vibrometry, 2017). The Doppler effect itself finds its origin when a light beam is backscattered on a vibrating surface and experiences a change in wave phase (https://en.wikipedia.org/wiki/Doppler_effect, 2017). The backscattered laser beam is captured by the laser scanning vibrometer, and the phase change will be the function of the magnitude of the vibration of the Smartpeg. The response signal is processed and points to maximum detected resonance frequency that will be used to compute the

ISQ value by means of the algorithm used by Osstell methodology. The calculated ISQ value is compared to ISQ values generated by the newest version of the Osstell device, Osstell IDx®, using a laboratory setup that enables to capture and measure, by means of laser Doppler vibrometry, the generated electromagnetic excitation of an implant-mounted Smartpeg® transducer, evoked by a the Osstell IDx device. The coefficients implemented in the formulae were confidently supplied under the agreement that publication will not be done. This computed ISQ value will be compared to the ISQ value, obtained by the Osstell IDx device in the same laboratory setup.

Methods

Test implants

Test implants originating from various manufacturers were investigated. Straumann sandblasted, large-grit, acid-etched (SLA)® tissue level standard implants (Straumann AG, Basel, Switzerland) with the following diameter: length configurations were 3.3–12 mm (RN connection), 3.3–4.1 mm (RN connection), and 4.8–8 mm (WN connection), Ankylos Cell Plus® surfaced B-implant types (Dentsply Implants, Mannheim,

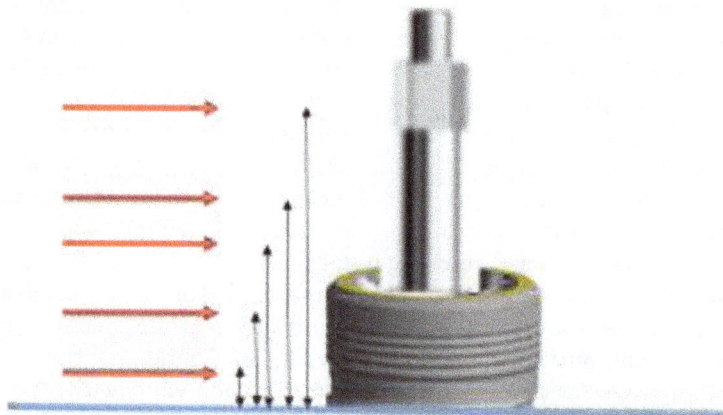

Fig. 1 Concept for study of deflection and stiffness aspects of implant-Smartpeg complex by laser Doppler vibrometry. Intentional partial imbedding of implants allows to detect both the deflection of implant and Smartpeg separately at different vertical levels by changing the position of the laser beam

Germany) with the following diameter: length configurations used were 4.5–8 mm and 4.5–9.5 mm, and Biomet 3i Full Osseotite® Tapered Certain implants (Biomet 3i, Barcelona, Spain) with a 4-mm diameter/13-mm length were investigated.

Preparatory procedures

Test implants were imbedded using Duromod B® dual component polyurethane resin (Dumont Instruments, Brussels, Belgium) in a silicon mould with a bar-shaped recipient (approximal dimensions (length × width × height): 16 cm × 2.5 cm × 3 cm)). Per bar, five implants were imbedded using system-specific implant mounts allowing correct vertical positioning. After resin polymerization, all implants were given an identification number in order to allow transfer of the measurement outcomes to the datafile.

Smartpeg connection

A fresh implant system-specific Smartpeg® (Integration Diagnostics AB, Säveden, Sweden) transducer was connected to each implant using a manual torque controlling device set at 8 Ncm (Tochnichi, Ota-Ku, Tokyo, Japan). For Straumann implants, Smartpeg type # 04 and, for Ankylos implants, Smartpeg type # 16 were used. For 3i Tapered Certain implants, Smartpeg type # 15 was used.

Laboratory setup for indirect measurements

Smartpeg excitation was performed by using the Osstell IDx device. The cabled probe of the Osstell IDx was positioned towards the most coronal part of the Smartpeg

by the aid of a stand (Mitutoyo 70105N, Mitutoyo, Santo Amaro, Brazil) (Fig. 2). The measured ISQ value was noted and input in the datafile.

The speed of vibration, $v(t)$, of an excited Smartpeg was measured by means of a portable laser vibrometer (laser class 2) (Polytec PDV 100, Polytec, Irvine, CA, USA), generating a focusable laser beam ($\lambda = 640$ nm), mounted on a tri-pod with a three-way tilting head (Manfrotto, Cassolo, Italy) allowing for easy and precise laser beam orientation in X, Y, and Z directions. The measurement range was set at 20 mm/s with a sensitivity of 5 mm/s. The generated laser beam was orientated towards a flat surface of the hexed part of an implant-mounted Smartpeg. Correct positioning of the laser beam orientation was by visual inspection of laser dot position on a flat surface of the Smartpeg hexagon and by using the reflection index on the laser scanning vibrometer device.

Laboratory setup for direct ISQ determination

The Smartpeg excitation mode was exactly performed as described above. Notation of the maximum resonance frequency for indirect measurements is followed by notation of direct ISQ value on the display of Osstell IDx device. Positioning of the probe was not changed during indirect and direct recordings for a given test implant.

Measurements and calculations

Each resin block contained five identical implants with attached Smartpegs of a given implant type with a specific diameter and length configuration. Correct positioning of the Osstell probe towards the Smartpeg

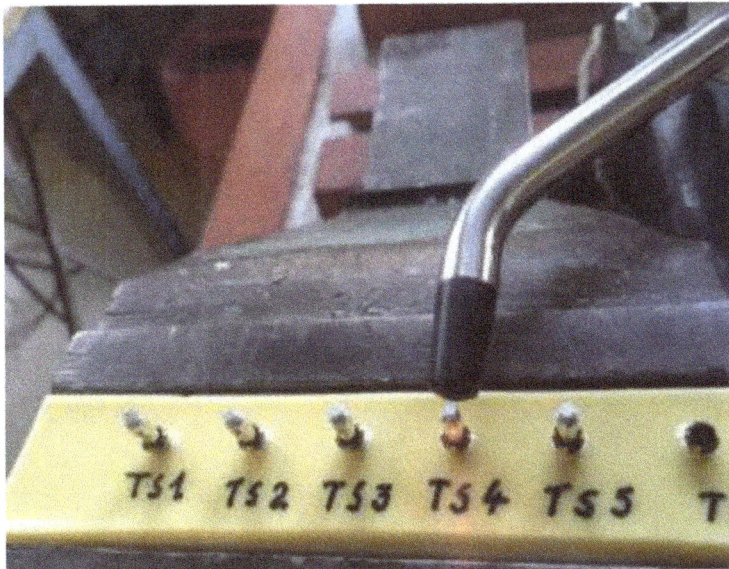

Fig. 2 Clamped Osstell probe orientated towards a Smartpeg mounted on a test implant. Note the red laser beam dot on the flat surface of the Smartpeg hexagon part

magnet part was confirmed by the auditory signal generated by the Osstell device. Correct positioning of the vibrometer laser beam was checked by the visual reflection indicator on the vibrometer display.

The output signal of the laser Doppler vibrometer was linked through an ADC/frontend interface (3160-A-4/2 (Bruëll & Kjaër, Nærum, Denmark) to a laptop with signal processing software (Bruëll & Kjaër Pulse Labshop, Bruëll & Kjaër Nærum, Denmark) to convert the speed of resonance $v(t)$ into a resonance frequency $v(f)$ using the autospectrum function.

The software enabled to analyze the continuously monitored input signal from the laser vibrometer. The measurement period was set at 31.25 ms. The time signal $v(t)$ was processed through a fast Fourier transformation ("FFT") analysis $V(f)$, resulting in a frequency span ranging between 0 and 12.58 kHz with 400 frequency intervals, resulting in a frequency resolution of 32 Hz. The FFT analysis generates a so-called autospectrum, based on the following formulae:

$$S_v(f) = \sqrt{V(f) \cdot V^*(f)}$$

with $V^*(f)$ being the complex conjugate of $V(f)$.

The final generated autospectrum pointed the maximum resonance frequency value based on an average of 1000 measurements per detection session (Fig. 3). This

recorded maximum resonance vibration frequency was noted in the datafile. The measurement was done in fivefold, and a mean value of all five measurements was computed, serving as the value to be input in the Osstell algorithm. Secondly, the "direct" ISQ value generated by the Osstell device was also noted in the datafile. After completion of measurements for each out of the five implants in each resin blocks, measurements were repeated in fourfold. In total, five measurements were made for each test implant.

In total, for each given implant type with a given diameter/length configuration, 25 measurements for indirect and 5 measurements for direct ISQ computing were performed.

Statistics

The SPSS statistical software package 22.0 (IBM SPSS, Chicago, USA) was used. A Shapiro-Wilk test was used to verify distribution normality for both direct and indirect determined ISQ values. The paired sample t test and the Wilcoxon signed rank test were used to evaluate the match between direct and indirect ISQ values. The Pearson product-moment correlation coefficient was used to assess the strength of the linear relationship between direct and indirect determined ISQ values. A 0.05 p value was used as type I error.

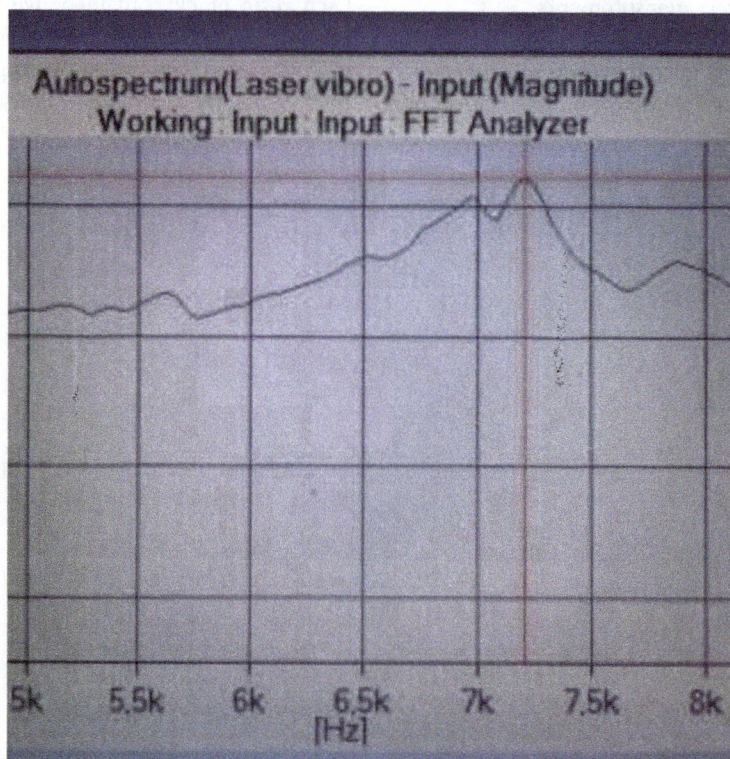

Fig. 3 Example of a typical autospectrum pointing to a 1 maximum RF based on 1000 measurements in case of a Straumann test implant

Results

Mean values (± SD) of recorded maximum RF values, calculated indirect ISQ values, and direct recorded ISQ values for Ankylos (A) and Straumann (S) test implants are shown in Table 2.

Normality of indirect (calculated) versus direct generated ISQ values

Using the Shapiro-Wilk test for indirect ISQ ($p = 0.05$) and direct ISQ ($p = 0.02$), we can conclude that both indirect and direct ISQ measures are not drawn from a normal distribution (data not shown). Both variables show a negative skewness and kurtosis (skewness indirect ISQ = − 6.22; skewness direct ISQ = − 0.491; kurtosis indirect ISQ = − 0.786; kurtosis direct ISQ = − 0.850).

Match between indirect (calculated) versus direct generated ISQ values

The mean indirect ISQ value is on average 0.535 IDSQ units higher than the direct ISQ value although this is not significantly different from 0 (paired t test $t = 2.018$, df = 19, $p = 0.058$). This is confirmed by the Wilcoxon signed rank test ($Z = 1.867$, $p = 0.062$). Figure 4 graphically represents the match between both outcome variables for all test implants. Differences are noted between Ankylos and Straumann implants and furthermore

between the different length-diameter clusters of the Straumann implants.

Correlation between indirect (calculated) versus indirect generated ISQ values

The Pearson product-moment correlation between indirect and direct ISQ values equals 0.990 with $p = 0.000$ indicating a significantly high linear relationship between both measures.

Discussion

The focus of this in vitro study was to develop a laboratory method, intended for future research of aspects of implant-Smartpeg complex stiffness and its possible influence on the overall RFA-based implant stability determination. In the past, other laboratory methodologies have been engineered to investigate implant deflection and/or lateral displacement by means of transducers. A setup using a motorized load transducer enabling to impact imbedded implant through a customized mounted abutment in combination with a micrometer gauge is described [18]. Furthermore, induction of resonant vibration on imbedded implants by an impulse-forced hammer, detection of the vibration signal by an acoustic microphone, and subsequent signal processing by fast Fourier transformation are described [19].

Table 2 Mean values (± SD) of recorded maximum RF values, calculated indirect ISQ values, and direct recorded ISQ values for Ankylos (A) and Straumann (S) test implants

Batch #	Implant system	Implant length (mm)	Implant diameter (mm)	Mean measured resonance freq (kHz)	SD measured resonance freq (kHz)	Mean indirect ISQ	SD indirect ISQ	Mean direct ISQ	SD direct ISQ
26	A	9.5	4.5	8607.60	0.894	89.19	0.006	90	0
27	A	9.5	4.5	8000.00	0	85.02	0	85	0
28	A	9.5	4.5	8032.00	0	85.24	0	85	0
29	A	9.5	4.5	8256.00	0	86.77	0	85.8	1.0954
30	A	9.5	4.5	8256.00	0	86.77	0	87	0
40	S	12	3.3	5180.00	3.346	65.63	0.025	65	0
41	S	12	3.3	5180.00	2.828	65.62	0.0212	65	0
42	S	12	3.3	5180.00	2.828	65.62	0.0212	65	0
43	S	12	3.3	5180.00	2.828	65.62	0.0212	65	0
44	S	12	3.3	5038.40	2.190	64.54	0.0168	64	0
ts1	S	4.1	10	7257.60	26.773	79.95	0.1814	80	0
ts2	S	4.1	10	7251.20	17.5271	79.90	0.1187	80	0
ts3	S	4.1	10	7225.60	14.3108	79.93	0.0968	80	0
ts4	S	4.1	10	7206.40	14.3108	79.60	0.0968	80	0
ts5	S	4.1	10	7232.00	0	79.77	0	80	0
55	S	4.8	8	7070.80	17.922	78.68	0.1209	75	0
56	S	4.8	8	7100.00	30.4302	78.88	0.2055	79	0
57	S	4.8	8	6857.60	21.4196	77.24	0.1441	77	0
58	S	4.8	8	7375.20	41.8473	80.7448	0.2842	77	0
59	S	4.8	8	7115.20	31.5150	78.9835	0.2129	78	0

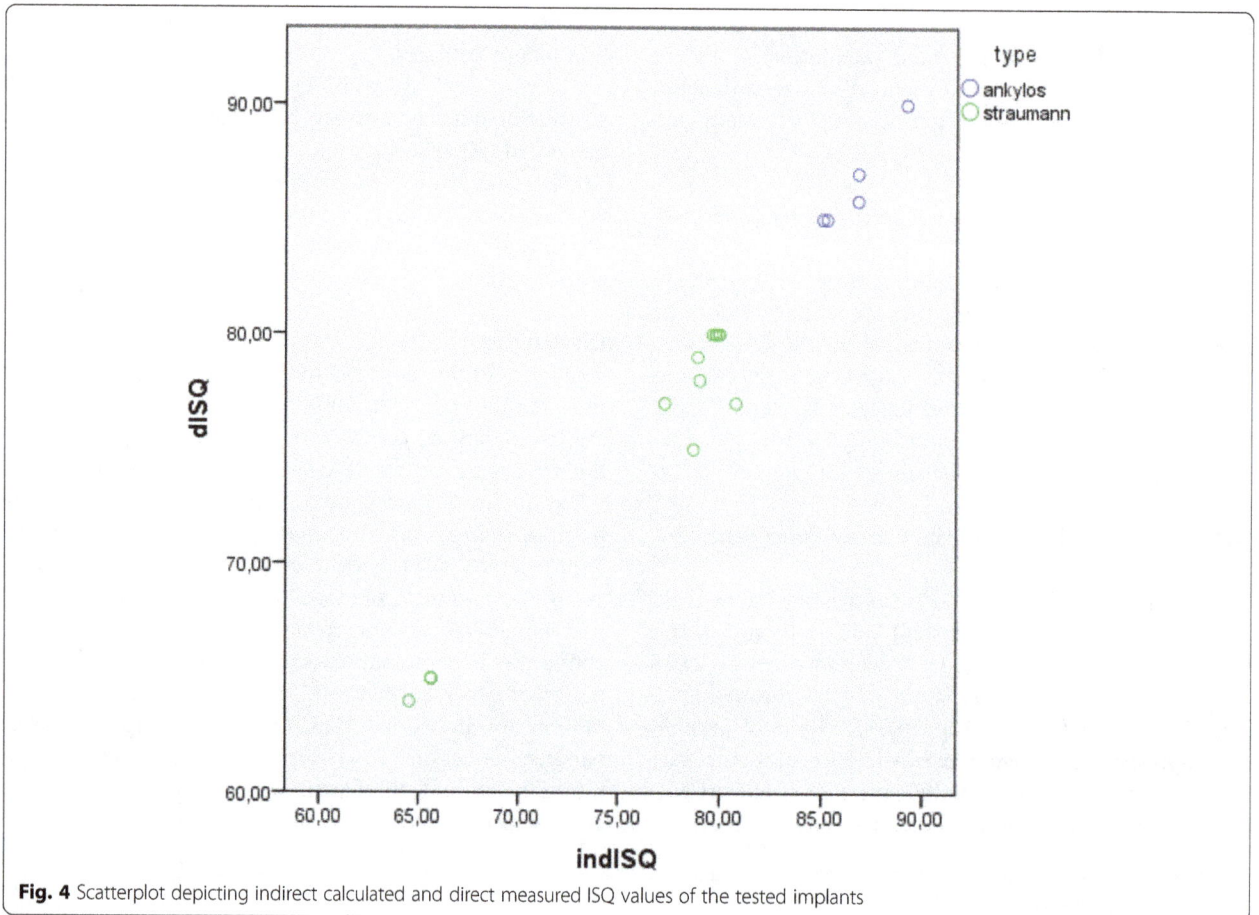

Fig. 4 Scatterplot depicting indirect calculated and direct measured ISQ values of the tested implants

By means of the above-described laboratory setup, quantitative measurement of maximum resonance frequency was performed after Smartpeg stimulation with subsequent indirect calculation of ISQ values using the Osstell algorithm. These indirect computed ISQ values were compared to directly determined ISQ values through the Osstell IDx device. The comparison of the indirect and direct ISQ datasets enabled to evaluate the correctness of the laboratory procedure by using the algorithm proposed by Osstell. Since the signal processing software provided a maximum resonance frequency based on 1000 recorded excitation measurements for each single analysis with a frequency resolution of 32 Hz, a measurement technique with high power could be obtained. The calculated ISQ values matched well with the directly generated ISQ values recorded by the IDx device. The difference between indirect and direct ISQ was rejectable from a clinical point of view.

Conclusions

In conclusion, the present study demonstrated that the algorithm applied and provided by Osstell to calculate ISQ values is correct, making the laboratory procedure valuable for future research focused on stiffness aspects of the implant-Smartpeg complex and its possible influence on the overall RFA measurement. Vice versa, the present study demonstrates the correctness of the actual applied algorithm for calculation of ISQ values by Osstell Mentor and Osstell IDx devices. From a clinical perspective, this study adds proof to the finding of ISQ values obtained by original Osstell devices, at least for Straumann tissue level SLA-surfaced implants, that are biased and underestimated. This implies that comparison of implant stability in terms of ISQ for identical implant systems between different studies has to be done with caution and need to be corrected when used for comparisons in systematic reviews.

Authors' contributions

SD has made substantial contributions to conception, laboratory engineering design, analysis and interpretation of data, and giving the final approval of the manuscript version to be published. NG has made substantial contributions to conception and in vitro design in view of currently available literature, data acquisition, and preparation of the manuscript. GV has made substantial contributions to the statistical analysis, data interpretation, and giving the final approval of the manuscript to be published. KVM has made substantial contributions to software engineering and fast Fourier transformation data processing. DM has made substantial contributions to drafting the manuscript and revising it critically for important intellectual content and giving the final approval of the manuscript version to be published. BVV has made substantial contributions to drafting the manuscript and revising it critically for important intellectual content and giving the final approval of the manuscript version to be published. All authors read and approved the final manuscript.

Competing interests
Stijn Debruyne, Nicolas Grognard, Gino Verleye, Korneel Van Massenhove, Dimitrios Mavreas, and Bart Vande Vannet declare that they have no competing interests.

Author details
[1]Department of Mechanics, Research Group Propolis, School of Engeneering Sciences, Katholieke Hoge School Brugge-Oostende, Ostend, Belgium. [2]Kliniek Royal, Koningstraat 41, 8400 Ostend, Belgium. [3]CHIR-Unit Dentistry–ORHE, Department of Orthodontics, Faculty of Medicine and Pharmacy, Vrije Universiteit Brussel, Laarbeeklaan 103, 1090 Brussels, Belgium. [4]Department of Communication Sciences, Ghent University, Korte Meer 7-9-11, 9000 Ghent, Belgium. [5]Katholieke Hoge School Brugge-Oostende, Ostend, Belgium.

References
1. Adell R, Lekholm U, Brånemark PI. Surgical procedures. In: Brånemark PI, Zarb GA, Albrektsson T, editors. Tissue integrated prothese. Osseointegration in clinical dentistry. Chigaco: Quintessence; 1985. p. 211–32.
2. Strid K. Radiographic procedures. In: Brånemark P-I, Zarb G, Albrektsson T, editors. Tissue integrated prothese. Osseointegration in clinical dentistry. Chigaco: Quintessence; 1985. p. 187–98.
3. Johansson P, Strid K. Assessment of bone quality from cutting resistance during implant surgery. Int J Oral Maxillofac Implants. 1994;5:279–88.
4. Sullivan D, Sherwood R, Collins T, Krogh P. The reverse torque test: a clinical report. Int J Oral Maxillofac Implants. 1990;5:179–85.
5. Olivé J, Aparicio C. The periotest as a measure of osseo-integrated implant stability. Int J Oral Maxillofac Implants. 1990;5:309–400.
6. Van Steenberghe D, Tricio J, Naert I, Nys M. Damping characteristics of bone-to-implant interfaces. A clinical study with the Periotest device. Clin Oral Implants Res. 1995;6:31–9.
7. Meredith N, Shagaldi F, Alleyne D, Sennerby L, Cawley P. The application of resonance frequency analysis to study the stability of titanium implants during healing in the rabbit tibia. Clin Oral Impl Res. 1997;8:234.
8. Meredith N, Alleyne D, Cawley P. Quantitative determination of the stability of the implant-tissue interface using resonance frequency analysis. Clin Oral Implants Res. 1997;24:568–72.
9. Aparicio C, Lang NP, Rangert B. Validity and clinical significance of biomechanical testing of the implant/bone interface. Clin Oral Impl Res. 2006;17(suppl 2):2–7.
10. Barewal R, Oates T, Meredith N, Cochran D. Resonance frequency measurement of implant stability in vivo on implants with a sandblasted and acid-etched surface. Int J Oral Maxillofac Implants. 2003;18:641–51.
11. Bischof M, Nedir R, Szmuckler-Moncler S, Bernard JP, Samson S. Implant stability of delayed and immediately loaded implants of delayed and immediately loaded implants during healing. A clinical RFA study with SLA ITI implants. Clin Oral Impl Res. 2003;15:529–39.
12. Huwiler M, Pjetursson D, Bosshardt D, Salvi G, Lang NP. Resonance frequency analysis in relation to jawbone characteristics qnd during early healing of implant installation. Clin Oral Impl Res. 2006;18:275–80.
13. Han J, Lulic M, Lang NP. Factors influencing resonance frequency analyis assessed by Osstell Mentor during implant issue integration: II: implant surface modifications and implant diameter. Clin Oral Implants Res. 2010;6:605–11.
14. Bornstein M, Hart C, Halbritter S, Morton D, Buser D. Early loading of nonsubmerged titanium implants with a chemically modified sand-blasted and acid-etched surface: 6-month results of a prospective case series study in the posterior mandible focusing on peri-implant crestal bone changes and implant stability quotien (ISQ) values. Clin Implant Dent Relat Res. 2009;11(4):338–47.
15. Guler A, Sumer M, Duran I, Sandikci E, Telcioglu N. Resonance frequency analysis of 208 Straumann dental implants during the healing period. J Oral Impl. 2013;39(2):161–7.
16. Valderrama P, Oates T, Jones A, Simpson J, Schoolfield J, Cochran D. Evaluation of two different resonance frequency devices to detect implant stability: a clinical trial. J Periodontol. 2007;2:262–72.
17. Tözüm T, Bal B, Turkyilmaz I, Gülay G, Tulunoglu I. Which device is more accurate to determine the stability/mobility of dental implants? A human cadaver study. J Oral Rehabil. 2010;37:217–24.
18. Pagliani L, Sennersby L, Petersson A, Verrochi D. The relationship between resonance frequency analysis (RFA) and lateral displacement of dental implants: an in vitro study. J of OralRehabilitation. 2013;40:221–7.
19. Haw-Ming H, Ching-Lai C, Ching-Ching Y, Sheng-Yang L. Factors influencing the resonance frequency of dental implants. J Oral Maxillofac Surg. 2003;61:1184–8.

26

Mechanical and degradation properties of advanced platelet-rich fibrin (A-PRF), concentrated growth factors (CGF), and platelet-poor plasma-derived fibrin (PPTF)

Kazushige Isobe[1], Taisuke Watanebe[1], Hideo Kawabata[1], Yutaka Kitamura[1], Toshimitsu Okudera[1], Hajime Okudera[1], Kohya Uematsu[2], Kazuhiro Okuda[3], Koh Nakata[4], Takaaki Tanaka[5] and Tomoyuki Kawase[6*] (iD)

Abstract

Background: Fibrin clot membranes prepared from advanced platelet-rich fibrin (A-PRF) or concentrated growth factors (CGF), despite their relatively rapid biodegradability, have been used as bioactive barrier membranes for alveolar bone tissue regeneration. As the membranes degrade, it is thought that the growth factors are gradually released. However, the mechanical and degradable properties of these membranes have not well been characterized. The purpose of this study was to mechanically and chemically characterize these membranes.

Methods: A-PRF and CGF clots were prepared from blood samples collected from non-smoking, healthy donors and were compressed to form 1-mm-thick membranes. Platelet-poor plasma-derived fibrin (PPTF) clots were prepared by adding bovine thrombin to platelet-poor plasma. A tensile test was performed at the speed of 1 mm/min. Morphology of the fibrin fibers was examined by SEM. A digestion test was performed in PBS containing trypsin and EDTA.

Results: In the tensile test, statistical difference was not observed in Young's modulus, strain at break, or maximum stress between A-PRF and CGF. In strain at break, PPTF was significantly weaker than CGF. Likewise, fibrin fiber thickness and crosslink density of PPTF were less than those of other membranes, and PPTF degraded faster than others.

Conclusions: Although the centrifugal conditions are different, A-PRF and CGF are prepared by essentially identical mechanisms. Therefore, it is conceivable that both membranes have similar mechanical and chemical properties. Only PPTF, which was prepared by a different mechanism, was characterized as mechanically weaker and enzymatically more degradable.

Keywords: Platelet-rich fibrin, Concentrated growth factors, Platelet-poor plasma, Young's modulus, Fibrin fiber, Degradability

Background

Platelet-rich fibrin (PRF), a self-clotted preparation of platelet-concentrated, blood-derived biomaterials, is prepared solely by contact activation of intrinsic coagulation pathways through centrifugation without addition of coagulation factors [1, 2]. Therefore, the preparation protocol is drastically simplified, and the resulting clot can be handled easily with forceps. PRF is further modified to two types: A-PRF, an advanced type that is expected to contain greater numbers of white blood cells [3] and concentrated growth factors (CGF), which is prepared under a facilitated intrinsic coagulation cascade [4]. Since these preparation protocols are similar and share the same principle of clot formation, A-PRF and CGF clots are not easy to differentiate either macroscopically or microscopically.

In clinical settings, both A-PRF and CGF preparations have been applied as barrier membranes and/or as carriers of growth factors to facilitate wound healing and tissue regeneration. However, their mechanical properties as

---

* Correspondence: kawase@dent.niigata-u.ac.jp
[6]Division of Oral Bioengineering, Institute of Medicine and Dentistry, Niigata University, Niigata, Japan
Full list of author information is available at the end of the article

barrier membranes have not been investigated sufficiently. For example, there is no available evidence as to which membrane is mechanically tougher. In addition, because the fibrin membranes degrade gradually at the implantation site in vivo, it is poorly understood how their mechanical properties change during the degradation process.

Degradability is also closely related to growth factor release, a phenomenon that is a key parameter in the efficacy at the implantation site. Recently, it has been demonstrated that growth factors are concentrated in A-PRF/CGF clots and released with time [5–10]. These experimental systems simulated the initial phase of growth factor release by simple diffusion; however, the simulation experiments were performed using conventional culture media in the absence of serum or proteases, which is not an appropriate simulation system of in vivo conditions. Therefore, it is apparent that growth factor release by degradation of fibrin fibers [11] is not well simulated. In the data obtained from our previous [12] and preliminary studies, fibrin clots can be maintained without substantial degradation under similar protease-free conditions for longer than a week. However, clinicians have frequently claimed based on their clinical experiences that fibrin clots applied to surgical sites, e.g., socket after tooth extraction, are almost completely degraded within a week or two. This observation is supported by several clinical review articles [13, 14].

In this study, we hypothesized that the mechanical properties of the fibrin membrane are closely related to its degradability. We compared these characteristics among A-PRF, CGF, and PPTF membranes through tensile and digestion tests.

Methods

Preparation of A-PRF and CGF clots

Blood samples were collected from four non-smoking, healthy, male volunteers with ages ranging from 27 to 56 years. Although having lifestyle-related diseases and receiving medication, these donors had no hindrance in daily life. The study design and consent forms for all procedures performed with the study subjects were approved by the ethical committee for human subjects at Niigata University School of Medicine in accordance with the Helsinki Declaration of 1975 as revised in 2008.

As described previously [6, 15, 16], blood samples (~9.0 mL) collected without anticoagulants using vacuum plain glass tubes (A-PRF+; Jiangxi Fenglin Medical Technology Co. Ltd., Fengcheng, China) or conventional vacuum plain glass tube (Plain BD Vacutainer Tube; Becton, Dickinson and Company, Franklin Lakes, NJ, USA) from the same donors were immediately centrifuged by an A-PRF centrifugation system (A-PRF12; DRAGON LABORATORY Instruments Ltd., Beijing, China) or a Medifuge centrifugation system (Silfradent

S. r. l., Santa Sofia, Italy). After eliminating the red blood cell (RBC) fractions, the resulting A-PRF and CGF clots were compressed using a stainless-steel compression device and preserved between wet gauze until mechanical testing (usually for a maximum of 3 h).

Preparation of PPP clots

To prepare platelet-poor plasma (PPP), peripheral blood (~9.0 mL) was collected using syringes containing A-formulation of acid-citrate-dextrose (ACD-A) (1.0 mL; Terumo, Tokyo, Japan) and immediately fractionated by the conventional double-spin method [17, 18]. The supernatant was collected as the PPP fraction. To prepare fibrin clots, bovine thrombin (Liquid Thrombin MOCHIDA Softbottle, Mochida Pharmaceutical Co. Ltd., Tokyo, Japan) was added to the PPP at a final volume percentage of 2.5% (v/v) at ambient temperature in glass chambers. The resulting PPP clots, which is designated as platelet-poor, thrombin-activated fibrin (PPTF), were compressed and preserved between wet gauze until mechanical testing (usually for a maximum of 3 h).

Determination of water content in fibrin clots

After excess amounts of exudate were quickly absorbed by the dry gauze, wet weights of freshly prepared A-PRF, CGF, and PPTF clots were measured using an electric balance. After compression with the stainless compressor, their weights were measured again. The compressed clots were then dried by heating at 140 °C for 30 min and were weighed in a pre-heated moisture analyzer (MA35; Sartorius Corporate Administration GmbH, Goettingen, Germany).

Mechanical testing

The mechanical properties of gel sheets were measured at a stretching speed of 1 mm/min with a desktop universal testing machine (EZ test; Shimadzu, Kyoto, Japan), of which maximum load cell capacity was 500 N under standard ambient conditions at 25 ± 3 °C and $50 \pm 25\%$ RH. The samples were gripped by clamps at each end (using slip-proof rubber sheets to prevent slippage) such that the initial apparent gauge length (the distance between clamp faces) was set to 10 mm for all the samples tested.

Young's modulus, maximum tensile strength, and tensile strain at break were obtained from the stress-strain plot. Stress was calculated by dividing the force by the initial tissue cross-sectional area, assuming a rectangular geometry (Table 1). The modulus for each sample was determined from the slope of the stress-strain curve during the apparent strain of 50–150% where the curve was almost linear while the sample had a sag during the apparent strain of 0–50%. The strain was recalculated to eliminate the sag when the Young's modulus and the maximum strain at break.

According to the definition in the Handbook of Polymer Testing [19], "Young's modulus" is the modulus of elasticity in tension and defined as ratio of stress difference to the corresponding strain difference (stress/strain). In this study, the initial elongation property (slope) was evaluated to determine Young's modulus. "tensile strain at break" is defined as tensile strain at the tensile stress at break, if it breaks without yielding. "Maximum tensile stress" sustained by the test specimen during a tensile test represents tensile strength.

Digestion test

A-PRF/CGF/PPTF clots (1 mm thick) were compressed in the stainless-steel compressor [16] and were punched out (φ8 mm) using a biopsy punch (Kai Corp., Tokyo, Japan). After repeatedly rinsing the disks with PBS to eliminate as much serum as possible, the disks were immersed into 4 mL of 0.05% trypsin plus 0.53 mM EDTA (Invitrogen, Carlsbad, CA, USA) in a 35-mm dish inside a CO_2 incubator. Fibrin is well known to be specifically degraded by plasmin in vivo; however, because it takes a long time to determine degradation using plasmin in vitro [12] and because fibrin could be degraded also by other proteases in vivo, we used trypsin plus EDTA, which is usually used in cell culture, in this study.

After pipetting the digestion solution, 50 μL of the digestion solution was collected every 20 min and was stored at –20 °C until protein measurement. Protein levels, which can be considered primarily as levels of digested fibrin fiber, were then determined by a BCA protein assay kit (Takara Bio, Kusatsu, Japan). The protein levels at the time point when the initial fibrin disks were completely digested overnight were evaluated at 100%.

Scanning electron microscopy (SEM)

The PRF clots that were compressed in a stainless-steel compressor, were fixed with 2.5% neutralized glutaraldehyde, dehydrated with a series of ethanol solutions and *t*-butanol, freeze-dried, and then were examined under a scanning electron microscope (TM-1000; Hitachi, Tokyo, Japan) with an accelerating voltage of 15 kV, as described previously [16].

Statistical analysis

The data were expressed as mean ± standard deviation (SD). For multi-group comparisons, statistical analyses were conducted to compare the mean values by one-way analysis of variance (ANOVA) followed by Dunn's multiple-comparison test (SigmaPlot 12.5; Systat Software, Inc., San Jose, CA, USA). Differences with P values < 0.05 were considered significant.

Results

The main purpose of this study was to compare A-PRF with CGF preparations to find possible differences in mechanical properties. As shown in Table 1, the sizes of A-PRF clots compressed to membranes were 8.6 ± 1.2 mm (W) × 27.5 ± 3.5 mm (L) and very similar to those of CGF clots (8.4 ± 0.8 mm × 27.6 ± 2.5 mm). As reference, PPTF membranes were also prepared by adding $CaCl_2$ to liquid PPP preparations using a molding glass chamber. The size of PPP membranes prepared by adding thrombin, designated PPTF in this study, was 8.3 ± 1.2 mm × 31.8 ± 2.1 mm. Furthermore, when subjected to the tensile test, both membranes could be stretched two to four times their original length. As shown in Table 2, the water content of A-PRF clots was very similar to that of CGF clots. However, PPTF clots contained significantly less amounts of water than both A-PRF and CGF clots.

Surface microstructures of various fibrin clots, including A-PRF and CGF clots, were compared, as shown in Fig. 1. Based on SEM examinations, CGF clots contained thicker fibrin fibers than A-PRF clots. PPP clots prepared by adding $CaCl_2$ were composed mainly of relatively thin fibers. In contrast, PPTF clots were easily distinguishable from the other three clot types and were composed of highly crosslinked fibers that were the thinnest observed.

Individual membrane types were examined by a tensile test and were characterized by three parameters: (1) Young's modulus, (2) strain at break, and (3) maximum stress in the stress-strain curves. As shown in Fig. 2, no significant differences in both Young's modulus and maximum stress were observed among A-PRF, CGF, and PPTF membranes. However, in strain at break, PPTF membranes were significantly inferior to CGF membranes.

Degradability of individual membrane types was examined in PBS containing trypsin and EDTA. As shown in

Table 1 Similarity in size and stretching property of A-PRF and CGF membranes

	Size (W × L mm)	Stretching (times longer)	Number
A-PRF	8.6 ± 1.2 × 27.5 ± 3.5	2–4	9
CGF	8.4 ± 0.8 × 27.6 ± 2.5	2–4	9
PPTF	8.3 ± 1.2 × 31.8 ± 2.1	2–4	3

Table 2 Comparison of water content of A-PRF, CGF, and PPTF clots

	Wet weight (g)	Dry weight (g)	Water content (%)
A-PRF	1.905 ± 0.416	0.043 ± 0.014*	97.8 ± 0.7*
CGF	1.753 ± 0.302	0.035 ± 0.009*	98.0 ± 0.6*
PPTF	1.774 ± 0.287	0.066 ± 0.004	96.2 ± 0.7

$N = 5$
*$P < 0.05$ compared with PPTF

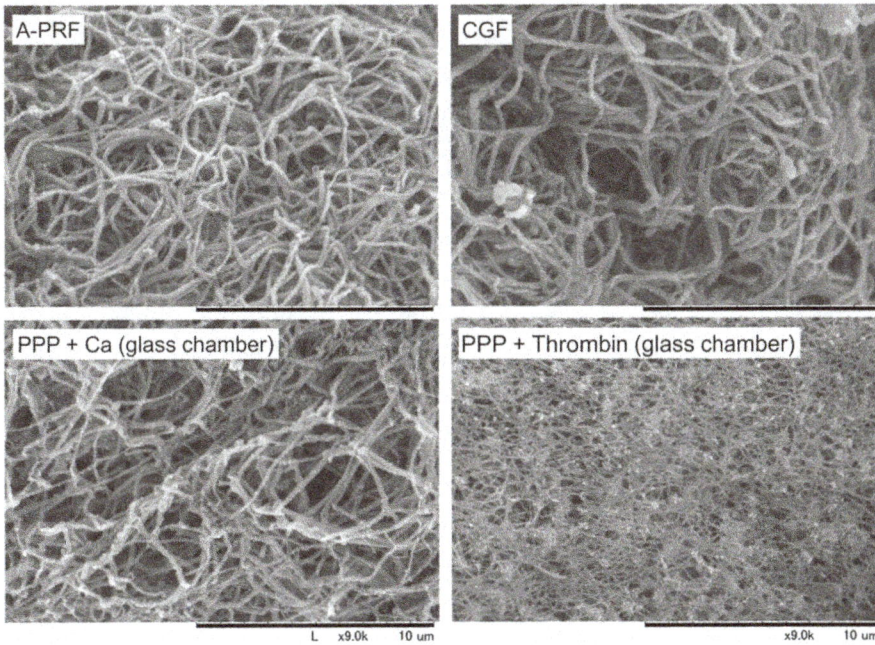

Fig. 1 Surface microstructures of A-PRF, CGF, and fibrin clots prepared by PPP + CaCl$_2$ and PPTF (fibrin clots prepared by PPP and thrombin). Similar observations were obtained from other three independent blood samples. *Scale bar* = 10 μm. *Note*: the same magnification (×9000) was used in all the SEM images shown here

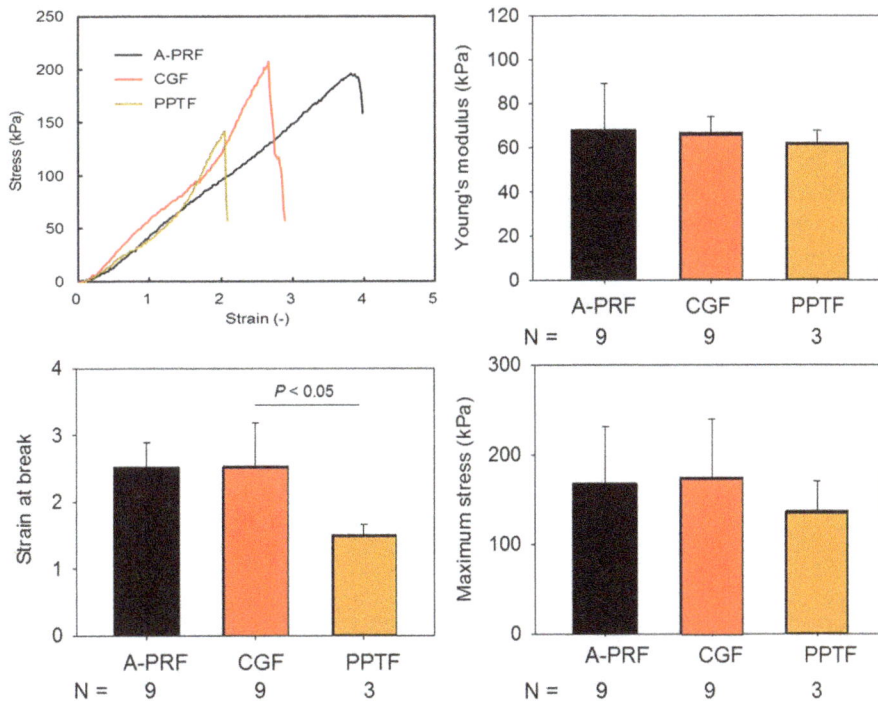

Fig. 2 Representative stress-strain curves for A-PRF and CGF membranes and mechanical properties (Young's modulus, strain at break, and maximum stress) of A-PRF, CGF, and PPTF membranes. *N* = 3–9

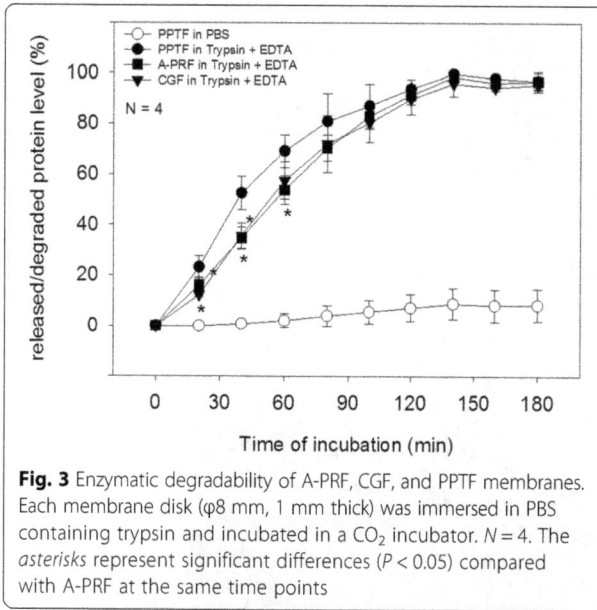

Fig. 3 Enzymatic degradability of A-PRF, CGF, and PPTF membranes. Each membrane disk (φ8 mm, 1 mm thick) was immersed in PBS containing trypsin and incubated in a CO_2 incubator. $N = 4$. The *asterisks* represent significant differences ($P < 0.05$) compared with A-PRF at the same time points

[20], these structural characteristics can be correlated to their degradability. As expected, we demonstrated that PPTF membranes degraded faster than other self-clotted fibrin membranes and A-PRF and CGF degradation rates were almost identical. However, it has not yet been clarified if those structural characteristics are correlated to mechanical properties.

In the tensile test, we again found no significant difference in any parameters evaluated among A-PRF, CGF, and PPTF membranes. However, in the strain at break, PPTF membranes were broken by a significantly weaker tensile force. The order of this parameter from high to low was CGF ≈ A-PRF > PPTF. As described above, the order of degradability was PPTF > CGF ≈ A-PRF, which is the reverse of the mechanical strength. Despite higher crosslink density, fibrin fibers formed in PPTF clots were substantially thinner and therefore they are probably not capable of bearing higher tensile forces. The manufacturer explains that the difference between PRF and CGF is related to the centrifugation techniques; programmed switching between acceleration and deceleration facilitates both conversion of fibrinogen to fibrin and their polymerization more efficiently than centrifugation at fixed speeds. However, as far as we examined, CGF is identical to A-PRF in terms of mechanical and degradable properties.

Growth factor release is a key function of these fibrin clots for tissue regeneration. Our previous study [16] demonstrated that CGF membranes compressed by the stainless steel compression device contain significantly higher levels of growth factors even after releasing approximately 85% of exudate. Repeated rinsing with PBS failed to completely remove the growth factors from CGF membranes. The rinsed CGF membranes retained angiogenic effects in ex vivo and in vitro experimental systems. Considered together, these data imply that significant amounts of the growth factors are secured in CGF membranes, specifically in fibrin fibers. Similar

Fig. 3, PPTF membranes degraded significantly faster than A-PRF and CGF membranes. This disparity in degradability was observed at 20 and 40 min.

Discussion

In this study, we found no apparent differences between A-PRF and CGF clot microstructures, especially in fibrin fiber thickness or crosslink density. However, in PPTF clots, which were prepared through direct conversion of fibrinogen by thrombin, fibrin fiber thickness and their crosslink density were substantially thinner and higher, respectively, than those of either A-PTF or CGF clots. This finding was supported by the water content data, which revealed that significantly less amounts of water were contained in PPTF clots. These data are summarized along with the centrifugal conditions in Table 3.

Since the ratio of surface area to volume is known to be a significant factor for degradation of polymer material

Table 3 Summaries of preparation procedures, relative mechanical, degradation, and related properties of A-PRF, CGF and PPTF

		A-PRF	CGF	PPTF
Centrifugal conditions		$198\,g \times 8$ min	$692\,g \times 2$ min[a] $547\,g \times 4$ min $692\,g \times 4$ min $855\,g \times 3$ min	$580\,g \times 8$ min (1st)[b] $1060\,g \times 8$ min (2nd)
Anticoagulants		None	None	ACD-A
Coagulation factors		None	None	Thrombin
Mechanical strength		Tough	Tough	Moderate
Serum retention		High	High	Medium
Degradation		Moderate	Moderate	Fast
Fibrin fibers	Thickness	Thick	Thick	Thin
	Crosslink density	Low	Low	High

[a]The centrifugal force was automatically changed by the specific program of centrifuge
[b]PPP was prepared by the double-spin method

functions were found in A-PRF and PPTF membranes. Therefore, it is thought that two distinct mechanisms are involved in controlled release of growth factors in exudate-depleted fibrin membranes: growth factors adsorbed to fibrin fibers and growth factors caged in platelets aggregated on fibrin fibers.

The initial phase of growth factor release from fibrin clots is mainly attributed to simple diffusion. In contrast, the late phase, i.e., the delayed growth factor release, is probably due to degradation of fibrin fibers and platelet membranes. We think that these combined releasing mechanisms determine how long the individual fibrin clot types last for tissue regeneration. This complex process of growth factor release from PRF (CGF) membranes should be investigated more carefully by developing appropriate experimental conditions.

Conclusions

In the mechanical parameters and degradability we tested, CGF membranes were almost identical to A-PRF membranes. In contrast, PPTF membranes were mechanically weaker and highly degradable. Therefore, we conclude that all of these fibrin membranes are tough enough to serve as barrier membranes; however, we should pay attention to their degradability and choose an appropriate membrane type depending on the purpose of treatment and the condition of wounds or bone defects.

Abbreviations
ACD: Acid citrate dextrose solution; A-PRF: Advanced platelet-rich fibrin; CGF: Concentrated growth factors; PPTF: Platelet-poor plasma-derived, thrombin-activated fibrin; PRP: Platelet-rich plasma

Authors' contributions
KI, TW, TT, and TK conceived and designed the study, performed the experiments, and wrote the manuscript. HK, YK, TO, KU, and KO performed the experiments and data analysis. YK, HO, and KN participated in manuscript preparation. All authors read and approved the final version of the manuscript.

Competing interests
Kazushige Isobe, Taisuke Watanebe, Hideo Kawabata, Yutaka Kitamura, Toshimitsu Okudera, Hajime Okudera, Kohya Uematsu, Kazuhiro Okuda, Koh Nakata, Takaaki Tanaka, and Tomoyuki Kawase state that they have no competing interest.

Author details
[1]Tokyo Plastic Dental Society, Kita-ku, Tokyo, Japan. [2]Division of Dental Implantology, Niigata University Medical and Dental Hospital, Niigata, Japan. [3]Division of Periodontology, Institute of Medicine and Dentistry, Niigata University, Niigata, Japan. [4]Bioscience Medical Research Center, Niigata University Medical and Dental Hospital, Niigata, Japan. [5]Department of Materials Science and Technology, Niigata University, Niigata, Japan. [6]Division of Oral Bioengineering, Institute of Medicine and Dentistry, Niigata University, Niigata, Japan.

References
1. Choukroun J, Diss A, Simonpieri A, Girard MO, Schoeffler C, Dohan SL, Dohan AJ, Mouhyi J, Dohan DM. Platelet-rich fibrin (PRF): a second-generation platelet concentrate. Part V: histologic evaluations of PRF effects on bone allograft maturation in sinus lift. Oral Surg Oral Med Oral Pathol Oral Radiol Endod. 2006;101:299–303.
2. Kawase T. Platelet-rich plasma and its derivatives as promising bioactive materials for regenerative medicine: basic principles and concepts underlying recent advances. Odontology. 2015;103:126–35.
3. Choukroun J. Advanced PRF, & i-PRF: platelet concentrates or blood concentrates? J Periodont Med Clin Practice. 2014;1:3.
4. Corigliano M, Sacco L, Baldoni E. CGF- una proposta terapeutica per la medicina rigenerativa. Odontoiatria. 2010;1:69–81.
5. Ghanaati S, Booms P, Orlowska A, Kubesch A, Lorenz J, Rutkowski J, Landes C, Sader R, Kirkpatrick C, Choukroun J. Advanced Platelet-Rich Fibrin (A-PRF)– a new concept for cell-based tissue engineering by means of inflammatory cells. J Oral Implantol. 2014: in press.
6. Masuki H, Okudera T, Watanebe T, Suzuki M, Nishiyama K, Okudera H, Nakata K, Uematsu K, Su CY, Kawase T. Growth factor and pro-inflammatory cytokine contents in platelet-rich plasma (PRP), plasma rich in growth factors (PRGF), advanced platelet-rich fibrin (A-PRF), and concentrated growth factors (CGF). Int J Implant Dent. 2016;2:19.
7. Fujioka-Kobayashi M, Miron RJ, Hernandez M, Kandalam U, Zhang Y, Choukroun J. Optimized Platelet Rich Fibrin With the Low Speed Concept: Growth Factor Release, Biocompatibility and Cellular Response. J Periodontol. 2016;88:112–21.
8. Kobayashi E, Fluckiger L, Fujioka-Kobayashi M, Sawada K, Sculean A, Schaller B, Miron RJ. Comparative release of growth factors from PRP, PRF, and advanced-PRF. Clin Oral Investig. 2016;20:2353–60.
9. Passaretti F, Tia M, D'Esposito V, De Pascale M, Del Corso M, Sepulveres R, Liguoro D, Valentino R, Beguinot F, Formisano P, Sammartino G. Growth-promoting action and growth factor release by different platelet derivatives. Platelets. 2014;25:252–6.
10. Schar MO, Diaz-Romero J, Kohl S, Zumstein MA, Nesic D. Platelet-rich concentrates differentially release growth factors and induce cell migration in vitro. Clin Orthop Relat Res. 2015;473:1635–43.
11. Mosesson MW. Fibrinogen and fibrin structure and functions. J Thromb Haemost. 2005;3:1894–904.
12. Kawase T, Kamiya M, Kobayashi M, Tanaka T, Okuda K, Wolff LF, Yoshie H. The heat-compression technique for the conversion of platelet-rich fibrin preparation to a barrier membrane with a reduced rate of biodegradation. J Biomed Mater Res B Appl Biomater. 2015;103:825–31.
13. Hartshorne J, Gluckman H. A comprehensive clinical review of Platelet Rich Fibrin (PRF) and its role in promoting tissue healing and regeneration in dentistry. Part II: preparation, optimization, handling and application, benefits and limitations of PRF. Int Dent. 2016;6:34–48.
14. Wang J, Wang L, Zhou Z, Lai H, Xu P, Liao L, Wei J. Biodegradable polymer membranes applied in guided bone/tissue regeneration: a review. Polymers (Basel). 2016;8:115.
15. Kobayashi M, Kawase T, Okuda K, Wolff LF, Yoshie H. In vitro immunological and biological evaluations of the angiogenic potential of platelet-rich fibrin preparations: a standardized comparison with PRP preparations. Int J Implant Dent. 2015;1:31.
16. Kobayashi M, Kawase T, Horimizu M, Okuda K, Wolff LF, Yoshie H. A proposed protocol for the standardized preparation of PRF membranes for clinical use. Biologicals. 2012;40:323–9.
17. Nakajima Y, Kawase T, Kobayashi M, Okuda K, Wolff LF, Yoshie H. Bioactivity of freeze-dried platelet-rich plasma in an adsorbed form on a biodegradable polymer material. Platelets. 2012;23:594–603.
18. Okuda K, Kawase T, Momose M, Murata M, Saito Y, Suzuki H, Wolff LF, Yoshie H. Platelet-rich plasma contains high levels of platelet-derived growth factor and transforming growth factor-beta and modulates the proliferation of periodontally related cells in vitro. J Periodontol. 2003;74:849–57.
19. Hawley S. Particular requirements for plastics. In: Brown R, editor. Handbook of polymer testing. New York: Marcel Dekker, Inc; 1999. p. 313.
20. Makadia HK, Siegel SJ. Poly Lactic-co-Glycolic Acid (PLGA) as Biodegradable Controlled Drug Delivery Carrier. Polymers (Basel). 2011;3:1377–97.

Permissions

All chapters in this book were first published in IJID, by Springer; hereby published with permission under the Creative Commons Attribution License or equivalent. Every chapter published in this book has been scrutinized by our experts. Their significance has been extensively debated. The topics covered herein carry significant findings which will fuel the growth of the discipline. They may even be implemented as practical applications or may be referred to as a beginning point for another development.

The contributors of this book come from diverse backgrounds, making this book a truly international effort. This book will bring forth new frontiers with its revolutionizing research information and detailed analysis of the nascent developments around the world.

We would like to thank all the contributing authors for lending their expertise to make the book truly unique. They have played a crucial role in the development of this book. Without their invaluable contributions this book wouldn't have been possible. They have made vital efforts to compile up to date information on the varied aspects of this subject to make this book a valuable addition to the collection of many professionals and students.

This book was conceptualized with the vision of imparting up-to-date information and advanced data in this field. To ensure the same, a matchless editorial board was set up. Every individual on the board went through rigorous rounds of assessment to prove their worth. After which they invested a large part of their time researching and compiling the most relevant data for our readers.

The editorial board has been involved in producing this book since its inception. They have spent rigorous hours researching and exploring the diverse topics which have resulted in the successful publishing of this book. They have passed on their knowledge of decades through this book. To expedite this challenging task, the publisher supported the team at every step. A small team of assistant editors was also appointed to further simplify the editing procedure and attain best results for the readers.

Apart from the editorial board, the designing team has also invested a significant amount of their time in understanding the subject and creating the most relevant covers. They scrutinized every image to scout for the most suitable representation of the subject and create an appropriate cover for the book.

The publishing team has been an ardent support to the editorial, designing and production team. Their endless efforts to recruit the best for this project, has resulted in the accomplishment of this book. They are a veteran in the field of academics and their pool of knowledge is as vast as their experience in printing. Their expertise and guidance has proved useful at every step. Their uncompromising quality standards have made this book an exceptional effort. Their encouragement from time to time has been an inspiration for everyone.

The publisher and the editorial board hope that this book will prove to be a valuable piece of knowledge for researchers, students, practitioners and scholars across the globe.

List of Contributors

Demos Kalyvas, Andreas Kapsalas, Sofia Paikou and Konstantinos Tsiklakis
Department of Oral and Maxillofacial Surgery, School of Dentistry, National and Kapodistrian University of Athens, Greece, Thivon 2 str, 11527 Athens, Greece

Kazuhiro Okuda
Division of Periodontology, Institute of Medicine and Dentistry, Niigata University, Niigata, Japan

Koh Nakata
Bioscience Medical Research Center, Niigata University Medical and Dental Hospital, Niigata, Japan

Takaaki Tanaka
Department of Materials Science and Technology, Niigata University, Niigata, Japan

Tomoyuki Kawase
Division of Oral Bioengineering, Institute of Medicine and Dentistry, Niigata University, Niigata, Japan

Stijn Debruyne
Department of Mechanics, Research Group Propolis, School of Engeneering Sciences, Katholieke Hoge School Brugge-Oostende, Ostend, Belgium

Nicolas Grognard
Kliniek Royal, Koningstraat 41, 8400 Ostend, Belgium
CHIR-Unit Dentistry– ORHE, Department of Orthodontics, Faculty of Medicine and Pharmacy, Vrije Universiteit Brussel, Laarbeeklaan 103, 1090 Brussels, Belgium

Dimitrios Mavreas and Bart Vande Vannet
CHIR-Unit Dentistry–ORHE, Department of Orthodontics, Faculty of Medicine and Pharmacy, Vrije Universiteit Brussel, Laarbeeklaan 103, 1090 Brussels, Belgium

Gino Verleye
Department of Communication Sciences, Ghent University, Korte Meer 7-9-11, 9000 Ghent, Belgium

Korneel Van Massenhove
Katholieke Hoge School Brugge-Oostende, Ostend, Belgium

Moustafa N. Aboushelib
Dental Biomaterials Department, Faculty of Dentistry, Alexandria University, Champollion st, Azarita, Alexandria, Egypt

Rehab Shawky
Oral Surgery Department, Faculty of Dentistry, Alexandria University, Alexandria, Egypt

Torsten Wassmann
Department of Prosthodontics, University Medical Center Goettingen, Robert-Koch-Strasse 40, 37075 Goettingen, Germany

Ralf Buergers
Department of Prosthodontics, University Medical Center Goettingen, Robert-Koch-Strasse 40, 37075 Goettingen, Germany
Department of Prosthetic Dentistry, Regensburg University Medical Centre, Regensburg, Germany

Stefan Kreis and Michael Behr
Department of Prosthetic Dentistry, Regensburg University Medical Centre, Regensburg, Germany

C. J. Butterworth and S. N. Rogers
Department of Oral & Maxillofacial Surgery, University Hospital Aintree, Lower Lane, Liverpool L9 7AL, UK

Kohya Uematsu
Division of Dental Implantology, Niigata University Medical and Dental Hospital, Niigata, Japan

Gintaras Juodzbalys
Department of Oral and Maxillofacial Surgery, Lithuanian University of Health Sciences, LT-46383 Kaunas, Lithuania

Frank Schwarz
Department of Oral Surgery and Implantology, Carolinum, Johann Wolfgang Goethe-University Frankfurt, D-60596 Frankfurt am Main, Germany

Murat Ulu
Faculty of Dentistry, Oral and Maxillofacial Department, İzmir Katip Celebi University, İzmir, Turkey

Erdem Kılıç and Alper Alkan
Faculty of Dentistry, Oral and Maxillofacial Department, Bezmialem University, İstanbul, Turkey

Eduardo Anitua
Private practice in oral implantology, Clínica Eduardo Anitua, Vitoria, Spain
University Institute for Regenerative Medicine and Oral Implantology – UIRMI (UPV/EHU Fundación Eduardo Anitua), Vitoria, Spain
BTI Biotechnology Institute, Vitoria, Spain
Eduardo Anitua Foundation, C/Jose Maria Cagigal 19, 01007 Vitoria, Spain

Mohammad Hamdan Alkhraisat
University Institute for Regenerative Medicine and Oral Implantology – UIRMI (UPV/EHU Fundación Eduardo Anitua), Vitoria, Spain
BTI Biotechnology Institute, Vitoria, Spain

Laura Piñas
Universidad Europea de Madrid, Madrid, Spain

S. Wentaschek and S. Hartmann
Department of Prosthetic Dentistry, University Medical Center of the Johannes Gutenberg University Mainz, Augustusplatz 2, 55131 Mainz, Germany

C. Walter and W. Wagner
Department of Oral and Maxillofacial Surgery - Plastic Surgery, University Medical Center of the Johannes Gutenberg-University Mainz, Augustusplatz 2, 55131 Mainz, Germany

Masazumi Yoshitani and Atsuro Yokoyama
Division of Oral Functional Science, Department of Oral Functional Prosthodontics, Graduate School of Dental Medicine, Hokkaido University, Kita-13, Nishi-7, Kita-ku, Sapporo 060-8648, Japan

Yoshiyuki Takayama
Removable Prosthodontics, Hokkaido University Hospital, Hokkaido University, Kita-14, Nishi-5, Kita-Ku, Sapporo 060-8648, Japan

P. W. Kämmerer and D. G. E. Thiem
Department of Oral and Maxillofacial Surgery, Facial Plastic Surgery, University Medical Centre Rostock, Schillingallee 35, 18057 Rostock, Germany

A. Alshihri
Department of Prosthetic and Biomaterial Sciences, King Saud University, Riyadh, Saudi Arabia
Harvard School of Dental Medicine, Boston, MA, USA

G. H. Wittstock, B. Al-Nawas and M. O. Klein
Department of Oral and Maxillofacial Surgery, Plastic Surgery, University Medical Centre Mainz, Mainz, Germany

R. Bader
Department of Orthopedics, University Medical Centre Rostock, Rostock, Germany

Bartosz Maska, Suncica Travan and Erika Benavides
Department of Periodontics and Oral Medicine, School of Dentistry, University of Michigan, 1011 N University Ave, Ann Arbor, MI, USA

Guo-Hao Lin
Department of Periodontics and Oral Medicine, School of Dentistry, University of Michigan, 1011 N University Ave, Ann Arbor, MI, USA
Department of Surgical Sciences, School of Dentistry, Marquette University, 1801 W Wisconsin Ave, Milwaukee, WI, USA

Abdullah Othman
Department of Periodontics and Oral Medicine, School of Dentistry, University of Michigan, 1011 N University Ave, Ann Arbor, MI, USA
Department of Periodontology & Dental Hygiene, University of Detroit Mercy, 2700 Martin Luther King Jr. Blvd, Detroit, MI, USA

Shabnam Behdin
Department of Periodontics and Oral Medicine, School of Dentistry, University of Michigan, 1011 N University Ave, Ann Arbor, MI, USA
Department of Periodontics, School of Dental Medicine, Case Western Reserve University, 2124 Cornell Rd, Cleveland, OH, USA

Yvonne Kapila
Department of Periodontics and Oral Medicine, School of Dentistry, University of Michigan, 1011 N University Ave, Ann Arbor, MI, USA
Department of Orofacial Sciences, School of Dentistry, University of California San Francisco, 513 Parnassus Ave, S612D, San Francisco 94143, CA, USA

Sergio Alexandre Gehrke
Biotecnos Research Center, Calle Cuareim, 1483, CP: 11.100, Montevideo, Uruguay
University Catholica San Antonio de Murcia (UCAM), Murcia, Spain

Leana Kathleen Bragança
Implant Dentistry, Seville University, Seville, Spain

Eugenio Velasco-Ortega
General Dentistry, Seville University, Seville, Spain
Implant Dentistry Master, Seville University, Seville, Spain

José Luis Calvo-Guirado
International Dentistry Research Cathedra, Faculty of Medicine and Dentistry, San Antonio Catholic University of Murcia (UCAM), Murcia, Spain

Diederik F. M. Hentenaar and Gerry M. Raghoebar
Department of Oral and Maxillofacial Surgery, University of Groningen, University Medical Center Groningen, 9700 RB Groningen, The Netherlands

Henny J. A. Meijer
Department of Oral and Maxillofacial Surgery, University of Groningen, University Medical Center Groningen, 9700 RB Groningen, The Netherlands
Center for Dentistry and Oral Hygiene, University of Groningen, University Medical Center Groningen, Groningen, The Netherlands

Yvonne C. M. De Waal and Hans Strooker
Center for Dentistry and Oral Hygiene, University of Groningen, University Medical Center Groningen, Groningen, The Netherlands

Arie-Jan Van Winkelhoff
Center for Dentistry and Oral Hygiene, University of Groningen, University Medical Center Groningen, Groningen, The Netherlands
Department of Medical Microbiology, University of Groningen, University Medical Center Groningen, Groningen, The Netherlands

Silvio Valdec, Pavla Pasic, Bernd Stadlinger and Martin Rücker
Clinic of Cranio-Maxillofacial and Oral Surgery, Center of Dental Medicine, University of Zurich, University Hospital Zurich, Plattenstrasse 11, 8032 Zürich, Switzerland

Alex Soltermann
Institute of Surgical Pathology, University Hospital Zurich, Zurich, Switzerland

Daniel Thoma
Clinic of Fixed and Removable Prosthodontics and Dental Material Science, Center of Dental Medicine, University of Zurich, Zurich, Switzerland

Tommaso Grandi and Luigi Svezia
Private practice, Via Contrada 323, 41126 Modena, Italy

Giovanni Grandi
Department of Obstetrics, Gynecology and Pediatrics, University of Modena and Reggio Emilia, Modena, Italy

Nicola Sgaramella, Ivo Ferrieri, Giovanni Corvo, Gianpaolo Tartaro and Salvatore D'Amato
Multidisciplinary Department of Medical and Dental Specialties, Oral and Maxillofacial Surgery Unit, AOU - University of Campania "Luigi Vanvitelli", Naples, Italy

Mario Santagata
Multidisciplinary Department of Medical and Dental Specialties, Oral and Maxillofacial Surgery Unit, AOU - University of Campania "Luigi Vanvitelli", Naples, Italy
Piazza Fuori Sant'Anna 17, 81031 Aversa, Italy

Holger Kirsten
Institute for Medical Informatics, Statistics, and Epidemiology (IMISE), Haertelstraße 16-18, 04107 Leipzig, Germany
LIFE Research Center for Civilization Diseases, University of Leipzig, Philipp-Rosenthal-Straße 27, 04103 Leipzig, Germany

Rainer Haak
Department of Cariology, Endodontology and Periodontology, University of Leipzig, Liebigstraße 12, Haus 1, 04103 Leipzig, Germany

Ausra Ramanauskaite
Department of Oral Surgery, Westdeutsche Kieferklinik, Universitätsklinikum Düsseldorf, D-40225 Düsseldorf, Germany
Clinic of Dental and Oral Pathology, Lithuanian University of Health Sciences, Kaunas, Lithuania

Constanze Olms and Pia Baumgart
Department of Dental Prosthodontics and Materials Science, University of Leipzig, Liebigstraße 12, Haus 1, 04103 Leipzig, Germany

Giuseppe Allocca, Diana Pudylyk, Fabrizio Signorino and Carlo Maiorana
Center for Edentulism and Jaw Atrophies, Maxillofacial Surgery and Dentistry Unit, Fondazione IRCCS Cà Granda – Ospedale Maggiore Policlinico, University of Milan, Via Commenda 10, 20122 Milan, Italy

Giovanni Battista Grossi
Oral Surgery, Maxillofacial Surgery and Dentistry Unit, Fondazione IRCCS Cà Granda – Ospedale Maggiore Policlinico, University of Milan, Via Commenda 10, 20122 Milan, Italy

Toshihisa Toyoda, Kazushige Isobe, Tetsuhiro Tsujino, Yasuo Koyata, Fumitaka Ohyagi, Taisuke Watanabe, Masayuki Nakamura, Yutaka Kitamura and Hajime Okudera
Tokyo Plastic Dental Society, Kita-ku, Tokyo, Japan

Koh Nakata
Bioscience Medical Research Center, Niigata University Medical and Dental Hospital, Niigata, Japan

Tomoyuki Kawase
Division of Oral Bioengineering, Institute of Medicine and Dentistry, Niigata University, Niigata, Japan

Paul S. Rosen
Clinical Professor of Periodontics, Baltimore College of Dental Surgery, University of Maryland Dental School, Baltimore, MD, USA
Private Practice limited to Periodontics and Dental Implants, 907 Floral Vale Boulevard, Yardley, PA 19067, USA

Herman Sahlin
Neoss Ltd, Gothenburg, Sweden

Rudolf Seemann
University Clinic of Craniofacial, Maxillofacial and Oral Surgery, Vienna, Austria

Ari S. Rosen
University of Delaware Newark, Delaware, USA

Sven Marcus Beschnidt
Private practice, Baden-Baden, Germany

Claudio Cacaci
Private practice, Munich, Germany

Kerem Dedeoglu
Private practice, Istanbul, Turkey

Detlef Hildebrand
Private practice, Berlin, Germany

Helfried Hulla
Private practice, Strass in Steiermark, Austria

Gerhard Iglhaut
Private practice, Memmingen, Germany
Department Oral and Maxillofacial Surgery/Plastic Surgery, University Hospital Freiburg, Center for Dental Medicine, Freiburg, Germany

Gerald Krennmair
Private practice, Marchtrenk, Austria

Markus Schlee
Private practice, Forchheim, Germany
Department of Maxillofacial Surgery, Goethe University Frankfurt, Frankfurt, Germany

Paul Sipos
Private practice, Amstelveen, Netherlands

Tetsurou Torisu and Hiroshi Murata
Department of Prosthetic Dentistry, Graduate School of Biomedical Science, Nagasaki University, 1-7-1 Sakamoto, Nagasaki 852-8588, Japan

Mihoko Tanaka
Department of Prosthetic Dentistry, Graduate School of Biomedical Science, Nagasaki University, 1-7-1 Sakamoto, Nagasaki 852-8588, Japan
Centre for Periodontology and Implantology Leuven, IJzerenmolenstraat 110, B-3001 Heverlee, Belgium

Emrah Soylu
Faculty of Dentistry, Oral and Maxillofacial Department, Erciyes University, Kayseri, Turkey

Mehmet Kürkçü
Faculty of Dentistry, Oral and Maxillofacial Department, Cukurova University, Adana, Turkey

David E. Simmons, Pooja Maney, Austin G. Teitelbaum, Susan Billiot and A. Archontia Palaiologou
Department of Periodontics, Louisiana State University Health Sciences Center School of Dentistry, 1100 Florida Avenue, New Orleans, LA 70119, USA

Lomesh J. Popat
Tulane University SPHTM, 1440 Canal St, Suite 2001, New Orleans, LA 70130, USA

Demos Kalyvas, Andreas Kapsalas and Sofia Paikou
Department of Oral and Maxillofacial Surgery, School of Dentistry, National and Kapodistrian University of Athens, Greece, Thivon 2 str, 11527 Athens, Greece

Konstantinos Tsiklakis
Oral Diagnosis & Radiology Clinic, School of Dentistry, National and Kapodistrian University of Athens, Greece, Thivon 2 str, 11527 Athens, Greece

Collaert Bruno
Centre for Periodontology and Implantology Leuven, IJzerenmolenstraat 110, B-3001 Heverlee, Belgium

Reinhilde Jacobs
OMFS IMPATH, Department of Imaging & Pathology, University of Leuven, Kapucijnenvoer 33, BE-3000 Leuven, Belgium
Oral and Maxillofacial Surgery, University Hospitals Leuven, Kapucijnenvoer 33, BE-3000 Leuven, Belgium

Kathrin Becker
Department of Orthodontics, Westdeutsche Kieferklinik, Universitätsklinikum Düsseldorf, D-40225 Düsseldorf, Germany

Kazushige Isobe, Masashi Suzuki, Taisuke Watanabe, Yutaka Kitamura, Taiji Suzuki, Hideo Kawabata, Masayuki Nakamura, Toshimitsu Okudera and Hajime Okudera
Tokyo Plastic Dental Society, Kita-ku, Tokyo, Japan

Koh Nakata
Bioscience Medical Research Center, Niigata University Medical and Dental Hospital, Niigata, Japan

Index